# FATAL CIVIL AIRCRAFT ACCIDENTS

## THEIR MEDICAL AND PATHOLOGICAL INVESTIGATION

BY

PETER J. STEVENS

*O.B.E.*, M.D. (B'ham), M.R.C.Path., D.C.P. (Lond.), D.T.M. & H. (Eng.)

*Consultant Pathologist, Regional Plastic Surgery and Jaw Injuries Centre, Queen Victoria Hospital, East Grinstead; Late Consultant in Pathology, Royal Air Force Institute of Pathology & Tropical Medicine, Halton*

WITH A FOREWORD BY

GROUP CAPTAIN J. B. VEAL, *C.B.E.*, A.F.C.

*Director General of Safety and Operations, Board of Trade*

BRISTOL: JOHN WRIGHT & SONS LTD.
1970

*Distribution by Sole Agents:*
*United States of America: The Williams & Wilkins Company, Baltimore*
*Canada: The Macmillan Company of Canada Ltd., Toronto*

ISBN 0 7236 0253

PRINTED IN GREAT BRITAIN BY JOHN WRIGHT & SONS LTD.
AT THE STONEBRIDGE PRESS, BRISTOL BS4 5NU

This book

is dedicated to

ALL THOSE FRIENDS AND COLLEAGUES,

WHOSE COMMON CAUSE IS

THE PROMOTION OF SAFETY IN AVIATION

## PREFACE

The majority of fatal accidents to British registered aircraft that have occurred since 1960 have had a medical and pathological investigation carried out by a Royal Air Force pathologist. I was involved directly with most of them up to October 1967 while in charge of Aviation Pathology at Halton; the remainder were investigated by other members of the Department.

This book, which is an abridged version of my M.D. Thesis, brought up to date with respect to references and tables of accident statistics, is an account of the experience thus gained, a review of the relevant literature and a discussion of the place of medical and pathological investigation of fatal flying accidents at the present time and in the future. Special emphasis is laid upon the need for this to be a routine part of every investigation; only thus can be reduced the chance of important evidence being lost—evidence that could serve one of the prime purposes of accident investigation which is to provide the basis for measures to improve flight safety.

The subject matter is dealt with in three main sections; public transport aviation accidents; light aircraft accidents; and glider accidents. A fourth section is devoted to the problems of the multi-passenger aircraft accidents as a special type of mass disaster. Most of the accidents discussed are identified in the text only by their file number in the records of the Departments.

The co-operation of H.M. Coroners and their pathologists during my investigations of aircraft accidents has been very much appreciated as has the interest of those civilian colleagues who have sent us material when it was not possible for a Royal Air Force pathologist to attend the autopsies.

For the interest and encouragement of successive Chief Inspectors of Accidents, especially Group Captain J. B. Veal, *C.B.E.*, A.F.C., and their staff in the Accidents Investigation Branch I am particularly grateful. In recent years I have been fully accepted as a member of the accident investigation teams by all inspectors and investigating officers concerned. Group Captain Veal allowed me access to the archives of the Accidents Investigation Branch, Mr. G. Acock allowed me to use material from his researches into the history of the Branch, and Mr. R. C. Warren, *O.B.E.*, checked the accuracy of the technical aspects of those accidents where they have been discussed in some detail.

I am indebted to Dr. L. Buley, Chief Medical Officer of the International Civil Aviation Organization, Mr. J. Templeton of the Air Registration Board and Mr. E. Martin, Civil Aviation Department, Board of Trade; they have provided me with much information and many reports.

It is a pleasure to thank my friends and colleagues Squadron Leaders S. W. Tarlton and D. A. Montgomery and Wing Commander A. J. C. Balfour who have worked with me at various times in the Department of Aviation Pathology for their help and for allowing me to use some of their cases. I must pay a tribute to my predecessor (and successor) Group Captain J. K. Mason; but for his example I doubt that this book would have been written. He was good enough to allow me to use the few civilian accidents with which he was concerned during the period of this study.

The help and co-operation of the Directors and the staff of J. H. Kenyon Ltd., Funeral Directors, London, during the investigation of most of the accidents abroad is warmly acknowledged; their efforts contributed in large measure to the successful investigation of these accidents. Dr. F. E. Lipscomb, *C.B.*, *C.B.E.* (Air Vice-Marshal, ret'd), helped with the preparation of many of the illustrations; photographs were prepared by Messrs. J. Watkin, N. Chandler, and R. B. Lovell of the Photographic Department of Princess Mary's Royal Air Force Hospital, Halton; Mrs. M. Pearce, Mrs. P. Seager, Mrs. H. J. Figg and Miss S. Denton shared the typing of the drafts; to all these I offer my sincere thanks.

I am grateful to Mr. J. Pragnell of Irving Air Chute of Great Britain, for his assistance in the preparation of *Figs*. 54, 55, and 57 and to those who gave permission for the reproduction of illustrations as individually acknowledged.

To Air Vice-Marshal W. P. Stamm, *C.B.E.*, Q.H.S., Royal Air Force senior Consultant Pathologist, I am especially indebted for his advice and constant encouragement over the years. Dr. Lipscomb, Air Vice-Marshal Stamm, and Wing Commander K. E. A. Underwood-Ground read the draft of this work; I benefited greatly from their discerning and constructive criticism.

The Director General of the Royal Air Force Medical Services kindly gave permission for publication. I must make it clear, however, that any expression of opinion herein given is mine and does not necessarily represent the view of the Ministry of Defence or the Board of Trade.

*January*, 1970 P.J.S.

## CONTENTS


*Chapter* *Page*

PREFACE . . . . . . . . . . . . v

FOREWORD . . . . . . . . . . . . xi

1. GENERAL INTRODUCTION . . . . . . . . . 1
   Accidents: Epidemiological Aspects 1; History of Civil Aircraft Accident Investigation in Britain 2; Establishment of a Royal Air Force Department of Aviation Pathology 5; Aviation Pathology in other Countries 6

*SECTION I*

*PUBLIC TRANSPORT ACCIDENTS*

2. INTRODUCTION . . . . . . . . . . . . 7
   Accident Trends 7; The Case Material 11; The Aims of the Pathologist's Investigation 11

3. NATURAL DISEASE IN THE OPERATING CREW . . . . . . 12
   I—As a Main Cause for an Accident 12; General Considerations, Coronary Artery Disease, Isolated Focal Myocarditis, Other Diseases associated with Acute Incapacitation; II—Natural Disease as a Contributory Cause for an Accident 26; Reduced Efficiency of a Pilot; The Incidence of Natural Disease in Airline Pilots 27

4. IMPAIRED EFFICIENCY OF A PILOT DUE TO INTOXICATION . . . . 29
   Alcohol 29; Drugs 31; Carbon Monoxide Intoxication 31

5. A NON-MEDICAL CAUSE FOR AN ACCIDENT . . . . . . 42
   Sabotage 42

6. PATHOLOGICAL EVIDENCE OF EVENTS PRIOR TO AN ACCIDENT . . . 49

7. RECONSTRUCTION OF EVENTS AT IMPACT AND IMMEDIATELY AFTER AN ACCIDENT . . . . . . . . . . . . 52
   Survival and Escape 52; Safety Equipment 58; Lap Belts, The Orientation of Seats

8. GENERAL CONCLUSIONS . . . . . . . . . . 61

*SECTION II*

*LIGHT AIRCRAFT ACCIDENTS*

9. INTRODUCTION . . . . . . . . . . . . 62
   Accident Trends 62; The Case Material 63; The Aims of the Pathologist's Investigation 63

*Chapter* *Page*

10. Natural Disease in the Pilots . . . . . . . . . 65
Coronary Artery Disease 65; Other Conditions 68; Suicide 76; The Incidence of Accidents Caused by Natural Disease 77; The Incidence of Natural Disease in Private Pilots 77; Conclusions 78

11. Impaired Efficiency of the Pilot Due to Intoxication . . . . 79
Alcohol 79; Drugs 81; Carbon Monoxide Intoxication 82

12. Reconstruction of Events at Impact . . . . . . . . . 84
Safety and Survival 84; The Injury Potential of Lap Belts, Analysis of Survival Aspects 89; Protective Helmets, Shoulder Harnesses

13. General Conclusions . . . . . . . . . . . . . . 96

*SECTION III*
*GLIDER ACCIDENTS*

14. Introduction . . . . . . . . . . . . . . . . 97
History of the Sport of Gliding 97; Glider Accident Trends 98; Case Material 99

15. Natural Disease in Glider Pilots . . . . . . . . . . 100

16. Reconstruction of Events During an Accident . . . . . 111
The Cause of a Structural Failure 111; A Failed Attempt to Escape in Flight 112

17. Survival and Safety Equipment . . . . . . . . . . 116

18. General Discussion . . . . . . . . . . . . . . 117
Medical Standards for Glider Pilots 117

*SECTION IV*

*THE FATAL AIRLINER ACCIDENT AS AN EXAMPLE OF MASS DISASTER: MEDICOLEGAL ASPECTS AND THE ORGANIZATION OF THE INVESTIGATION*

19. Introduction . . . . . . . . . . . . . . . . 121
The Major Aircraft Accident in Perspective 121

20. The Various Authorities, Official Bodies, and Groups Concerned with the Investigation of an Accident . . . . . . 123
The International Civil Aviation Organization 123; The National Commission of Inquiry 125; The Local Legal Authority's Inquiry 125; The Police and the Initial Rescue Operations 128; Local Pathologists and their Facilities 129; The Relatives of the Deceased 130; The Airline 132; Illustrative Case Histories 132; Discussion 139

*Chapter* *Page*

21. THE IDENTIFICATION OF THE BODIES OF THE DEAD—I . . . . . 140

General Comments 140; Visual Identification 142; Personal Property 144; Clothing, Documents, Jewellery and other Personal Effects, Medical Evidence 148; Radiography 149; Finger-prints 150; Serology 151

22. THE IDENTIFICATION OF THE DEAD—II . . . . . . . . . 152

Dental Evidence 152; Introduction, Dental Nomenclature, Comparison of Dental Records with Dental Evidence in Cadavers, Inconsistencies between the Chart of a Known Person and the Findings in a Cadaver, Difficulties encountered with Molars, Recent Extractions, Anatomical Abnormalities, Distinctive Prostheses and Restorations, Dental Radiographs, Dental Evidence of Age, Coincidence of Unusual Findings in Two Bodies, Conclusions

23. THE IDENTIFICATION OF THE DEAD—III . . . . . . . . 173

Process of Identification by Exclusion 173; The Count of the Bodies Recovered 175; The Organization of an Information Service 176; Miscellaneous Techniques in the Work of Identification 179

24. CERTIFICATION OF DEATH AND THE DISPOSAL OF THE DECEASED . . . 184

25. FINAL CONCLUSIONS . . . . . . . . . . . . . . 186

APPENDIX . . . . . . . . . . . . . . 189

Gliding: Detailed Statistics, 1950–68

REFERENCES . . . . . . . . . . . . . . 193

INDEX . . . . . . . . . . . . . . 203

# FOREWORD

As Chief Inspector of Accidents in the Ministry of Aviation, and subsequently the Board of Trade, from 1963 to 1968 it was my good fortune for much of that time to be able to invoke the help of Wing Commander Peter Stevens as the pathologist member of our aircraft accident investigating team. It is perhaps one of the hazards of a doctor's life that he is apt to be called at any time of the day or night; the calls to participate in aircraft accident investigations are no exception, with the added possibility of a journey to the other side of the world and the prospect of joining in post-mortem examinations immediately upon arrival.

I am very happy to have the opportunity, in writing this Foreword, to acknowledge the extremely important and enthusiastic contribution which Peter Stevens and his pathologist colleagues from the R.A.F. Institute of Pathology and Tropical Medicine and physiologists and psychologists from the R.A.F. Institute of Aviation Medicine have made over the years to the investigation of aircraft accidents, often in very difficult circumstances.

Air transport has now become the normal method of travel for medium and long distances, and in some countries for even relatively short journeys. Although aircraft accidents still make banner headlines, international statistics show that a constantly increasing level of safety is being attained whatever base of comparison is chosen. The most spectacular—fatalities per 100 million passenger-kilometres—has shown a tenfold improvement during the period 1945–68, reducing from 3·09 to 0·32. But improving statistical levels of safety are cold comfort to those involved in the tragic consequences of an aircraft disaster and clearly can provide no justification for complacency, particularly when with the constantly increasing size of aircraft a single accident could result in the death of many hundreds of people. Thus the efficient investigation of accidents becomes increasingly important so that the knowledge gained may be applied to the prevention of other accidents or the amelioration of those that unfortunately may continue to occur.

Statistics indicate that human factors are the direct or indirect cause of between 50 and 60 per cent of aircraft accidents; the significant contribution that the medically qualified investigator can make in these circumstances is readily apparent. On occasion the evidence found from the pathologist's investigation may be startling and give a direct and certain lead to the discovery of the cause of an accident or provide corroboration of the technical finding; however, the accumulation of what might be termed 'negative evidence', ruling out any probability of a medically based human factor, may in fact be equally valuable in tending to establish the validity of some other probable cause.

With the predominantly international nature of British air transport it was perhaps natural that we should pioneer the inclusion of an aviation pathologist in the team sent to assist in the investigation of accidents to our transport aircraft abroad. It has been found by experience to result in much more effective medical investigation in many cases than there would otherwise have been. It has also demonstrated internationally the value of methodical autopsies and positive identification in aircraft accident inquiries and has encouraged other countries to follow our example.

Success has not been easy and, in the peculiarly sensitive atmosphere which is so frequently associated with the aftermath of a serious accident, it has often needed tremendous tact and persistence to penetrate national barriers. That so much has been achieved is in itself apt recognition of the contribution which Peter Stevens and his colleagues have made in the general field of accident investigation and thus to improving safety.

*February*, 1970 J.B.V.

# FATAL CIVIL AIRCRAFT ACCIDENTS

## *Chapter 1*

## GENERAL INTRODUCTION

### ACCIDENTS: EPIDEMIOLOGICAL ASPECTS

ACCIDENTS are the man-made epidemic of the machine age (British Medical Association, 1965a). Although the total death-rate from accidents to people under 45 years of age may not have changed from 1904 to 1964 (Gissane, 1966), the decline in importance of infectious diseases as causes of death has resulted in accidents becoming increasingly prominent; they are now third on the list of causes of death in Britain (Osmond-Clarke, 1967) and fourth in the U.S.A. (Halpin, 1969).

Nearly one and a quarter million persons are injured in accidents in Britain annually (H.M. Chief Inspector of Factories, 1966, 1967; British Medical Association, 1964; *British Medical Journal*, 1966). These published figures may be low; the true figure may approach five million (British Medical Association, 1965a). Deaths from accidents total about 18,000 annually (Registrar-General, 1965, 1966); approximately 4 per cent of these deaths result from industrial accidents, 46 per cent from accidents in the home, and 50 per cent from transportation accidents. In the U.S.A. more than 100,000 persons die each year from accidents (U.S. Public Health Service, 1966), and Stapp (1966) reported that during the twenty years following the Second World War there were nearly three and a half times as many deaths due to accidents in the U.S. Armed Forces as were due to all other causes combined, including enemy action.

Although road traffic accounts for the majority of deaths from transportation, deaths on the railways and from aviation are considerable. Train accidents have tended to decrease in number over the last 30 years (Ministry of Transport, 1965); in recent times the numbers of passengers killed on the railways have averaged less than 50 each year (Ministry of Transport, 1967), whereas an average of nearly 150 people were killed annually in accidents to British registered aircraft in the period 1961–68. The chance of being killed rather than injured in a road accident is approximately 1 in 12; in a train accident it is only between 1 in 75 and 1 in 140. Aviation has a much higher death/injury ratio; the chance of being killed rather than injured in an aircraft accident is about 2:1

(Hawkes, 1956). Indeed, this is a matter of increasing concern as reported by the National Transportation Safety Board, U.S.A. (1969a) in a comment on the rising ratio of fatal to total aviation accidents.

It is impossible to prevent accidents without analysis of their causes; their potential for causing death and injury cannot be reduced if it is not known precisely what injuries are sustained and how they are produced. It is rational, therefore, that accidents should be the subject of routine and comprehensive scientific investigation.

Research into road traffic accidents and road safety did not commence on a substantial scale until after the Second World War (Road Research Laboratory, 1963). Only in very recent years has the steadily mounting mortality and morbidity of road accidents stimulated both detailed accident investigation and planned research in which medical participation has been prominent. Such studies have been carried out in Britain at the Road Research Laboratory, Crowthorne (Hobbs, 1967; Grattan, Hobbs, and East, 1967; Grattan and Jeffcoate, 1968), and by units such as the Birmingham University Accident Investigation Team established in 1964 and the Road Injuries Research Group at the Birmingham Accident Hospital. Many similar groups have been established in the U.S.A. during the last two decades and the American literature in this field is now considerable.

In the field of aviation the technical aspects of both military and civil flying accidents have been thoroughly investigated from the early days of flying; however, in common with road traffic, it is only in recent years that the medical aspects of accidents have been the subject of routine and detailed study.

## HISTORY OF CIVIL AIRCRAFT ACCIDENT INVESTIGATION IN BRITAIN

When aviation first developed in Britain on a large scale during the First World War, the very considerable loss of men and machines of the Royal Flying Corps led to the setting up of a specialist branch to deal with the investigation of certain flying accidents. Following the formation of the Air Ministry in January, 1918, the Accidents Investigation Branch, as it was then called (now generally referred to by its initials, A.I.B.), was reorganized on a civilian basis within the new Department of Civil Aviation (Acock, 1967). The A.I.B. retained its responsibility for Service accident investigation for a time, but later relinquished it to the Air Ministry; it continued to provide, however, and still provides, expert assistance to the Royal Air Force when required, particularly in obscure accidents, cases of structural failure in the air, fire in the air, and accidents from which useful lessons of general importance to aviation might be learned (Brown, 1966).

In 1920 the Air Navigation Act provided for the routine investigation of civil flying accidents and in 1922 the Air Navigation (Investigation of Accidents) Regulations were published. This legislation caused certain flying accidents to be notifiable to the Ministry and provided for a preliminary investigation of an accident to be carried out by an 'Inspector of Accidents' and for a 'formal investigation' to be held should the Secretary of State deem it expedient.

The first civil flying accident investigation report on file is dated 31 May, 1919; this accident was not a fatal one. Since then the A.I.B. has investigated nearly 1250 civil accidents of which almost 1000 have occurred in the United Kingdom; the remainder have involved British registered aircraft overseas. The first formal investigation, now known as a 'Public Inquiry', was held in 1925; the subject was the accident to the Imperial Airways DH34 which crashed on Christmas Eve, 1924, and resulted in the death of the pilot and seven passengers (Air Ministry, 1925). In 1937 the A.I.B. was considerably enlarged and Wing Commander Vernon Brown (now Air Commodore Sir Vernon Brown) was appointed the first Chief Inspector of Accidents. During the Second World War the A.I.B. concentrated on the investigation of Service accidents. These occurred in large numbers and the staff of the A.I.B. was increased and the methods of investigation were brought more into line with the requirements of the modern aircraft of the day (Brown, 1966).

In 1951 the Civil Aviation (Investigation of Accidents) Regulations were promulgated to replace those of 1922; these were superceded by new Regulations in July, 1969. As did those of 1951, the new Regulations empower the Chief Inspector of Accidents to investigate any aircraft accident to a British registered aircraft or to a foreign registered aircraft in the United Kingdom. He may carry out such an investigation himself or cause one of his inspectors to do so. The Chief Inspector or one of his staff of inspectors is required to report his conclusions about the cause of the accident to the Board of Trade and to add any observations or recommendations he thinks appropriate with a view to the preservation of life and the avoidance of similar accidents in the future.

Before 1961, the investigation of a civil aircraft accident was essentially a technical one; comprehensive studies of medical aspects were sporadic. An inspector of accidents in the early years was an engineer; now he is usually a very experienced ex-airline pilot and he is assisted in an investigation by an aircraft engineer called an 'Investigating Officer'. These men have tended to concentrate on the circumstances of an accident and the examination of the aircraft wreckage.

It was not until the late 1950's that it became the general practice for coroners to order post-mortem examinations following transportation accidents but they did so occasionally in earlier years. For example, an autopsy and toxicological analysis of the organs of Driver Martin were undertaken following the inexplicable railway accident at Shrewsbury in October, 1907 (Hamilton, 1967a), and reports in the files of the A.I.B. show that from time to time between the two world wars the medical aspects of a fatal aircraft accident were similarly investigated. It is not always clear what stimulated the study of the medical aspects of a given accident; it may have been an unusually interested Coroner, a particularly keen pathologist asked by a Coroner to perform an autopsy, or because good reason to suspect illness or impaired function in the pilot was uncovered by the inspector. In one accident in 1929 a passenger who survived said that the pilot had become ill in the air but an autopsy revealed no pathology or evidence of illness in the pilot.

As early as 1921 a detailed autopsy was carried out on a pilot of an aircraft that was at first seen to be in a dive and then on fire. The post-mortem examination revealed that the pilot had tuberculosis of the spine, had had a haemorrhage into a cold abscess and that this appeared to have been causing pressure upon the spinal cord and the roots of the nerves to the lower limbs. The possibilities were, therefore, firstly, that the haemorrhage into the abscess had been spontaneous, had resulted in partial or complete paralysis of one or both lower limbs, and had caused the pilot to lose control of the aircraft with the fire occurring during the ensuing dive. Alternatively, the fire may have been the primary event and the haemorrhage into the pre-existing spinal lesion a result of injuries received on impact with the ground. Obviously the latter explanation was the more acceptable having regard to all the circumstances; but at least full consideration was given to the medical aspects.

In most of the reports that show that an autopsy was performed on the pilot, it is recorded that no pre-existing disease was found. The circumstances of many fatal accidents suggested that the pilots had simply lost control of their machines; this was given frequently as the cause without further explanation. It is true that many similar accidents occurred without the pilots being killed; it was known that these had not resulted from physical incapacitation of the pilots and it is at least probable that most of the fatal accidents were due to inexperience and incompetence of the pilots rather than their acute incapacitation. It is equally probable that some accidents were due to illness but that this was not discovered because the possibility was not fully investigated on a routine basis.

The first accident in which alcohol was recorded as having been a possible contributory factor in an accident occurred early in 1930. This, however, was purely on the circumstantial evidence of the pilot having been seen drinking before flying. There was no evidence from any eye-witness that he had been the worse for drink and no post-mortem examination appears to have been carried out. After another accident later the same year, witnesses reported the pilot and his passenger to have been apparently in good health and sober; a pathologist's report stated that the bodies at autopsy smelt strongly of alcohol. In 1933 there were two more accidents in which circumstantial evidence suggested that the pilots had taken a good deal of alcohol prior to crashing their aircraft on take-off but in neither case are there reports of post-mortem examinations. In 1936 still stronger circumstantial evidence that alcohol was a factor in an accident was negated by a report of the post-mortem examinations carried out on the pilot and his passenger three days after the accident; the pathologist reported, 'I found no signs of inordinate drinking', but he gave no further details.

Human factors clearly played a part in a number of accidents and it must be admitted that post-mortem examinations in several would have been unlikely to have contributed more than was obtained from the pilots' histories. For example, in 1930 a young Royal Air Force pilot obtained a 10-hour leave pass from Halton Hospital, where he was recovering from leg injuries received in an aircraft accident some months previously. He went to a nearby airfield, hired an aeroplane and spent the day flying. On one trip he flew over the hospital and 'beat it up'. Shortly afterwards he appeared to lose control of the machine and it crashed; both the pilot and his passenger were killed. The recklessness and irresponsibility of this pilot in flying when the physical disability in his lower limbs would be likely to impair his efficiency at the controls of the aircraft, seems a sufficiently obvious contributory cause for the accident; it is not surprising that an autopsy was considered unnecessary.

Brown (1966) recorded that during the Second World War the accident rate reached alarming proportions. The possible importance of hypoxia, carbon monoxide contamination of cockpits, pilot fatigue, and failure of dark adaptation caused him to seek medical help in their assessment as contributory factors for accidents. He warmly acknowledged the value of the Service medical contribution in this field; this contribution did not derive, however, from routine pathological investigations into fatal accidents, nor from pathological studies on those killed in particular accidents.

The 524th accident report in the A.I.B. files is the first to describe an accident the cause of which was believed to be an attack of coronary artery insufficiency in the pilot. This accident occurred in mid-1948, and on the basis of the autopsy evidence combined with the witnessed manœuvres of the aircraft prior to impact (*see* Chapter 10) the pathologist stated, 'I hold the considered opinion that the accident may well have resulted from the deceased having been the subject of a cardiac (anginal) attack while flying' (Heggie, 1968).

The worst air disaster to occur in the United Kingdom happened near Cardiff in 1950. A Tudor 5 aircraft was carrying a group of supporters returning from a rugby football match in Ireland and it crashed on the approach to the airfield; 80 of the 83 persons on board were killed. This accident was the subject of a public inquiry (Ministry of Civil Aviation, 1950a); it appeared to have been caused by the pilot pulling back the control column too forcefully causing the aircraft to stall on the approach to land. Some 'Riddabron', a non-antihistamine antispasmodic, was found among the pilot's possessions and the possible significance of his history of mild asthma was given some consideration during the inquiry. But so far as it has been possible to determine, no post-mortem examinations were carried out on the pilot or his crew.

The first report of a pathological investigation into an aircraft accident recorded in the British medical literature was that of Teare (1951). He discussed the problems encountered in dealing with mass casualties (28 persons had been killed) and the causes of lethal injury in the casualties; he attributed a number of ruptured aortae to acute flexion over seat belts and argued the case for rearward-facing seats.

In 1954 the disasters to two Comet I's occurred. These were the subject of the utmost concern to the British Government, aircraft industry, and airlines, for so much depended on the success or failure of the Comets, the world's first jet civil transport aircraft. Only human wreckage was recovered initially following these accidents and the question arose whether an examination of the bodies of the victims would provide clues to the causes of the disasters. The extent to which autopsies helped, the subsequent experimental work, and the final correlation of medical and technical evidence was fully reported by Armstrong, Fryer, Stewart, and Whittingham (1955), Stewart, Spells, and Armstrong (1955), and Fornari (1955).

## ESTABLISHMENT OF A ROYAL AIR FORCE DEPARTMENT OF AVIATION PATHOLOGY

As a direct consequence of the Comet accidents and the medical aspects of their investigation, a Department of Aviation Pathology was established at the Royal Air Force Institute of Pathology and Tropical Medicine in 1955 (Stamm, 1968). Mason (1962a) gave a detailed account of his experience while in charge of this Department during the late 1950's and fully discussed the role of an aviation pathologist in the context of fatal military aircraft accident investigation.

During the years from 1960 to 1967 there was a continuous decrease in the volume of military aviation in Britain, accompanied by improving accident rates and a steady fall in the absolute number of both non-fatal and fatal military aircraft accidents. In 1961 a Ministry of Aviation Committee report dealing with civil aircraft accident investigation acknowledged the potential value of 'aero-medical specialists' attending the scene of a major accident, for both their help in the assessment of safety factors and their contribution to the determination of the cause of the accident or the elimination of possible causes. The report recommended that aero-medical specialists participate in accident investigation whenever possible. In the latter part of 1961 there were special features about one or two large passenger aircraft accidents which resulted in requests from the A.I.B. for a Royal Air Force aviation pathologist to help. The accident near Ndola, Rhodesia, in which the Secretary-General of the United Nations Organization, Mr. Dag Hammarskjöld, was killed occurred about the same time; the Rhodesian authorities also sought the assistance of the Royal Air Force.

Two years later, Tweedie (1963), an ex-Chief Inspector of Accidents, wrote that the team from A.I.B. was 'often' accompanied by 'aero-medical experts' and that the investigators frequently needed to concern themselves with 'the grim facts of human injury' in order to reach a solution to the accident or to provide 'specialized data upon which future safety measures may be taken'. It can now be claimed that, in the case of fatal aircraft accidents, it is *routine* practice for the A.I.B. team to include a pathologist from the R.A.F. Department of Aviation Pathology.

## AVIATION PATHOLOGY IN OTHER COUNTRIES

Leeper (1968) recorded that the first aviation fatality in the U.S.A. was autopsied in 1908 but that thereafter and until 1954, in the U.S.A. as in Britain, the pathological investigation of fatal flying accidents was sporadic. Stimulated also by the British Comet disasters and by the British plan to form a special department to study the pathological aspects of fatal flying accidents, a conference was held in March, 1955. From this developed the Joint Committee on Aviation Pathology (a body comprised of representatives of the flying Armed Services of the U.S.A., Britain, and Canada) and the Department of Aerospace Pathology at the Armed Forces Institute of Pathology, Washington. This Department started with a main interest in military accidents but in due course came to provide, as does the Royal Air Force, valuable assistance in the field of civil aircraft accident investigation.

An aviation pathology service has been developed in Australia (Brown and Lane, 1966), and Anderson (1968) has shown how Canada, though a country with 'limited aero-medical resources' has approached the problem of medical participation in fatal aircraft accident investigation. In Germany the air force have developed a Department of Aviation Pathology based at Fürstenfeldbruck on similar lines to ours at Halton; in recent years it has been providing an increasing amount of assistance in German civil accident investigation (Krefft, 1967). However, in most other countries little is apparently being done at the present time to establish any form of aviation pathology service.

## *SECTION I*

# *PUBLIC TRANSPORT ACCIDENTS*

---

## *Chapter 2*

## INTRODUCTION

### ACCIDENT TRENDS

In its annual surveys of accidents the Civil Aviation Department of the Board of Trade defines public transport flights as all scheduled and non-scheduled passenger- and freight-carrying operations. Data extracted from the surveys of recent years published by the Ministry of Aviation (1962, 1963, 1964, 1965) and, more recently, the Board of Trade (1966, 1967, 1968a, and 1970) are presented in *Table I* and refer to United Kingdom

*Table I.*—British Public Transport Aviation Accident Data: 1961–9

| | 1961 | 1962 | 1963 | 1964 | 1965 | 1966 | 1967 | 1968 | 1969* |
|---|---|---|---|---|---|---|---|---|---|
| Total Accidents | 13 | 10 | 13 | 13 | 22 | 16 | 19 | 11 | 4 |
| No. fatal† | 4(3) | 4(2) | 0(0) | 1(1) | 3(3) | 3(2) | 4(4) | 4(4) | 1(1) |
| Fatal accident rate‡ | 0·67 | 0·69 | 0 | 0·16 | 0·47 | 0·29 | 0·58 | 0·43 | § |
| No. killed | 102 | 124 | 0 | 83 | 64 | 224 | 228 | 60 | 2 |

* First six months only.
† Figures in brackets are the number investigated by the staff of the Department of Aviation Pathology, R.A.F. Institute of Pathology, Halton.
‡ Expressed as the number of fatal accidents per 100,000 aircraft hours flown.
§ Figure not available.

operators' aircraft engaged in public transport service. The annual total of accidents has ranged from 10 to 22; no more than 4 of these have been fatal in any one year.

The safety of aviation can be assessed from fatal accident statistics; these can be presented in several ways. Rates may be calculated for fatal accidents or total fatalities relative to hours or miles flown by aircraft or the numbers of passengers carried. *Fig.* 1 shows the changes in three such rates for world-wide scheduled passenger air services from 1950 to 1968. It would appear from all these graphs that flight safety is improving, but the extent of the improvement implied by each differs. The fatality rate expressed as the number of fatalities (passengers) per 100 million passenger-miles flown suggests that scheduled passenger aviation was six times as safe in 1968 as compared with 1950.

This is a figure which impresses potential passengers; it does not, however, reflect truly the reduced chance of a fatal aircraft accident. The chance that an individual will be involved in a fatal flying accident is more closely related to the chance that a particular aircraft will crash than to the number of passengers it carries. The chance that an aircraft will crash is affected more by the hours it is at risk than the miles it travels, which is dependent largely upon its speed. The number of fatal aircraft accidents per 100 million miles flown and the number of fatal aircraft accidents per 100 thousand hours flown by aircraft, suggest

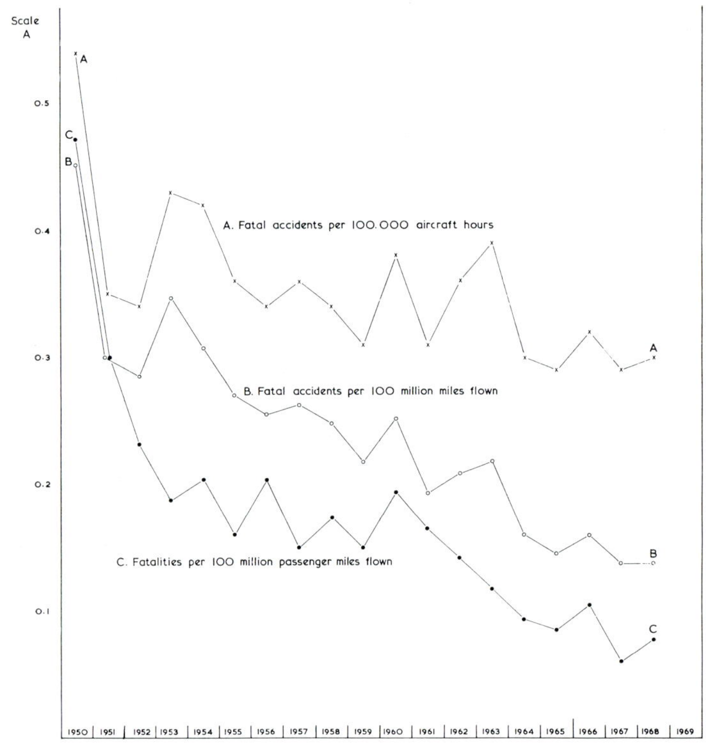


*Fig.* 1.—Aviation safety statistics: Three accident rates for world-wide scheduled passenger air services: 1950–68.

that the improvement in flight safety over the same period was threefold and double respectively. These rates, therefore, are all misleading to some extent; the speed, range, and passenger-carrying capacity of the aircraft concerned in any operation under review, so affect such statistics that they must be used with great caution in assessing the relative safety of any particular type of aviation or any particular organization's flying activities (Fryer, 1965a; Dressler, 1966).

According to Dressler the accident rate per stage-flight (a stage-flight or flight segment includes one take-off and landing irrespective of the hours or distance flown) is the least misleading figure for general purposes. However, the rate most usually calculated and used in the published statistics of past years is the fatal accident rate that is defined as the number of fatal accidents per 100 thousand flying hours; for assessing general trends in public aviation safety, this statistic seems reasonably satisfactory. In the United Kingdom it has not exceeded 0·69 in recent years and in 1963 was nil.

In the introduction to each annual survey, the Board of Trade has referred to the extreme caution that must be exercised in making deductions based on annual figures, for 'aircraft accidents are too varied in nature and indeed too few in number to provide a reliable basis for statistical comparison between different years and different types of accident.' A more realistic appraisal of accident trends is achieved by studying rates calculated for longer periods as this reduces the fluctuations due to chance. *Table II*

*Table II.*—Comparison of Fatal Accident Rates of British and World-wide Scheduled Passenger-carrying Services (I.C.A.O., 1969; Board of Trade, 1970)

| Quinquennium | Fatal Accidents per 100,000 Hours Flown | |
|---|---|---|
| | *U.K.* | *World-wide** |
| 1950–1954 | 0·48 | 0·42 |
| 1951–1955 | 0·45 | 0·38 |
| 1952–1956 | 0·48 | 0·38 |
| 1953–1957 | 0·61 | 0·38 |
| 1954–1958 | 0·53 | 0·36 |
| 1955–1959 | 0·36 | 0·34 |
| 1956–1960 | 0·25 | 0·34 |
| 1957–1961 | 0·29 | 0·34 |
| 1958–1962 | 0·24 | 0·34 |
| 1959–1963 | 0·19 | 0·35 |
| 1960–1964 | 0·23 | 0·35 |
| 1961–1965 | 0·32 | 0·33 |
| 1962–1966 | 0·27 | 0·33 |
| 1963–1967 | 0·22 | 0·32 |
| 1964–1968† | 0·30 | 0·30 |

* Excluding Communist China and U.S.S.R.
† Preliminary figures.

shows the average fatal accident rate in quinquennia for all countries (derived from figures published by the International Civil Aviation Organization (I.C.A.O.), 1969) compared with those for the United Kingdom. The British figures have not differed markedly from those of world-wide aviation, although the much larger numbers involved in the world-wide statistics still further reduce fluctuations due to chance.

These statistics, then, give an impression of steadily improving safety in public transport aviation, an impression which is fortified by Stanojlovic (1967), who reported that:—

i. Annually in the period 1920–6, 1 in 4 commercial pilots was killed. This decreased to 1 in 50 in 1932 and by 1966 was 1 in 1600.

ii. Two hundred million people travelled safely on the worlds' scheduled air services in 1966 and insurance companies at that time gave a passenger a better than 40,000 to 1 chance of making an airline journey in safety.

However, as is apparent in *Table I*, fatal public transport accidents which involved British aircraft killed an average of just over 110 persons each year during the period 1961–8, although only two persons died in such accidents in the first six months of 1969. *Fig.* 2 shows that improved flight safety as judged by a falling fatal accident rate has

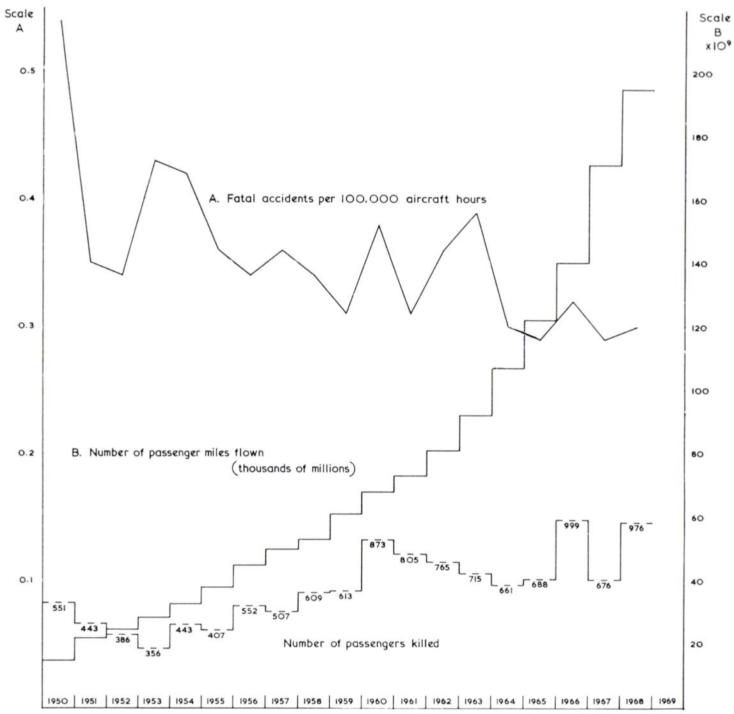


*Fig.* 2.—Combined graph and histograms showing that the increase in volume of public transport aviation during the period 1950–68 was accompanied by a trend towards an increasing annual total of deaths due to aircraft accidents despite an accompanying decline in fatal accident rate.

been accompanied, nevertheless, by a mounting toll of human life due to aircraft accidents. This has resulted from the ever expanding volume of aviation arising from larger aircraft and increasing mileage flown, and it would appear that these trends will continue. Lundberg (quoted by Brown, 1966) estimated that 15,000 people will be killed each year on the worlds' scheduled flights in the 1980's and that there will be one major accident nearly every day. This may or may not be taken as a cause for alarm; it certainly leaves no room for complacency.

Improvement in flight safety can derive from many sources; as suggested in the introduction to this monograph, one source is the comprehensive investigation of all aspects of each accident to discover its main and contributory causes and to study in detail the factors influencing individual safety and survival when this is appropriate. Investigation of the series of fatal accidents here reported shows that a medical and pathological analysis of the relevant evidence is required if the fullest reconstruction of an accident is to be achieved and all the flight safety implications appreciated.

## THE CASE MATERIAL

Eighteen accidents were investigated; all except 3 occurred during public transport flights as defined by the Board of Trade. These 3 involved public transport aircraft which were being flown for the purposes of flight testing or route familiarization. Ninety-six operating and cabin crew and 647 passengers died in these accidents. Fourteen accidents were wholly fatal; 32 persons survived from the other 4. Sixteen of the accidents investigated were to British registered aircraft; 1 was American and 1 Swedish. Eleven accidents occurred abroad, 7 in the United Kingdom.

## THE AIMS OF THE PATHOLOGIST'S INVESTIGATION

Each investigation was undertaken to find any medical evidence which might reveal:—

i. Natural disease or abnormality such as could cause impaired function in the operating crew and provide, therefore,—

*a.* A *possible* medical cause for the accident, or

*b.* A *probable* medical cause for the accident.

ii. A possible or probable non-medical cause for the accident.

iii. The probable events in the aircraft prior to the accident, or

iv. The probable events at impact and immediately after the accident, particularly so far as these related to the questions of survivability and escape.

The main sources of medical evidence were the detailed autopsies on the bodies of all those that were killed. The post-mortem findings had to be correlated with the medical histories of the aircrew, the laboratory examinations of specimens taken at post-mortem, and the evidence in the victims' clothing and at the scene of the accident. Further, and most important, the medical and pathological evidence had to be correlated with, and interpreted in the light of, that found by the non-medical investigators.

# *Chapter 3*

# NATURAL DISEASE IN THE OPERATING CREW

## I—AS A MAIN CAUSE FOR AN ACCIDENT

### General Considerations

A pilot who is a captain of a public transport aircraft must hold an airline transport pilot's (A.L.T.P.) licence and a pilot who acts as co-pilot must have either an A.L.T.P. or a commercial pilot's licence (C.P.L.). These licences are issued for a period of 5 years but are only valid if they contain an up-to-date certificate of medical fitness which has to be renewed every 6 months. It seems probable that a pilot whose livelihood depends upon his retention of a valid licence to fly will maintain himself as physically fit as possible. However, incipient chronic disease can develop and not be detected at the periodic medical examinations and acute illnesses can occur between examinations; either type of condition can be a causative factor in a fatal flying accident.

The assessment of whether natural disease or abnormality discovered in a pilot could be the cause for the accident in which he has been killed is initially a theoretical exercise and involves answering two questions:—

i. Could the disease or condition discovered conceivably cause sudden, severe, or complete incapacitation such that a man might lose control of his aircraft or collapse onto the dual controls of his machine or in some other way interfere with a co-pilot's assumption of effective control?

ii. Could the condition be held to be one that might possibly affect the pilot's state of health or level of efficiency such as to make him unduly liable to commit an error of skill or judgement in the handling of his machine, particularly if some form of mechanical or other emergency had already occurred?

The concept that an accident could be caused by the sudden incapacitation of a vehicle operator is simple enough and well recognized, both in the field of aviation (Townsend and Stembridge, 1958; Robie, Lovell, and Stembridge, 1959; Jackson, 1962a,b; Stevens, 1963; Urschel, 1963) and on the ground (Simpson, 1939; Tannenbaum, 1958). There is evidence from many countries that about 1 in 1000 road traffic accidents is caused by the acute illness of a driver (Herner, Smedby, and Ysander, 1966). In 41 such accidents in Sweden, no persons other than the drivers were killed. In contrast, a transport aircraft accident thus caused will frequently result in much greater loss of life. However, the modern transport aircraft carries two or more pilots. Except at certain critical stages of flight, in particular the take-off and landing phases, sudden incapacitation of one pilot should not be particularly hazardous. Incapacitation of the only pilot in an aircraft is, of course, extremely serious at any stage of flight.

## CORONARY ARTERY DISEASE

The medical condition most likely to be the cause of serious sudden incapacitation is acute coronary insufficiency. This is true both for the general population (Simpson, 1947, 1953) and for aviators (Jackson, 1962b). Benson (1937) reported the first case of a pilot who had suffered a heart attack in flight; there was no accident for he flew for a further 20 minutes to reach his destination and landed safely, but he died an hour later. White (1940) described a similar incident; a pilot suffered a heart attack, managed to land safely, but died some 3 hours later. It was not until 1948 that the first aircraft accident attributed to an attack of coronary insufficiency in a pilot appears to have occurred. This was not reported in the medical literature but is on the files of the Accidents Investigation Branch of the Board of Trade (Warren, 1967; Heggie, 1968). The pilot was flying a light aircraft at the time and the accident is described in Chapter 10.

Mason, Townsend, and Jackson (1963) reported 13 cases of death at the controls of an aircraft and, in an addendum, mentioned that a further 7 had been brought to their notice; only 1 of their 13 cases involved an airline pilot and this was 1 of the 4 described by these authors which did not result in an accident. The captain landed the aircraft, a Super Constellation which was not carrying passengers on that flight; the co-pilot, sensing that reverse thrust was not being applied, glanced at the pilot, a man of 39 years, and saw him collapsed in his seat, dead (Mason, 1963a).

Reighard and Mohler (1968) quoted an unpublished report by Orlady and Carter stating that 16 deaths occurred in airline pilots during flight between 1951 and 1966 but that only 1 of these resulted in a fatal accident. At least 20 cases have occurred since 1963, of which 5 have involved airline pilots: 1 occurred in 1964 when a pilot landed his fully laden passenger aircraft at Kennedy Airport, New York, taxied to dispersal, collapsed and died as he shut down the engines (Peffers, 1964); and 3 cases occurred at O'Hare, Illinois, and Hector, California, during 1964 and 1965, but no accident resulted. The fifth case did result in an accident; it occurred at Ardmore, Oklahoma, in 1966 (Civil Aeronautics Board, 1967) and 83 people were killed. Buley (1969) collected 17 cases of death or terminal collapse of airline pilots while at the controls of aircraft from 1961 to March, 1968, from reports made by 17 nations; in 5 instances accidents resulted and in 4 the cause of the pilot's collapse was coronary artery disease; in 5 of the other 12 an accident was narrowly avoided, and in all 12 coronary artery disease was proved at autopsy (4 cases) or alleged to have been the cause of collapse although autopsy findings were not known (8 cases).

Should a pilot killed in an aircraft accident be found at autopsy to have severe narrowing of the coronary arteries, this would provide a hypothetical cause for the accident. Adequate appraisal of the significance of such pathology can rarely be made at the mortuary table. The appearances in many who die from acute coronary insufficiency are of coronary artery narrowing only (Knight, 1965; Baroldi and Manion, 1967); Baroldi (1965) found no thrombosis or histological abnormality in 53 per cent of 116 cases of 'unexpected "coronary" heart death'. Unless the patient survives his episode of coronary insufficiency for from 2 to 4 hours or more, even the most modern techniques (Knight, 1965, 1967) will not reveal evidence of an infarct (or 'idiopathic coagulation necrosis', as Baroldi (1965) and Baroldi and Manion (1967) prefer to call the condition; they do not believe that myocardial 'infarcts' are true infarcts). It is possible, if not probable, that coronary artery disease found in a pilot following an accident is most often incidental; Mason (1963b) showed that severe coronary artery disease is common even in medically highly selected and apparently fit men; often such a man will be killed in an accident for which sudden incapacitation on his part has not been the cause, and Scheinman (1968) made a plea for 'extreme conservatism in implicating coronary artery disease in an otherwise unexplained aviation accident'.

Should a pilot be found to have not only gross narrowing of his coronary arteries but complete occlusion by thrombus at one point, this would be more strongly suggestive that his sudden incapacitation may have been the cause for the accident. However, even then, two other possibilities must be considered. Firstly, the thrombosis could have been a terminal event and an integral part of a 'heart attack' occurring in a pilot struggling unsuccessfully to cope with some emergency due to a technical fault in his aircraft. Secondly, it is known that many persons who have no history of ever having had a heart attack of any sort, are found at autopsy to have evidence of old myocardial infarcts. Knight (1965) has pointed out that in a number of cases of sudden death evidence of a myocardial infarct several hours old is found; this has apparently been silent and compatible with normal activity and efficiency up to the moment of collapse and death. It could have happened, therefore, by coincidence that some other cause for an accident had supervened despite the pilot having had a silent myocardial infarct. *A hypothetical explanation for an accident, therefore, based on post-mortem findings can only become a theoretical explanation for an accident with a degree of probability if there is supporting evidence, and little or no conflicting evidence.*

In the accident at Ardmore (Civil Aeronautics Board, 1967) referred to above, the evidence for incapacitation of the pilot appeared overwhelming. The aircraft was approaching to land. Local weather conditions caused the captain to make a late change in his choice of runway for landing. At an altitude of about 1200 feet he was making a right-hand turn to line up with the finally selected runway when the aircraft suddenly dived and crashed into high ground 350 feet below. The very gross coronary artery disease with some myocardial fibrosis found in the captain at autopsy suggested that loss of control as a result of an attack of acute coronary insufficiency may have precipitated the accident. The circumstances of the accident fitted the hypothesis; the co-pilot would have had too little time to regain control (6 seconds was estimated as the maximum); fractures of the co-pilot's upper limbs were more severe than those of the captain; the co-pilot's thumbs were fractured but not those of the captain. This evidence was regarded as consistent with the co-pilot grasping the control column at the time the aircraft struck the ground (Reals, Mohler, Doyle, and Gibbons, 1968). It transpired further, that the captain had concealed a history of diabetes for over 3 years and clinical heart disease for about 18 years. His angina pectoris had become increasingly severe during the previous few years and he had taken increasing dosages of nitroglycerin and similar drugs. At his periodical medical examinations for renewal of his licence no abnormality had been detected and he had not revealed his symptoms or treatment. In view of all the available evidence there is little doubt that this particular accident resulted from incapacitation of the pilot.

In the present series of fatal public transport accidents there is no instance in which a pilot was found to have coronary artery disease of sufficient severity for it to be considered a possible cause of the accident. However, the difficulty of assessing the significance of coronary artery disease in the context of a particular accident is matched by that of evaluating other pathological conditions, notably myocarditis; this series of public transport accidents does include 2 cases of this condition.

## Isolated Focal Myocarditis

Manion (1966) reviewed the development of the concept of myocarditis from its introduction into the medical literature by Sobernheim (1837), through its association, in both acute and chronic form, with many infectious diseases as described by numerous authors in the second half of the nineteenth century, to the recognition of 'primary acute interstitial myocarditis' by Fiedler in 1899 (Baensch and Fiedler, 1900) in whose cases there were no clinical symptoms of other diseases nor were there changes in other organs. There followed many papers describing 'isolated' myocarditis—'without accompanying septic signs in other organs' (Sellentin, 1904); Scott and Saphir had collected 30 cases from the literature by 1929.

Then for a period the term 'myocarditis' fell into disrepute, partly because of its indiscriminate use on death certificates and partly because any chronic disease of the myocardium, whatever its nature, tended to be called 'chronic myocarditis'. Manion (1966) concluded that, although from the more recent literature there was still not complete agreement on what constituted 'myocarditis', it was probably best to accept the original meaning as given by Sobernheim (1837), 'an inflammation of heart muscle', and accept what all would agree as evidence of that inflammation, namely 'an exudative or proliferative cellular reaction' (Clawson, 1928) demonstrated microscopically.

Thus over a period of about a hundred years have arisen the terms 'isolated', 'Fiedler's', 'idiopathic', and 'interstitial' myocarditis, with the addition of adjectives such as 'focal' and 'diffuse' to indicate the extent of the microscopic changes in the heart muscle.

An indication of the prevalence of myocarditis was given by Saphir (1942) who found this condition in 240 hearts from 5626 routine autopsies and by Gore and Saphir (1947) who studied 1042 autopsies and found myocarditis in 25 per cent of cases with rheumatic fever and diphtheria, and in a high proportion of cases of rickettsial, streptococcal, meningococcal, spirochaetal, and other infections. In only 3 per cent of their cases was the myocarditis not associated with extracardiac manifestations of disease processes known to cause myocarditis.

Although Simpson (1947) did not list myocarditis as a cause of death in his review of over 6000 cases of sudden unexpected death, there is evidence that 'isolated myocarditis' can cause sudden unexpected death. Corby (1960) described 32 cases and said that the incidence of the condition in medicolegal autopsies carried out in the London area was 0·35 per cent and that this was in agreement with other published figures which varied between 0·2 and 0·4 per cent. However, he did not report that histological examinations of the myocardium were carried out in all medicolegal autopsies in the

London area. Twenty-eight of his series of 32 cases died suddenly in a manner similar to that often associated with coronary artery disease; 4 cases were accompanied by a relatively prolonged illness but were included because death was unexpected and otherwise unexplained at autopsy.

Corby (1960) found in each of his 32 cases that the myocardium was infiltrated by inflammatory cells, mostly lymphocytes and monocytes but with occasional polymorphonuclear leucocytes and eosinophils. He stated that some degree of muscle degeneration and necrosis was always present, although he described 1 case where 'the only finding in 4 blocks of heart was a small circumscribed area with interfibrillary infiltration of lymphocytes and somewhat small muscle-fibres'. He agreed with Saphir (1942) that the lesions of isolated myocarditis were essentially patchy; some sections in each of his cases were free from inflammation.

Gormsen (1955) reviewed 1378 cases of sudden natural death or death from unknown causes in persons between 2 and 89 years of age; he found 17 cases of myocarditis and claimed that the incidence of this condition was therefore 1·2 per cent. He called the majority of his cases 'isolated diffuse interstitial myocarditis' but some 'isolated granulomatous myocarditis'; some he said were incidental to severe acute infections and others 'cases of sequels to myocarditis'. The latter were cases of focal myocardial fibrosis associated with occasional mild inflammatory infiltrate.

Gormsen carried out detailed histological examinations of the myocardium in only those 117 of the 1378 cases for which no acceptable cause of death had been demonstrated at autopsy. In fact, he discovered evidence of myocarditis in 14·5 per cent of cases of otherwise unexplained death; in these he attributed death to the myocarditis discovered. The cause of the death in 28 of the 117 cases remained obscure after all examinations; it was, therefore, at least theoretically possible that some of those cases in which myocarditis was found died from the same cause or causes as the 28 cases of death from unknown cause and that the myocarditis discovered was incidental and not the true cause of death. Gormsen did not indicate how extensive were the inflammatory changes found in all his cases; in some, all sections examined showed the pathological changes but some were clearly 'focal', although he didn't use that term. In 16 cases he described an interstitial infiltration predominantly by lymphocytes; histiocytes were present in most instances as were a few plasma cells and neutrophil polymorphonuclear leucocytes.

Mason (1962b) described the case of a pilot who collapsed and died in his cockpit as he was preparing to take-off in his light aircraft. After a detailed post-mortem examination, death was ascribed to myocarditis; this was not 'isolated' in this instance as there were abnormal histological changes present in bowel mucosa, liver, pancreas, kidneys, and thyroid. The patient had had a history of an influenza-like illness with loss of weight, tachycardia, and a hypochromic anaemia a week or two before his death. Had he died from his illness a minute or so later an accident would have ensued; had the findings in the heart been incriminated as the cause of his collapse and therefore the accident, this conclusion would, in this instance, have been correct. In this case the heart muscle showed interfibrillary oedema, some congestion, a few tiny petechial haemorrhages, and occasional small collections of round cells, and the myocarditis was thought to be thyrotoxic.

Myocarditis can lead to death within 24–48 hours of sudden but not necessarily completely incapacitating onset of symptoms; I think it likely that this is the commonest type of history in those who die from myocarditis. Lowe and Broughton (1965) had such a case; death occurred approximately 36 hours following the onset of acute dyspnoea; diffuse inflammatory changes and patchy necrosis of myocardial fibres were present throughout every histological section from every block of myocardium examined. Whitehead (1965) reviewed 18 cases of isolated myocarditis from nearly 13,000 autopsies. He selected the cases on the basis that the pathology was confined or virtually confined to the heart and was directly responsible for death. Of the 18 cases none had dropped dead; 2 died within an hour or so of the onset of 'subacute' dyspnoea, cyanosis, and vomiting; only 2 appeared to have been completely and suddenly incapacitated—one by a Stokes-Adams attack (he lived several days to suffer several more such attacks) and the other was found dead in bed.

There is evidence that myocarditis may be an incidental finding when death occurs from some other unrelated cause. Schwartz and Mitchell (1962) reported a detailed study of the hearts of 137 unselected hospital deaths of people over the age of 35; they found an average of 7 per cent to have focal myocarditis; but they could not explain a sex incidence of 3 per cent in males and 11 per cent in females. They found that 26 per cent of the hearts they examined had small fibrous lesions scattered throughout the myocardium; some of these lesions were specks visible to the naked eye but others were detectable only on histological examination. The presence of these small fibrous areas could not be correlated with coronary artery disease although they did increase with age. In contrast large fibrous lesions could always be correlated with pre-existing coronary artery disease and therefore myocardial ischaemia. They considered that the small fibrous scars were the result of old inflammatory lesions—that is myocarditis.

Mason (1962c) described a case of myocarditis in a pilot in which there was no doubt that the condition had no connexion with his death; the latter resulted from the complications of his inadvertent ejection from a military aircraft. Mason (1962d) also reported the case of a pilot who was believed to have died from decompression sickness—he collapsed after a few minutes at an altitude of 35,000 feet in an unpressurized aircraft, became deeply comatose, and died about twelve hours later. The myocardium was oedematous and there was a focal but widespread infiltration with polymorphonuclear leucocytes. Fryer (1961) found that histological evidence of focal myocarditis was rare in decompression sickness; it was present in only 3 of the 17 cases he reviewed and in each instance the changes were minimal. The myocarditis in the case of decompression sickness may, therefore, have been incidental.

The incidental finding of focal myocarditis in military pilots following fatal aircraft accidents due to known and unrelated causes has been reported by others including Robie, Lovell, and Stembridge (1959) and Jackson (1962a).

I have studied sections taken from 10 standard blocks from the ventricular and atrial walls and the interventricular septum from hearts of 35 apparently healthy men between the ages of 18 and 52 years, killed in accidents which could not have been precipitated by their own collapse. Two of these had focal myocarditis; in each case it was undoubtedly an incidental finding unrelated to the man's accident or his death.

Tonge (1968) studied the myocardium in a series of 134 persons who died similarly from accidents which they themselves could not have caused. He prepared complete transverse sections at 1 ventricular level in 10 hearts, at 18 ventricular levels in 10 hearts and at 3 levels in the remaining 114 hearts. Of the hearts sectioned at 1 ventricular level, 40 per cent contained inflammatory lesions; of those sectioned at 3 levels 67 per cent had lesions; and of those sectioned at 18 levels 9 of the 10 hearts contained lesions.

It would seem, therefore, that very considerable caution should be exercised before focal myocarditis found at autopsy on a person killed in an accident is interpreted as the cause of that person's collapse and therefore the cause of the accident; but at least 1 fatal aircraft accident has been attributed to this condition (Department of Civil Aviation, Australia, 1962). The 2 accidents in which pilots were found to have focal myocarditis in the present series are detailed below:—

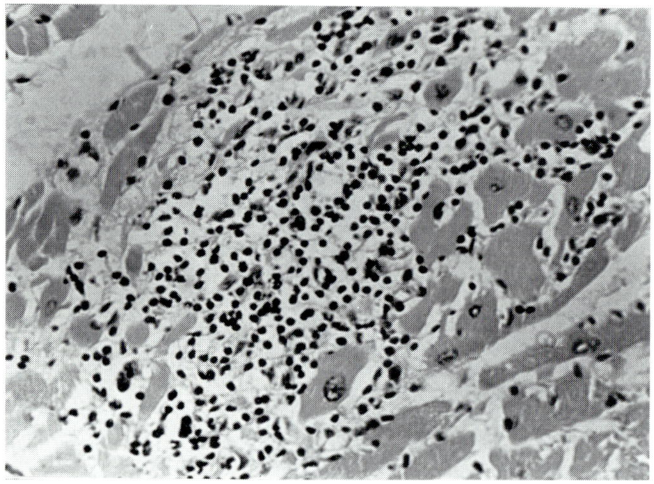

*Fig*. 3.—Moderately extensive focal myocarditis in a co-pilot. In some low-power fields three or four foci of inflammation could be seen; this is a high-power view of one focus. The infiltrate is predominantly lymphocytic, there are moderately severe degenerative changes in, and apparent actual loss of, muscle cells. H. & E. (× 120.) (*Reproduced from Stevens (1968a) by permission of the Editor 'Medicine, Science and the Law'*.)

## ACCIDENT NUMBER 219

The changes of focal myocarditis were found in the left ventricle (*Fig*. 3), the interventricular septum, and beneath the pericardium of the right ventricle of the heart of the co-pilot of a freight-carrying aircraft. The captain was making a ground-controlled approach to land and announced changing to a visual approach after the aircraft had descended clear of cloud and was lined up with the runway.

Eye-witnesses saw the descent continue normally to about 100 feet but then the aircraft began a slow turn to one side; the angle of bank increased and was maintained until the machine crashed into a factory roof about 1000 feet to the side of the runway. More than one-third of the 110 slides prepared from 18 representative blocks of the co-pilot's myocardium showed evidence of myocarditis; the changes appeared to be as extensive or more extensive than in some of the cases in which Gormsen (1955) and Corby (1960) attributed sudden death to focal myocarditis. This co-pilot's disease was, therefore, a hypothetical cause for the accident; it might have resulted in his sudden collapse and his fouling of the controls in a manner which prevented the captain from regaining control in the few seconds available.

A similar aircraft to the one which had crashed was taken to a safe height and repeated attempts were made to reconstruct, on the basis of the complete collapse of the co-pilot, a similar flight path to that taken by the crashed aircraft. This was done with and without fastened seat belts and with and without fastened shoulder harnesses. It was tried with the co-pilot and then with the captain at the controls at the time the simulated incapacitation of the co-pilot was initiated. From these experiments it appeared impossible, under any circumstances, to ascribe the accident to a sudden collapse of the co-pilot from his myocarditis. The hypothesis could not be substantiated and it was concluded that the myocarditis was an incidental finding.

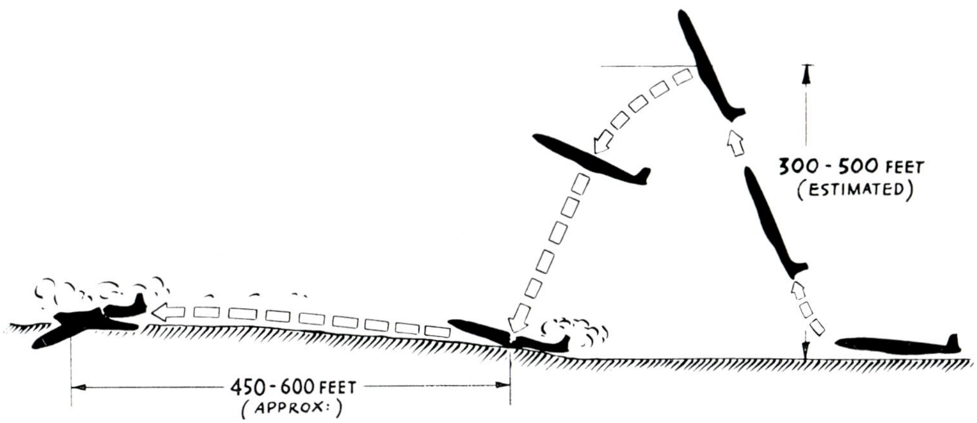


*Fig.* 4.—Diagrammatic representation of accident number 152. The angle of ascent is deliberately exaggerated to emphasize the circumstances of the accident; the angle of climb was probably no greater than 45° when the machine stalled. (*Reproduced from Stevens (1968a) by permission of the Editor 'Medicine, Science and the Law'.*)

## ACCIDENT NUMBER 152

This accident occurred to an aircraft which was seen to begin its take-off at night in a normal way; but the usual steep initial climb at an angle of about 20–25° became steeper, reaching about 45° by the time the machine was a few hundred feet up. The aircraft then stalled and crashed as depicted in *Fig.* 4; it broke in two and skidded several hundred feet in snow and mud and caught fire.

The operating crew consisted of a captain, a co-pilot, and a flight engineer. The captain was found to have focal myocarditis. Unfortunately the extent of the microscopic changes in the heart as a whole could not be assessed; this was one of my earlier cases and my practice of saving the whole heart for examination in the laboratory had not been adopted at that time. Although sections from one block of tissue taken from the left ventricle (*Fig.* 5) showed only a few small collections of lymphocytes scattered throughout the tissue, sections from a block of the interventricular septum showed some rather larger foci of chronic inflammatory cells with evidence of necrosis of muscle fibres (*Fig.* 6). There was, therefore, an unequivocal focal myocardial inflammation and the possibility that the pilot had collapsed at the controls had to be considered. There was both non-medical and additional medical evidence to be correlated with the finding of natural disease in the pilot as is summarized below.

### Pathological Evidence of the Cause of the Captain's Death and its Timing Relative to Ground Impact

There was no evidence found in the captain's body that he had been alive in the post-crash fire, although 21 of the 27 who died in this accident, including the co-pilot,

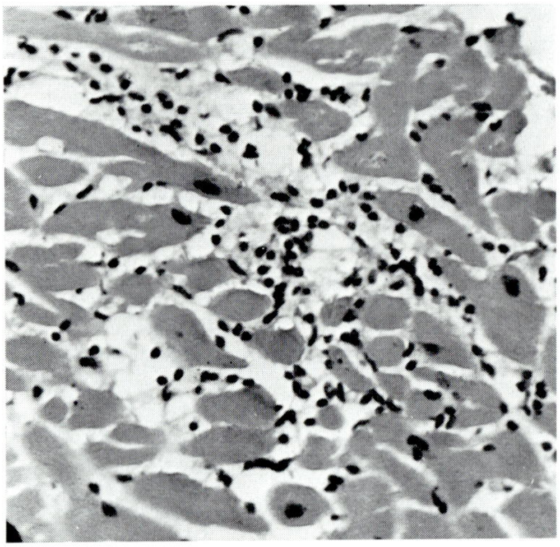

*Fig.* 5.—One of six small, widely separated foci of inflammatory infiltrate in a section of myocardium from the left ventricle of a pilot killed in accident number 152. H. & E. (× 120.)

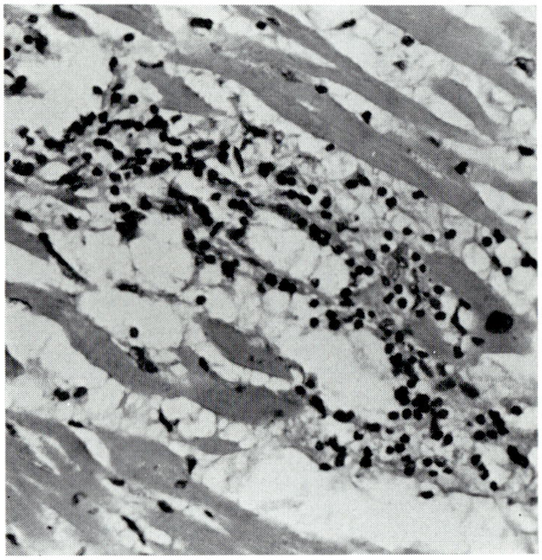

*Fig.* 6.—A rather larger focus of inflammation in the interventricular septum of the same case as *Fig.* 5. There is evidence here of necrosis of muscle-fibres. H. & E. (× 120.)

died from asphyxiation due to inhalation of products of combustion. These 21 all had gross oedema of lungs, evidence of swallowed or inhaled carbon (*Fig.* 7) and raised blood carboxyhaemoglobin levels.

The captain had injuries which were sufficient to explain his death at ground impact; a severe fracture of the base of the skull was accompanied by cerebral contusion and laceration and subarachnoid haemorrhage. There were, in addition, a number of less severe injuries including fractured legs. The cardiovascular system was found to be anatomically intact.

Histological preparations of the captain's lungs revealed both fat and bone-marrow emboli. Bone-marrow embolism and a moderate to severe degree of fat embolism, either alone or in combination, are specific evidence of bony injury occurring with an intact cardiovascular system which has continued to function for at least a sufficient length of time to permit the emboli to be transferred from the site of injury to the lungs (Mason, 1968a). It could be concluded, therefore, that the captain's

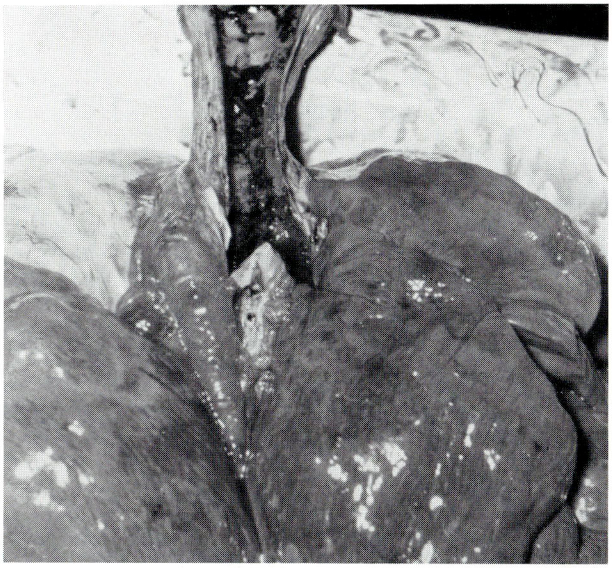

*Fig.* 7.—Swollen and oedematous lungs with carbon in the trachea showed that this air-crash victim had been alive for a period during the post-crash fire.

circulation was functioning at the time of ground impact when he received both lethal and non-lethal bony injury and that his circulation continued to function for a period of approximately 15 seconds, at least.

## Correlation and Interpretation of the Medical and Non-Medical Evidence

As stated above, the accident was precipitated, according to the evidence of reliable eye-witnesses, by an already steep climb becoming steeper and causing the aircraft to stall.

In 4 of the 32 cases of sudden death from focal myocarditis reported by Corby (1960), incapacitation was partial and accompanied by severe anginal pain without loss of consciousness; this preceded death by some hours. In view of the attitude of the aircraft during the climb, a pilot collapsing could only have fallen back in his seat; he could not have fallen forwards and thus fouled the controls, irrespective of whether he had had his shoulder harness fastened at the time. It had to be considered, therefore, whether, if the captain had been incapacitated by his myocarditis during take-off and had suffered severe angina pectoris without complete loss of consciousness, he may have tightened his grip upon the control column and inadvertently pulled it back. This could not be excluded completely but would be a most unlikely thing for an experienced captain to do while he remained conscious for he would be acutely aware of the danger to himself as well as to all on board.

Unexpected and sudden death due to focal myocarditis is likely to be due to interference with the normal conducting mechanism, thus causing cardiac arrest or ventricular fibrillation. I can find no evidence to show that such death is accompanied by other than immediate relaxation of muscles; I have found no records of cadaveric spasm in this type of death. Collapse, short of death, is of a syncopal nature. It was most likely, therefore, that if the captain had died or collapsed at the controls in the air he would have relaxed his grip upon the control column, and not pulled it back.

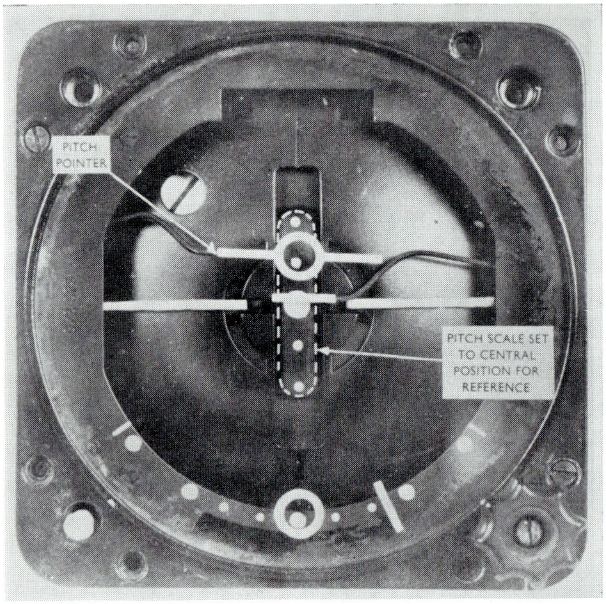
PITCH
POINTER
PITCH SCALE SET
TO CENTRAL
POSITION FOR
REFERENCE

*Fig.* 8.—The dial of an intact director horizon—one of a pilot's flight instruments. The white horizontal bar across the centre of the instrument face represents the horizon. The pitch pointer moves up and down and by its distance from the white horizontal line gives an indication of the angle of pitch, i.e., the angle of climb or descent. (*From Jones (1962); Crown Copyright, reproduced by permission of the Controller of Her Majesty's Stationery Office.*)

The effect upon the attitude of the aircraft if the pilot relaxed his hold on the control column would have depended upon the amount of trim applied to the elevator (this would normally have been set at about neutral during take-off) and the loading of the machine and its resultant centre of gravity. The chances were that if the pilot relaxed his grip on the control column it would not have resulted in the aircraft increasing its angle of climb, although this could not be claimed with certainty; the centre of gravity of the aircraft as loaded was not known (but the known distribution of passengers within the fuselage suggested that it would have been fairly far back) nor was it possible from an examination of the wreckage to determine the elevator trim setting. A more likely cause for the increased angle of climb was that the pilot pulled the control column back too far either deliberately or inadvertently for a reason other than incapacitation due to myocarditis.

An instrument known as a 'director horizon' was found in the wreckage and shown to be mechanically faulty. This had come from the captain's instrument panel. The face of an intact instrument is shown in *Fig*. 8. It is not appropriate to explain in detail the use of this type of instrument nor the considerable differences of opinion expressed by various pilots as to whether (and if so, how) the instrument should have been used during take-off. Suffice it to say, that there was strong evidence that both pilots had been taught to use the instrument to make the relatively steep climb immediately after

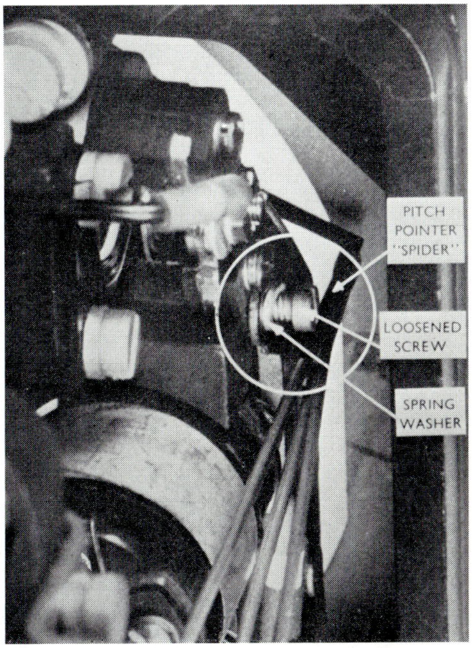


*Fig*. 9.—A view from the back of the partially dismantled director horizon from the captain's instrument panel from accident 152. The loosened screw in the position shown impeded the movement of the pitch pointer arm called a 'spider'. (*From Jones (1962); Crown Copyright, reproduced by permission of the Controller of Her Majesty's Stationery Office.*)

take-off required by the noise abatement regulations. To use the instrument in such a way, a pilot would achieve the desired angle of climb by pulling the control column back until the pitch pointer had travelled a certain distance upwards from the white horizontal bar representing the horizon on the instrument face.

*Fig*. 9 shows that the travel of the pitch pointer 'spider' in the instrument recovered from the wreckage is impeded by a loose dial mask retaining screw. Examination of the inside of the instrument suggested that the screw might not have been tightened securely when originally assembled and that it had become gradually unscrewed over a long period of time. At first, it was thought, the screw had not touched the spider during its movement, later it had just made contact but had allowed the spider to ride over it; finally, it was suggested, it had caused complete obstruction with the spider in a position which prevented the pitch pointer from showing more than an equivalent pitch attitude of $7\frac{1}{2}$ degrees (Jones, 1962).

### Discussion and Conclusions—Accident Number 152

The manufacturers of the director horizon are being sued by the airline concerned at the time of writing; the screw at the back of the instrument could only have become loose, it has been claimed, if it had not been properly secured during the assembly of the instrument. The importance of the medical evidence is apparent; that the utmost caution had to be taken in the interpretation of the medical evidence, in the light of all the circumstances of the accident and all the non-medical evidence, is equally clear. Only two theories could be advanced to explain the accident; in view of the pending litigation, the reader is left to decide for himself which is the more acceptable.

*First Theory*

The captain suffered a collapse due to myocarditis while the aircraft was in the initial climb after take-off. This collapse resulted in his clutching the control column and pulling it back thus increasing the angle of climb of the aircraft to the point of stall. The collapse, however, was not accompanied by cessation of his circulation; or, if the heart did stop functioning due to ventricular fibrillation, impact with the ground resulted in temporary resumption of normal pumping action. At ground impact, lethal and non-lethal bony injury occurred, and the pumping action of the heart with an intact circulatory system resulted in pulmonary bone-marrow and fat embolism. As death followed almost immediately, the captain did not inhale products of combustion in the ensuing fire as did his fellow crew. The state of the captain's director horizon was irrelevant, either having been caused in the crash or subsequent to the crash before expert examination, and the deductions based on the evidence in the instrument were erroneous.

*Second Theory*

The captain took off and judged the angle of the climb he induced in the aircraft by the information displayed on his director horizon. This instrument, being faulty, indicated a much lower angle of pitch than was in fact attained; a satisfactory angle of climb was achieved immediately but this the captain did not realize. Acting upon the false information given by his instrument the pilot pulled the control column further back; this caused a stall from which recovery was impossible from the height attained—about 500 feet. The focal myocarditis was an incidental finding, asymptomatic and completely unrelated to the cause of the accident.

## Other Diseases associated with Acute Incapacitation

Pathological conditions other than those which affect the heart may be a cause for sudden incapacitation or death. Jackson (1962a) suggested that acute infection could be a cause for sudden incapacitation; this received some support from Mason (1962e) who quoted Roberts (1957) and Neilson (1958) and discussed two cases of sudden death in aircrew which may have been due to influenza. Spontaneous pneumothorax has been discussed in the context of acute incapacitation by Robie and others (1959, quoted by Mason, 1962e), Stevens (1963), and, more recently, by Fuchs (1967a,b,c); most of these reports deal with military aviators and it is likely that this condition is of less importance in civil aviation than in military aviation which often involves flight at high altitude in aircraft pressurized to only a low differential and the use of positive-pressure oxygen breathing apparatus. The case reported by Flux and Dille (1969) involved a civilian pilot but he was flying a military type aircraft at a cockpit pressure equivalent of about 21,000 feet at the time.

Siegel and Mohler (1969) reported a fatal light aircraft accident the pilot of which had an acute suppurative appendicitis and peri-appendiceal abscess, but whether or not it was a contributory cause of the accident was not known. I have found no recorded cases of in-flight incapacitation due to perforated peptic ulcer or to acute renal colic. Payne (1962) drew attention to the danger of acute glaucoma as a cause of sudden blindness and consequent accident, though Catlett and Kidera (1968) considered that chronic glaucoma was not generally a cause for grounding commercial pilots as drug therapy and regular ophthalmic and tonometric surveillance were satisfactory.

Epilepsy is the second commonest cause of road traffic accidents due to illness of a driver (Herner, Smedby, and Ysander, 1966); it has been reported also in aviators. Rook (1947) investigated 500 cases of loss of consciousness (though not necessarily having occurred in flight) among pilots and other aircrew; he found that just over one-eighth of these were epileptic. A glider accident which was almost certainly due to the pilot having suffered an epileptic fit is described in Section III, and 6 cases of epilepsy, 2 of which occurred during flight, were described by Bennett (1964). Seipal and Wentz (1963) reported an instance of a pilot who had an epileptic fit while flying solo and recovered a half an hour later to find himself still safely airborne! Buley (1969) reported 42 cases of incapacitation of airline pilots in flight; organic disease was diagnosed in 24 instances and in 6 it was a form of epilepsy.

Cerebral haemorrhage due to the rupture of a berry aneurysm of an intracranial artery is a well-known cause for very severe headache and loss of consciousness. It occurs typically in apparently previously healthy persons and, although commonest between the ages of 40 and 60 years, may occur at any age (McDowell, 1959). No record of a case of an aircraft accident thus precipitated has been found in the literature.

There are other causes for loss of consciousness in flight; Mason (1968b) quoted Camps (1963) as publicizing hypoglycaemia as a cause for accidents on the ground, but cited several authors who had dismissed this as a prominent cause for aircraft accidents. Gibbons, Plechus, Chandler, and Ellis (1966) discussed alcohol-induced hypoglycaemia but failed to produce substantial evidence that it played a significant role in the causation of flying accidents. Franks (1959) and McCann and Schulze (1963) referred to the summation of adverse physiological factors as a cause of syncope; these are far more likely to operate in military aviators, however, than in airline pilots, though they may be of importance occasionally in pilots of light aircraft. Death at the controls of an aircraft and sudden unconsciousness in a passenger due to a colloid cyst of the third ventricle were reported by Nelson and Haymaker (1957); Berry and Stembridge (1958) recorded sudden loss of consciousness in a pilot at the controls of an aircraft as the first manifestation of an astrocytoma; and Dille and Pei (1964) described a case of unexplained vertigo and loss of consciousness in flight affecting a young pilot flying solo.

Invalidings from airlines' flying staff occur from time to time for a variety of potentially incapacitating illnesses including epilepsy, cerebral tumour, cerebral thrombosis, schizophrenia, asthma, Menière's disease and vertiginous attacks due to various causes (Peffers, 1961; Preston, 1968a). Many of these conditions could present their first serious symptoms during flight and result in an accident.

There is little doubt that flying accidents due to conditions such as those cited above will occur from time to time but they are likely to be infrequent. Their infrequency is all the more reason why they should be kept in mind during fatal accident investigation, for they are likely to be overlooked. Detailed medical histories of the crew must be sought and detailed autopsies with careful histological examination must be carried out on the crew if natural disease is not to be missed.

## II—NATURAL DISEASE AS A CONTRIBUTORY CAUSE FOR AN ACCIDENT

### Reduced Efficiency of a Pilot

It has been shown above that it is often difficult to assess accurately the significance of any potentially incapacitating natural disease found at autopsy in the pilot. It is even more difficult to assess the significance of disease capable only of causing reduced

*Table III.*—The Association of 'Pilot Error' and British Public Transport Aircraft Accidents: 1961–7

| | 1961 | 1962 | 1963 | 1964 | 1965 | 1966 | 1967 | Total |
|---|---|---|---|---|---|---|---|---|
| Total Accidents | 13 | 10 | 13 | 13 | 22 | 16 | 19 | 106 |
| Investigation complete at publication of annual survey | 9 | 7 | 12 | 12 | 16 | 14 | 12 | 82 (100%) |
| No. attributed to pilot error | 6 | 1 | 3 | 7 | 9 | 7 | 6 | 39 (47·6%) |

efficiency rather than incapacitation. In such circumstances the accident will appear to have been due to and, in fact, will have been due to a pilot's error of skill or judgement. *Table III* shows that in recent years between 10 and 55 per cent (average 47·6 per cent) of total public transport accidents have been attributed in part or entirely to 'pilot error'.

Harper (1964) and Dougherty and Harper (1968) studied the relationship between minor physical defects (that is, defects not such as to have prevented the granting of a licence to fly) in general aviation pilots, their ages and their involvement in accidents. They found that the risk of a pilot having an accident was increased by a physical defect of any kind; the average increased risk was 2·24, the range of relative risks for various types of defect from 1·78 to 4·65. Multiple defects increased the risk. Increasing age of a pilot increased the risk only in so far as physical defects increased with age. Mohler, Bedell, Ross, and Veregge (1969), also noted that increasing age itself did not have an adverse effect upon accident records. Harper (1964) did not imply that the physical defects were the cause *per se* of accidents, only that they appeared to have some relationship as contributory factors, a relationship which required study.

Preston (1968b) stated that cases are recorded of aircrews being partially incapacitated by food poisoning. He described a severe outbreak of gastro-enteritis among aircrew as a result of eating polluted oysters in flight; fortunately the symptoms in this instance did not occur until about 30 hours after ingestion of the offending material and all involved were off-duty when affected. Buley (1969) discussed 'multiple-cause' accidents and pointed out that transient pilot indisposition due to a common cause (such as an attack of gastro-enteritis) could occur at a time of unfavourable operational conditions or malfunction of equipment and result, at best, in 'an unusually high task load' for the other crew members, or, at worst, 'in demands beyond the capability of the depleted system'. Clearly, there are many factors which, if present in combinations of two or more, could cause an accident attributable to pilot error; those factors inherent in the pilot himself include fatigue, professional or social anxieties, physiological variations, as well as subclinical disease of any type.

The present series does not include an example of subclinical natural disease that has been one of several summating causes leading to an accident of 'pilot error' type; this may well be because of the investigators' inability to demonstrate the true causes of some of the unexplained or partially explained accidents.

## THE INCIDENCE OF NATURAL DISEASE IN AIRLINE PILOTS

The 18 public transport accidents reviewed resulted in the death of 44 pilots (modern airliners may have a crew of three pilots). Twenty of these pilots suffered disintegrative mechanical trauma with or without incineration; the presence or absence of natural disease could not be determined in these cases. In 17 instances complete autopsies were possible and in a further 7 the autopsies were deficient only in that an examination for intracranial pathology was precluded by partial or complete decapitation.

In 4 of the 24 autopsies carried out, moderately severe coronary artery disease was found; 3 were Grade 2—severe, and 1 was Grade 3 but with an adequate lumen (classification according to Mason, 1963b). In none was the coronary artery disease considered to have any bearing upon the cause of the accident. Mason (1963b) collected and reviewed several series which showed the incidence of coronary artery disease in aviators (mostly military) and controls. He concluded that despite their regular medical surveillance, professional aircrew were as subject to severe undetected coronary artery disease as the male population in general. The finding of a few pilots in this series with moderately severe coronary artery disease is not, therefore, surprising.

One case of respiratory allergy was found and 3 cases of myocarditis, 1 of which was doubtful although 2 were unequivocal. The pilot with evidence of respiratory allergy and the pilot with equivocal myocarditis were both killed in accident number 158; there was no suggestion that this accident was due to pilot illness. The other 2 cases of myocarditis have been fully discussed above.

The pathology found in this small series of pilots does not justify any criticism of the present system of medical selection of pilots or their surveillance at periodic examinations. No recognized routine clinical examination can detect coronary artery disease of moderate severity; in many cases no procedure except coronary artery angiography can demonstrate even gross coronary artery obstruction (FitzGibbon, 1967). The mortality associated with coronary angiography (Gensini, 1963) has been considerably reduced in more recent practice (FitzGibbon, 1967) but the procedure continues to have an appreciable morbidity with complications such as segmental obstruction of the brachial artery. It is doubtful, therefore, whether coronary angiography will ever become a routine investigation for all pilots, but the evidence suggests that it is safe enough to be used if there is a suspicion of coronary artery disease in a pilot; his career will, and his passengers' lives may, depend upon an accurate diagnosis (FitzGibbon, 1969).

In only 19 of the 41 road traffic accidents caused by acute illness of a driver reported by Herner, Smedby, and Ysander (1966) was there any possibility of a previous medical examination having indicated that the subject was unfit to drive. As pointed out in the *Lancet* (1957), it is impossible within the compass of present medical knowledge, to detect all physical disorders which could lead to an accident. The medical standards for airline pilots are probably as satisfactory as they can be at the present time, but, as Buley (1969) observed, the need to pursue 'refinements in aeromedical examination and certification techniques' should not be neglected.

## *Chapter 4*

# IMPAIRED EFFICIENCY OF A PILOT DUE TO INTOXICATION

## ALCOHOL

ON the majority of occasions on which they have been available since 1960, tissues from pilots' bodies have been examined for the presence of alcohol. In the earlier investigations this was done by a coarse screening method but later Nicholls' method (1960) was used. In most instances the values were nil or not in excess of 25 mg. per 100 ml.; when such a low level was found it was considered to be negligible with regard to the cause of the accident. Furthermore, it was appreciated that not all the reducing substance measured was necessarily ethyl alcohol nor could the possibility be excluded that small amounts of ethyl alcohol had been produced post-mortem.

Much has been written on the subject of the production of ethyl alcohol post-mortem. Muehlberger (1954) stated that levels of alcohol from 20 to 80 mg. per 100 ml., could be produced in bodies free from alcohol at the time of death and further that a loss of alcohol could occur from bodies with high levels. Blackmore (1968) quoted, among others, Gormsen (1954a,b) as stating that ethyl alcohol could be generated post-mortem; Plueckhahn (1967) as reporting that alcohol levels in excess of 200 mg. per 100 ml. could be produced in samples of post-mortem blood not treated with sodium fluoride; Wolthers (1958) as stating that false levels would not be found within 48 hours of death and Turkel and Gifford (1957) as suggesting that ethyl alcohol was not produced in the cadaver. Kalant (1968) quoted several additional authors who had demonstrated the production of ethyl alcohol in post-mortem tissues including Bonnichsen, Halstrøm, Møller, and Theorell (1953) who reported that a level as high as 240 mg. per 100 ml. could be found in blood within 24 hours of death; but he pointed out that it had been claimed in the *Journal of the American Medical Association* (1954) that samples taken within four hours of death were probably reliable. Several authors including Bowden and McCallum (1949) (quoted by Plueckhahn, 1968) and Gifford and Turkel (1956), have suggested that post-mortem samples of blood from the heart can give erroneous levels of blood alcohol. On the other hand, Plueckhahn (1968) reported that if blood samples were taken properly within 48 hours of death from intact heart chambers or from peripheral sites such as femoral vessels, reliable alcohol levels could be obtained; that alcohol in the stomach did not affect the level of alcohol in the blood from an intact heart—and he cited several authors who agreed with this view—but that alcohol levels estimated on autopsy blood collected from the pericardial sac or the pleural cavities were unreliable, irrespective of whether there was alcohol in the stomach.

Following a fatal military accident in 1966 I found 40 mg. per 100 ml. alcohol in the pilot's blood (a sample from the pleural cavity). A forensic science laboratory was asked to examine the material by a gas chromatographic technique; my result was confirmed (Curry, 1966). Nevertheless, all attempts to correlate this finding with the pilot's history failed; there was very strong evidence that he had not been drinking on the night before the accident which occurred at 10 a.m. The body had not been recovered for a day or so following the crash as this had occurred in relatively inaccessible country; it was concluded that there must have been post-mortem putrefactive production of ethyl alcohol.

The case of a pilot whose body was recovered from the sea several weeks after his accident is described in Chapter 11. The bladder was found intact; urine and specimens of highly putrefied internal organs were analysed for alcohol. Nicholls' method gave results of 30 mg. per 100 ml. in urine and over 200 mg. per 100 g. in the liver. The specimens were sent to a forensic laboratory for gas chromatographic analysis; the value of 200 mg. per 100 g. in the liver could not be confirmed but 50 mg. per 100 g. was found; the level in the urine was confirmed as approximately 30 mg. per 100 ml. (Robinson, 1965).

Some unidentified bacteria were cultured from the bladder in this case; their ability to live and grow in urine containing up to 150 mg. per 100 ml. of ethyl alcohol was investigated. These levels of alcohol did not inhibit growth of the organisms but the alcohol was not metabolized. Attempts were made to show that the organisms could produce alcohol; although a wide range of substrates was used no success was achieved. It was impossible in the circumstances to know whether the small quantity of alcohol in the urine had resulted from post-mortem putrefactive production of ethyl alcohol or whether it had resulted from post-mortem loss of alcohol which had originally been at a much higher level.

A specimen of liver from one of the pilots killed in accident number 151 was found to give a very high value for alcohol. The examination on successive days showed that the alcohol level continued to rise; again it was concluded that the specimen was completely unsatisfactory for alcohol estimation due to putrefaction.

In 1967, in considerable measure due to my insistence that a toxicological section was urgently needed for the Department of Aviation Pathology, a combined Home Office/Royal Air Force toxicology research unit was established at the Home Office Central Research Establishment, Aldermaston. From that time a gas chromatographic technique for the estimation of alcohol in tissues has been available to us. Several other cases have been found where raised post-mortem levels of alcohol have not been due apparently to ante-mortem ingestion of ethyl alcohol; in some instances these raised levels were found in specimens taken within 18 hours of death. These cases stimulated an investigation into the bacterial production of ethyl alcohol; the work was reported by Blackmore (1968). He found that many organisms commonly present in or on the body during life or following post-mortem contamination were capable of producing significant quantities of ethyl alcohol from carbohydrate or tissue. He concluded that ethyl alcohol was unlikely to be produced by bacterial contamination of urine and that urine was, therefore, the test substance of choice; that if blood was available, samples should be taken from left and right heart and from one peripheral site; that in the absence of urine and blood, muscle from three peripheral sites should be sampled. If the concentration of ethyl alcohol per 100 ml. of tissue water was the same in all three samples, then the result represented ante-mortem ingestion of ethyl alcohol.

There was no case in the present series of public transport aircraft accidents in which analysis of a pilot's tissues suggested that his efficiency may have been impaired due to alcohol. Alcohol does not appear to be an important factor either in accidents in this type of aviation or in military flying accidents (Davis, 1968), but it is of greater importance in light aircraft accidents as is discussed in Chapter 11.

## DRUGS

Tissues from most of the pilots were not subjected to screening for the presence of drugs. Comprehensive toxicological screening to detect in therapeutic concentration any drug of conceivable importance as the main or contributory cause for an accident is not at present a practicable proposition. It is hoped that as a result of a research programme recently commenced at the Home Office Central Research Establishment, Aldermaston, in co-operation with members of the staff of the Royal Air Force Institute of Pathology and Tropical Medicine, the ideal of such routine toxicological screening will be achieved in the near future.

The finding of a drug in the pilot of a crashed aircraft might be significant in a number of ways. Undisclosed illness such as epilepsy might be discovered; therapeutic dosage of a drug such as an antihistamine can produce important side effects and might be a contributory factor in causing an accident by reducing the efficiency of a pilot; at the very least, the presence of a drug would indicate that the pilot was less than perfectly fit. It is of interest, however, that, although for some considerable time it has been preached that flying and drugs do not mix, there are recent cautious suggestions that pilots might be allowed to continue to fly on certain drug therapy—such as thiazide hypotensives (Jonsson and Sundgren, 1969). For several years it has been my practice to test for salicylates in the urine whenever this has been available at autopsy on pilots killed in aircraft accidents. No positive result was found in specimens from airline pilots but salicylates were present in a pilot involved in a fatal light aircraft accident as recorded in Chapter 10.

## CARBON MONOXIDE INTOXICATION

Whenever blood was available at post-mortem its carbon monoxide content was estimated. In the earlier years the microgasometric method of Scholander and Roughton (1943) was used. From 1963 Bowden and Woodhall's modification (1963) of Whitehead and Worthington's differential protein precipitation method (1961) was preferred. Blood, however, was not always available. With the establishment of the research facility at Aldermaston, a gas chromatographic technique for the estimation of carbon monoxide in blood, muscle, and other tissues was adopted.

### ACCIDENT NUMBER 261

An aircraft carrying an operating crew of 3 pilots, 2 members of cabin crew and 83 passengers crashed into mountains at night some 30 miles from its airfield of destination abroad. The first impression was that there must have been an error in navigation and that the investigation would not prove a particularly interesting one from the medical and pathological aspects. As so frequently happens first impressions were wrong: the medical and pathological evidence were of prime importance and the account of this case will illustrate the need, not only for routine and thorough investigations, but for critical appraisal of every piece of evidence, every analytical result and, indeed every piece of non-medical evidence, however obvious its apparent significance.

Disintegration of the aircraft and the bodies of the occupants was extreme; it was possible to distinguish the human remains of only 86 different persons. The bodies of the pilots, all virtually eviscerated, were eventually recovered and specimens of their tissues collected for toxicological analysis. The values for carbon monoxide found by a gas chromatographic analysis were:—

| | | |
|---|---|---|
| Captain | lung | 18·6 per cent |
| | muscle | 19·9 per cent |
| First Officer | muscle | 11·0 per cent |
| Second Officer | muscle | 6·3 per cent |

THE VALIDITY OF THE ELEVATED CARBON MONOXIDE VALUES

Analysis of body tissues for carbon monoxide using gas chromatographic techniques was first described by Dominguez, Christensen, Goldbaum, and Stembridge in 1959. A bloody fluid was extracted from the tissue and divided into two; carbon monoxide was liberated from one aliquot and measured; the other was fully carboxylated and carbon monoxide similarly liberated and measured. The carbon monoxide saturation of the specimen was recorded as the first measurement expressed as a percentage of the second.

The possibility that the raised carbon monoxide saturations had been due to a technical artefact had to be considered. Dominguez, Halstead, and Domanski (1964) showed that spuriously raised carbon monoxide saturations could be obtained in old blood or decomposing tissue when a technique involving 100 per cent carboxylation of a sample was used, because methaemoglobin formed by denaturation of oxyhaemoglobin and reduced haemoglobin could not be carboxylated, whereas carboxyhaemoglobin was relatively stable. Hence there was a reduction of carbon monoxide binding capacity without a corresponding loss of carbon monoxide content; an apparently raised carbon monoxide percentage saturation resulted. Pretreatment of a specimen prior to carboxylation with a reducing agent such as sodium hydrosulphite enabled any methaemoglobin present to be carboxylated; it was thought this was due to reconversion of methaemoglobin to reduced haemoglobin. The precaution of treating specimens with a reducing agent was taken prior to analysis in the present case.

The possibility that the raised carbon monoxide saturations had been produced post-mortem had to be assessed. The specimens from the captain's body were obtained on the third day after the accident but not frozen until the tenth day. The bodies of the other two pilots, not having been identified at an early stage, were embalmed with many other unidentified bodies on the eighth day and repatriated to Britain on the tenth day; it was not until the twelfth day that the bodies of these two pilots were identified, specimens collected and frozen. The specimens were kept at − 20° C. until 48 hours before the analyses were commenced; thereafter they were stored at − 4° C. Laboratory analyses were carried out on all specimens on the twenty-first and succeeding days.

Sjöstrand (1952) showed that the addition of certain chemicals to blood *in vitro* resulted in an increase in carboxyhaemoglobin content. Gettler and Freimuth (1940) reported that after 35–200 days embalming fluid containing formalin increased carbon monoxide saturation of blood by a range of from 2·7 to 25 per cent. They compared saturation levels immediately after the addition of formalin with those found after storage, having shown in 3 cases that the addition of formalin had no immediate effect on the carbon monoxide saturation except that of dilution. Their technique involved 100 per cent carboxylation of a sample without prior treatment with a reducing agent and their detailed figures suggested that their increased values may have been spurious (*see* the work of Dominguez, Halstead, and Domanski (1964) referred to above). However, using the same technique Gettler and Freimuth (1940) found no increase in carbon monoxide in blood stored for from 14 to 84 days, either at room temperature or in the cold; they did record loss of up to 20 per cent carbon monoxide after storage for from 24 to 84 days from bloods with saturation levels that had ranged from 40 to 80 per cent initially. Blackmore (1969) has very recently reported that he could not confirm these findings; although there was no loss or production of carbon monoxide in blood haemolysates at 4° C., 20° C., or 37° C. within 4 days, he found sporadic production of carbon monoxide in such specimens after 21 days and nearly half of 45 specimens stored in clear tubes at 20° C. in daylight for 124 days 'differed significantly in carbon monoxide from when originally analysed'. He also recorded one case of probable production of carbon monoxide between death and sampling in a body refrigerated shortly after death, still clothed in garments designed for high thermal insulation. Finck (1966) quoted Gullbring and Ström (1956) as demonstrating that carbon monoxide increased in blood stored in acid-citrate-dextrose for 20 days but only to a level of 1·5 per cent.

The possibility that artefactual production of carbon monoxide had occurred post mortem in the present specimens was excluded with a fair degree of certainty. Blackmore (1967) carried out experiments which showed that with low concentrations of the type of embalming fluid used, no carbon monoxide was produced *in vitro;* with high concentrations, concurrent denaturation of carboxyhaemoglobin and loss of the capacity of the tissue for carboxylation occurred. He further showed that with his technique (Blackmore, 1970) he had achieved complete liberation of the carbon monoxide from the specimens he had analysed, and complete saturation in the preparation of the 100 per cent samples; that under his conditions measurement of peak height on the recorder gave satisfactory quantitation of liberated carbon monoxide; that there was close reproducibility in his results. He showed later that there was some loss of carbon monoxide from the captain's muscle on storage for some months at − 4° C.; the saturation value fell to 14·1 per cent.

The possibility that post-mortem contamination of the specimens with carbon monoxide from an external source had occurred was dismissed fairly readily. Asvall (1961) considered that such post-mortem absorption could occur but only in extraordinary circumstances such as the exposure of the body for a period of hours to a concentration of carbon monoxide in excess of 12 per cent; no such circumstances had existed in the present case. Gettler and Freimuth (1940) could not demonstrate absorption of carbon monoxide by dead animals, but Dominguez (1962) cautioned that when there had been an explosion carbon monoxide might be driven physically into the outer layers of exposed tissue; a specimen should always be trimmed and only material from the middle should be analysed; this precaution was adopted with the present specimens.

On the basis of the foregoing it was concluded that within the limits of current scientific knowledge, the values obtained accurately reflected the state of carbon monoxide intoxication of the 3 crew at the time of their death.

### The Source of the Carbon Monoxide: Theoretical Considerations

The endogenous production of carbon monoxide *in vivo* in healthy people has been proved (Sjöstrand, 1951) and raised levels have been shown in those suffering from a variety of pathological conditions involving haemolysis (Hallberg, 1955; Birke, Liljedahl, and Troell, 1957; Coburn, Williams, and Kahn, 1966). In all cases the levels reached were less than 2 per cent and there is no possibility that the present crew acquired their levels of carbon monoxide saturation from any such process.

A degree of carbon monoxide intoxication can occur during a brief period of life in a fire. The history of this accident gave no support to the hypothesis that there had been a pre-crash fire in flight. The aircraft had first struck a ridge of high ground with one wing; this had broken off causing a fire in the vicinity of the wing root. The time taken for the aircraft to 'fly' from the point of initial impact to the bottom of the gulley, where it distintegrated and killed all aboard, could not have been more than 15–20 seconds. In these circumstances it was inconceivable that the carbon monoxide found in the crew could have resulted from the fire which started at first impact.

The captain was a smoker, the others were not. Smokers often acquire carboxy-haemoglobin levels of from 2 to 3 per cent; Bowden and Woodhall (1963), using a differential protein precipitation technique, showed that heavy smoking could cause saturations as high as 8 per cent. No workers have suggested that cigarette smoking can raise carboxyhaemoglobin to levels in excess of 10 per cent.

It seemed almost certain, therefore, that all 3 pilots must have acquired their levels of intoxication as a result of breathing a contaminated cockpit atmosphere during the flight. A possible source of such contamination was the cockpit heater; heaters of the type installed in the aircraft have been reported defective from time to time with resulting release of carbon monoxide in the cockpit. A small point but one of some interest was that the captain's carbon monoxide level was the highest and the supernumerary pilot's the lowest; the heater itself was so located in the cockpit that the captain's seat was nearest to it, the supernumerary pilot's most distant. However, ducts distributed the heated air to both sides of the cockpit; the area of the cockpit which would be most contaminated would depend therefore upon the exact nature and location of any defect in the heater system.

The very similar levels in the captain's lung and muscle suggested that the intoxication may have been a gradual process. The validity of this deduction depends upon whether carbon monoxide becomes bound to myoglobin *in vivo* and, if so, the physical conditions which determine the state of equilibrium between carboxyhaemoglobin and carboxymyoglobin. Millikan (1936, 1939) discussed the *in-vitro* properties of myoglobin and, quoting Hill (1933), Roche (1933), and Theorell (1934), stated that myoglobin had a much greater affinity for oxygen than did haemoglobin but a much lower relative affinity for carbon monoxide; the relative affinity of myoglobin for carbon monoxide as compared with oxygen was 20, in the case of haemoglobin it was 500. Blackmore (1969) carried out some experiments using tissues from cases of coal gas poisoning; he failed to show that carboxymyoglobin had been formed *in vivo* in any of the material he examined, although he could produce carboxymyoglobin *in vitro* without difficulty.

It was concluded that the relative levels in the captain's muscle and lung provided unreliable evidence as to the length of time that he had been inhaling contaminated air.

### Significance of the Discovered Levels of Carbon Monoxide Intoxication with regard to the Accident

The significance of the carbon monoxide intoxication could be assessed only by consideration of the series of events which led to the disaster so far as they could be deduced, and the potential effects of the levels of intoxication upon the efficiency of the crew in the circumstances of the particular flight. The inspector of accidents acting as the British accredited representative to the Commission of Inquiry for this accident, summarized the important items of evidence discovered from his investigation of the operational aspects of the accident thus:—

i. A reconstruction of the aircraft's flight path during the hour prior to impact, prepared from the flight recorder (colloquially but quite incorrectly often referred to as the 'black box').

ii. The recorded radio transmissions between the aircraft and ground control during this time, from which was known, among other things, the captain's estimate of his time of arrival over the airfield of destination.

iii. The channel selector settings of the V.O.R. (very high frequency omni range) radio navigational instruments found in the wreckage.

iv. The format of the airline company's flight plan so far as this related to the time allotted to the procedural approach to land (that is, the final descent, approach, and landing after having arrived over the airfield).

From this evidence the following conclusions were drawn:—

i. The aircraft flew over Radio Beacon A at 20.03 hours (*Fig.* 10).

ii. Forty-five minutes before the accident, it began to turn off course north of Radio Beacon B. This probably resulted from difficulty in receiving a clear signal from the beacon and consequent inability to home on to, and fly directly over it (radio interference had been previously reported with this particular low frequency, non-directional beacon).

iii. Thirty-nine minutes before the accident, the aircraft turned to fly on a heading corresponding to that from Beacon B to Checkpoint P, thus taking a flight path parallel to, but some miles west of the airway.

iv. Twenty-four minutes prior to the accident there was a slight change of course taking the aircraft still further west of the airway.

v. One minute later, at 20.43 hours, the aircraft was abeam Radio Beacon C. (The arrow from Beacon C (a V.O.R. beacon) in *Fig.* 10 indicates the point on the flight path at which the aircraft's instruments would have shown the beacon to be at a bearing of 270°, i.e., the point at which the aircraft was abeam the beacon.)

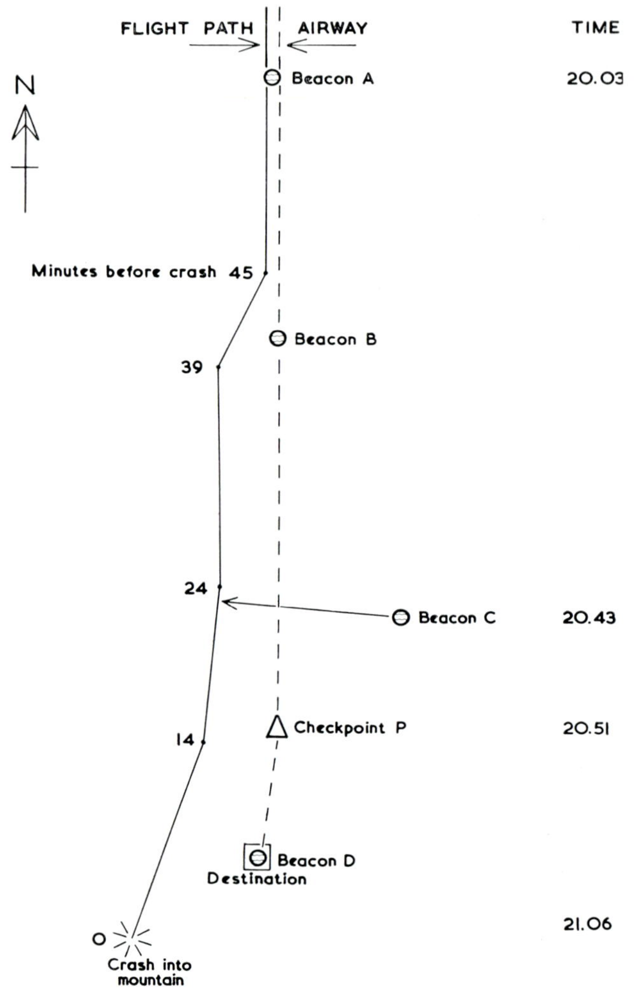


*Fig.* 10.—A reconstruction of the last hour's flight path of the aircraft involved in accident number 261, showing the deviation of the flight path from the airway.

vi. Not realizing that they were not flying along the airway, the crew elected to proceed by visual navigation and mistook the towns they were flying over for those they should have been flying over. They did not use their radio navigational instruments to obtain a bearing on Radio Beacon D located at their destination.

vii. At 20.51 hours the aircraft flew over a town which the crew visually mistook for Checkpoint P—a checkpoint for entering the area under the airfield's air traffic control, normally identified under non-visual conditions by radio compass bearings from beacons in the vicinity, such as C and D.

viii. About 1 minute later, 14 minutes before the crash, the aircraft again altered course, still further west.

ix. About the time they were passing several miles west of the airfield (that is about 6 or 7 minutes before the accident) the crew believed that they still had several more minutes to fly on the same heading before arriving over the airfield; this was because they had incorrectly included an additional 8 minutes allowed for the procedural approach in estimating their arrival over the airfield.

A study of the literature on the subject of the decrement in performance of physical and mental tasks at various levels of carbon monoxide intoxication (Killick, 1940; Lilienthal and Fugitt, 1946; Schulte, 1963; von Post-Lingen, 1964) shows that below a level of 25 per cent of carboxyhaemoglobin intoxication:—

i. A subject rarely experiences symptoms; he feels no malaise and has no headache.

ii. Physiological functions, e.g., resting pulse-rate, heart output, blood-pressure, and respiratory rate are not affected.

iii. Reaction time, muscle steadiness, and performance of skilled physical tasks are unaltered; speech remains coherent and quite normal.

However,

*a*. Tests of higher cerebral function such as the ability to sense the flicker in a rhythmically flashing light (von Post-Lingen, 1964), the ability to discriminate short intervals of time (Beard and Wertheim, 1967), simple choice discrimination, arithmetic, plural noun underlining, and 't' crossing tests, have demonstrated deterioration in the performance of persons having levels of carbon monoxide intoxication of even less than 20 per cent. Indeed, a level of as low as 5 per cent affects performance in some of these tests. Thus it is likely that 'complex psychological functions involving judgements, situational decisions and responses would be affected by exposure to levels of carbon monoxide which are sufficient to produce concentrations of carboxyhaemoglobin in the blood between 5% and 20%' (Schulte, 1963).

*b*. All the tests referred to in (*a*) above were carried out on otherwise healthy individuals at ground level. Carbon monoxide acts by inducing a state of relative hypoxia; the effect, therefore, of altitude must be taken into account. Gedye (1964) and Denison, Ledwith, and Poulton (1966) reported decrement in psychomotor skills with even the mild hypoxia that occurs at an altitude of 8000 feet, although Kelman, Crow, and Bursill (1969) were unable to confirm this. It is not easy to calculate the effect of altitude in terms of equivalence to an additional percentage of carbon monoxide saturation. The importance of the effect of altitude can be gained from the calculation that a pilot, breathing air, flying at a cabin altitude of 9000 feet above sea level, with a 15 per cent saturation level of carbon monoxide in his blood, would be experiencing the hypoxic effect of flying at over 16,000 feet without added oxygen (*Fig*. 11) (McFarland, Roughton, Halperin, and Niven, 1944).

The captain of this aircraft had only recently obtained command. He was flying at night to an airfield with which he was not particularly familiar and to which he had not previously flown at night. He had a co-pilot who, though many years his senior, had a flying history which readily explained why he was still flying as a co-pilot at the age of 58 years. It seemed possible, if not probable, that the captain could have been influenced in his actions by the co-pilot, who was known to prefer visual navigation to the use of instruments, and who was more familiar with the route than the captain.

Without question, correct flying techniques would have included the use of radio navigational aids in the approach to the airfield of destination, and this would have obviated the risks inherent in attempting visual navigation. The decision that was apparently made to attempt visual navigation was a remarkable lapse in the application of basic flying techniques and, incidentally, in the airline's regulations. It would be

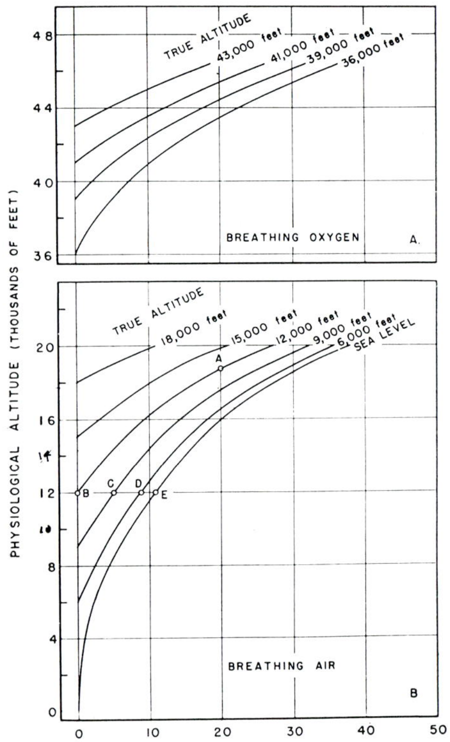


*Fig*. 11.—*Fig*. 6 from McFarland and others, 1944, showing 'the relationship between physiological altitude and per cent carboxy-haemoglobin at various true altitudes'. B, C, D, and E represent combinations of altitude and carbon monoxide intoxication giving an equivalent physiological altitude of 12,000 ft. (*Reproduced by permission of the Editor 'Journal of Aviation Medicine'*.)

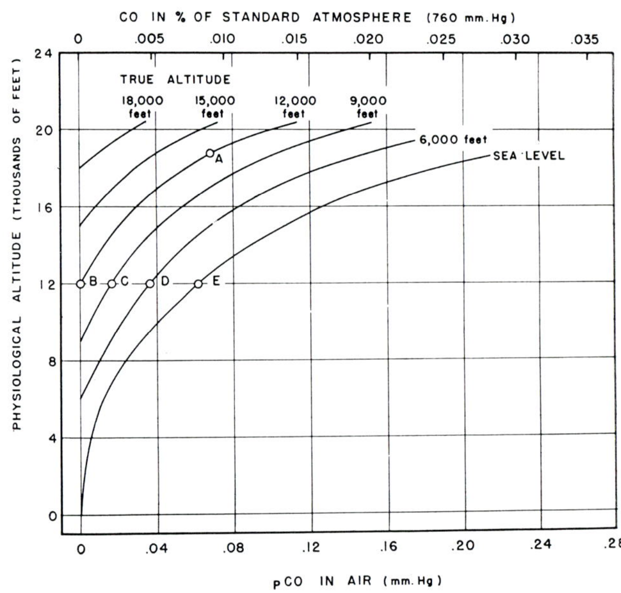


*Fig*. 12.—*Fig*. 8 from McFarland and others, 1944, showing 'the relationship between the altitude and the partial pressure of carbon monoxide in air at various true altitudes when equilibrium with the blood has been reached'. Points B, C, D, and E show a number of combinations of actual altitude and carbon monoxide concentration in the air which will result in a physiological altitude of 12,000 ft. (*Reproduced by permission of the Editor 'Journal of Aviation Medicine'*.)

anticipated that in completely normal circumstances a captain, particularly new to command and unfamiliar with the route, would resist any temptation to depart from standard procedure. Furthermore, it was extraordinary that the captain and possibly the other two pilots should apparently misunderstand or misinterpret the airline's flight plan and fail to appreciate at what time they should have had the airfield in sight. The transcripts of radio transmissions between the aircraft and the ground during the last hour indicated some confusion of thought on the flight deck. Several times a message from the aircraft mentioned the name of the location of a radio beacon incorrectly. Several times the captain was asked to confirm his estimated time of arrival over the airfield and, except for one occasion when the answer was an hour wrong, he confirmed his estimate which was clearly about 8 minutes later than it should

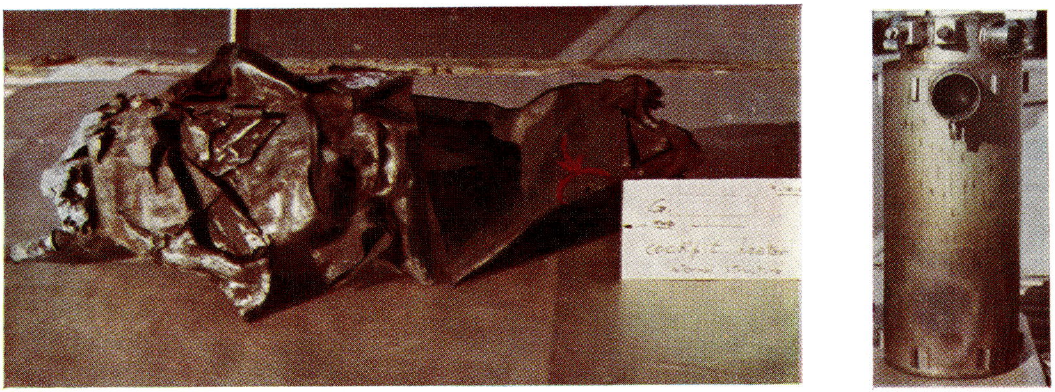

*Fig.* 13.—The damaged cockpit heater from the aircraft involved in accident number 261 is compared with an intact heater removed at random from a similar aircraft in service. The defect in the heater which antedated the accident is ringed in red. It had occurred in an area where the heated gases enter the annulus from the combustion chamber (*see Fig.* 14) and are particularly likely to damage the outer casing; this effect can be seen in the discoloration of the 'normal' heater. (*Reproduced by permission of the French Ministry of Transport.*)

have been. It seemed likely that the hypoxia resulting from the combined effect of the altitude at which they had been flying for nearly 2 hours and the carbon monoxide intoxication was the main cause for these errors of judgement.

### The Source of the Carbon Monoxide: Technical Evidence

A report in the above terms was submitted to the Commission of Inquiry through the British accredited representative. As a result, the technical investigators' attention was directed to the possible importance of the cockpit heater. A fresh search of the accident site was undertaken and despite the extreme disintegration of the aircraft, pieces of the heater were found. A pre-crash defect in the combustion chamber of the heater was discovered (*Fig.* 13).

It might be anticipated that the finding of this defect in the heater would complete the explanation of the accident and would be, in itself, acceptable proof of the correctness of the pathological findings and the deductions made therefrom. However, each piece of evidence, no matter how convenient or obvious its interpretation, requires thorough evaluation. The design of the cockpit heater is shown diagrammatically in *Fig.* 14. Cold air is forced into the intake and is heated as it passes through the jacket around the combustion chamber. A bleed from the main cold air intake provides the air intake for the combustion chamber. Pressure regulators, not shown in the diagram, ensure that there is a high differential between the outer jacket pressure and the combustion chamber pressure. A defect in the wall of the combustion chamber ought, therefore, to result in an inboard leak of fresh air into the combustion chamber and not to products of combustion into the heated air going to the cockpit.

The possibility that a Venturi effect, with suction of gases from the combustion chamber into the outer chamber, might occur with defects of particular size or shape had to be taken into account, as did the possibility that the heater had had an incorrect or defective burner fitted in the combustion chamber; repeated backfiring could result in retrograde dissemination of products of combustion up the combustion chamber

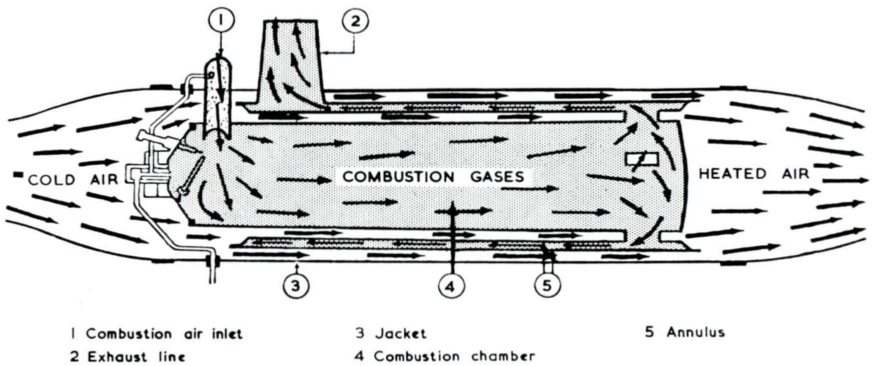


*Fig.* 14.—Diagram of the type of heater used in the aircraft involved in accident number 261. The gases from the combustion chamber could theoretically contaminate the heated air if there were a breach in the wall of the combustion chamber itself, the annulus or at the beginning of the exhaust line or if back-firing resulted in retrograde contamination down the combustion air inlet pipe. Although not shown clearly in this diagram the combustion air inlet is a bleed from the main cold air intake; there is no non-return valve in this system. Pressure regulators, not shown in the diagram, are designed to keep a pressure differential of 20 to 1 between the outer jacket containing the air being heated and the combustion chamber.

air intake. As there was no non-return valve in the bleed pipe from the cold air intake, contamination of the cold air before it passed into the outer jacket for heating could occur.

A very great deal of experimental work was carried out by the technical investigators. Using artificially damaged heaters, heaters returned for routine servicing and found similarly defective to the one in the crashed aircraft, and the burner recovered from the heater in the crashed aircraft, it appeared impossible in any way to achieve a contamination by carbon monoxide in excess of about 10–15 p.p.m. in the heated air passing to the cockpit from the heater. From the work of McFarland and others (1944) and, in particular, their graphs shown as *Figs.* 11 and 12, it can be seen that for a pilot to acquire a carboxyhaemoglobin level of 15 per cent at 9000 feet and thus a physiological altitude of just over 16,000 feet, he must breathe air contaminated with at least 75 p.p.m. of carbon monoxide. These figures accord with the statement by Lilienthal and Fugitt (1946) that 'inhalation of ambient air containing 0·008 per cent of carbon monoxide at 10,000 feet will, when equilibrium is reached, convert 10 per cent of the available haemoglobin to carboxyhaemoglobin'.

It could not be proved, therefore, that the discovered defect in the heater was the source of the carbon monoxide contamination of the cockpit atmosphere in this aircraft. It was finally concluded that the most likely source of carbon monoxide was a leak at a joint between the heater exhaust pipe and the main exhaust pipe. A leak at that site would certainly explain more satisfactorily the higher concentration of the carbon monoxide found in the captain as compared with the other pilots. It transpired that there had been a faulty joint in the exhaust line some weeks prior to the crash and this had been repaired. It was clearly quite possible that the repair had become defective. Unfortunately the relative part of the heater was never found but little doubt was felt by the investigators that a defective heater with carbon monoxide intoxication of the crew had been the main cause for this accident. The defect in the combustion chamber of the cockpit heater in this aircraft, discovered only as a consequence of the pathological investigation, prompted a check of similar heaters in current service. Several were found defective and potentially dangerous and although experiments had failed to show that the fail-safe differential pressure design could be ineffective, a notice was issued by the Air Registration Board (1968) laying down improved maintenance schedules for 'cockpit and cabin combustion type heaters and associated exhaust systems'.

## *Chapter 5*

# A NON-MEDICAL CAUSE FOR AN ACCIDENT

IN a military aircraft accident described by Mason (1962f) the medical evidence suggested that the pilot was in the passenger compartment when malfunction of the automatic pilot occurred; this later proved to be an accurate deduction. A case of raised carboxy-haemoglobin levels in the crew of an aircraft caused by contamination of the cockpit cabin atmosphere by a faulty heating system has been described in Chapter 4. In different circumstances, such a finding in the crew, and/or the passengers, might point to some other technical fault in the aircraft or the possibility of a fire in the air; although a radio distress signal would be expected if there were a fire in an aircraft in flight the radio might be put out of action for some reason almost as soon as the fire commenced.

## SABOTAGE

There have been at least 20 proved cases of sabotage to aircraft in flight during the last 21 years and a further 3 accidents that resulted from other criminal acts (*Table IV*). A number of unexplained accidents are also thought to have resulted from sabotage; an example is that which involved a Flying Tiger Airlines Constellation bound for Saigon carrying 96 military passengers and a crew of 11; it disappeared over the Pacific Ocean on 15 March, 1962, and there were unsubstantiated reports from eye-witnesses on ships that the aircraft disintegrated in flight.

There have been at least 3 other cases of attempted or planned sabotage. On 17 October, 1958, an aircraft engineer was killed when a bomb in his brief case exploded in the airport buildings at Wichita, Kansas; it was believed that he intended to take the bomb with him onto an aircraft. On 12 April, 1950, a man put his family and a bomb aboard an aircraft at Los Angeles, California; he repented in time and warned the baggage attendants. A Mexican planned his own death by putting a bomb in his luggage so that relatives could collect the insurance money; the bomb exploded in a parked aircraft and killed a number of airport employees on 9 May, 1958. The saboteur was arrested after a safe flight and in due course was sentenced to 30 years imprisonment—his luggage had been accidentally loaded into the wrong aircraft! The majority of cases of sabotage have been associated with attempted insurance fraud and, whenever there is the possibility or suspicion of sabotage, the insurance arrangements on the lives of the victims are important matters for close examination.

Four of the cases listed in *Table IV* involved the shooting of one or more members of the operating crew. In one instance a radioed transmission was received from an aircraft as follows: '. . . skipper's shot, we're being shot . . .' and immediately after this the radar target of the aircraft disappeared and the machine was later found to have crashed. The evidence supported the conclusion that this was as a result of the gunman shooting the crew (Doyle, 1968).

*Table IV.*—List of Aircraft Accidents and Incidents in Flight due to Sabotage, attempted Sabotage, or other Criminal Acts: 1949–June, 1969

| | Date | Airline | Aircraft | Location | Result | Comment | Source of Information |
|---|---|---|---|---|---|---|---|
| *Sabotage or Attempted Sabotage* | | | | | | | |
| 1 | 7.5.49 | Philippine Airlines | DC3 | The Philippines | Crashed: 13 killed | Time bomb planted by ex-convicts | Lloyd's List and Shipping Gazette, 1949a |
| 2 | 9.9.49 | Canadian Pacific Airlines | DC3 | Quebec, Canada | Crashed: 23 killed | Time bomb in baggage compartment | Lloyd's List and Shipping Gazette, 1949b; Flahiff, 1960 |
| 3 | 13.4.50 | British European Airways Corp. | Viking 1B | Over the English Channel | Landed safely: no casualties | Explosion in toilet | Ministry of Civil Aviation, 1950b |
| 4 | 24.9.52 | Compania Mexicana de Aviacion S.A. | DC3 | Mexico | Landed safely: 2 passengers injured | Bomb in suitcase in baggage hold | Lloyd's List and Shipping Gazette, 1952 |
| 5 | 11.4.55 | Air India | L-749A | South China Sea | Ditching attempted: 16 killed, 3 survivors | Bomb exploded in wheel well | International Civil Aviation Organization, 1957 |
| 6 | 1.11.55 | United Air Lines | DC6B | Colorado, U.S.A. | Disintegrated in flight: 44 killed | Bomb in baggage compartment | Civil Aeronautics Board, 1956 |
| 7 | 25.7.57 | Western Air Lines | CV240 | California, U.S.A. | Landed safely: saboteur killed | Explosion in toilet | Civil Aeronautics Board, 1958 |
| 8 | 19.12.57 | Air France | Armagnac | Central France | Landed safely | Bomb exploded in toilet | Lloyd's List and Shipping Gazette, 1957 |
| 9 | 8.9.59 | Compania Mexicana de Aviacion S.A. | DC3 | Mexico | Landed safely: minor injuries to 15, saboteur killed | Bomb carried by passenger | Lloyd's List and Shipping Gazette, 1959 |
| 10 | 6.1.60 | National Airlines | DC6B | North Carolina, U.S.A. | Disintegrated in flight: 24 killed | Dynamite explosion in passenger compartment | Civil Aeronautics Board, 1960 |
| 11 | 28.4.60 | Linea Aeropostal Venezolana | DC3 | Venezuela | Disintegrated in flight: 13 killed | Explosion in vicinity of cockpit | International Civil Aviation Organization, 1963 |
| 12 | 22.5.62 | Continental Air Lines | Boeing 707 | Missouri, U.S.A. | Disintegrated in flight: 35 killed | Explosion in rear toilet | Civil Aeronautics Board, 1962 |
| 13 | 7.5.64 | Pacific Air Lines | Fairchild F27 | California, U.S.A. | Crashed: 44 killed | Crew shot by demented passenger intent upon suicide | Civil Aeronautics Board, 1964 |
| 14 | 8.12.64 | Aerolineas Abaroa | C47 | Bolivia | Crashed: 15 killed | Explosion in baggage of heavily insured passenger | Lloyd's List and Shipping Gazette, 1964 and 1965 |
| 15 | 8.7.65 | Canadian Pacific Airlines | DC6B | British Columbia | Disintegrated in flight: 52 killed | Explosion in flight | Department of Transport, Canada, 1965 |
| 16 | 22.11.66 | Aden Airways | C47 | South Arabia | Disintegrated in flight: 30 killed | Believed due to explosion in passenger compartment | Lloyd's Weekly Casualty Reports 1966 |
| 17 | 29.5.67 | Aerovias Condor de Colombia | DC6 | Colombia | Landed safely | Explosion in flight | Lloyd's List and Shipping Gazette, 1967 |
| 18 | 12.10.67 | British European Airways | Comet 4b | Mediterranean | Disintegrated in flight: 66 killed | Explosion in passenger compartment | Board of Trade, 1968b |
| 19 | 11.12.67 | American Airlines | Boeing 727 | U.S.A. | Landed safely: no casualties | Explosion in baggage hold—small home-made bomb | Aviation Week and Space Technology, 1967 |
| 20 | 19.11.68 | Continental Air Lines | Boeing 707 | Gunnison, U.S.A. | Landed safely: no casualties | Explosion in toilet followed by fire. Passenger arrested on landing | Aviation Week and Space Technology, 1968 |
| *Other Criminal Acts* | | | | | | | |
| 1 | 16.7.48 | Cathay Pacific Airways | Catalina | Pearl river estuary 5 miles E. of Macao | Crashed: 25 killed, 1 survived | Pilot shot during attempt to hi-jack aircraft | Lloyd's List and Shipping Gazette, 1948 |
| 2 | 30.12.52 | Philippine Airlines | DC3 | Off Formosa | Landed safely : total casualties? | Pilot and purser shot during hi-jacking | Lloyd's List and Shipping Gazette, 1953 |
| 3 | 27.3.66 | Empresa Consolidada Cubana de Aviacion | Il-18 | Cuba | Crashed on landing | Pilot and passenger shot during attempt to hi-jack aircraft | Lloyd's List and Shipping Gazette, 1966 |

In 2 accidents in the present series the possibility of sabotage had to be considered seriously, although in each case it was eventually concluded that this had not been the cause of the accident.

## ACCIDENT NUMBER 151

This was the accident in which Mr. Dag Hammarskjöld, Secretary General of the United Nations Organization, and his party of 15 were killed in 1961. Their aircraft crashed in the bush 9 miles from the airfield at Ndola, Rhodesia. When an important political figure is a victim of an accident, suspicion of foul play is always aroused and

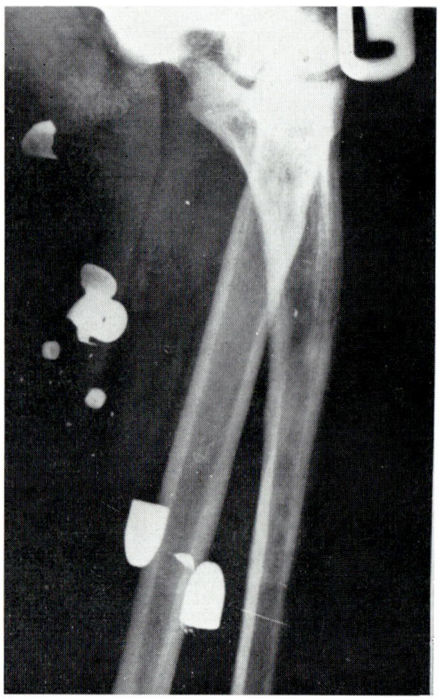

*Fig.* 15.—Radiograph of a victim from accident number 151 showing bullets, percussion caps, and a distorted cartridge case in the subcutaneous tissue. (*Reproduced from Stevens (1968a) by permission of the Editor 'Medicine, Science and the Law'.*)

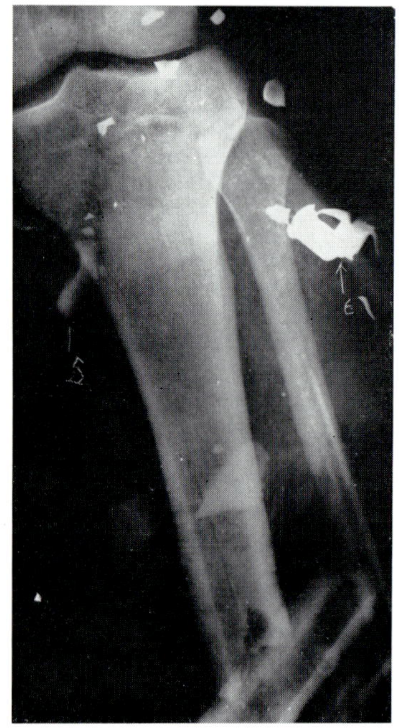

*Fig.* 16.—Radiograph from another victim of accident number 151, showing a cartridge case embedded in the skin and subcutaneous tissue.

within a few hours of this particular disaster certain Heads of State announced their personal conviction that the accident had resulted from some form of sabotage.

Most of the bodies were incinerated and presented a difficult problem in identification, a subject which is dealt with in some detail in Section IV. All bodies and fragments of bodies were radiographed; metallic objects were demonstrated in films of 6 bodies. In 2 of these the foreign objects included bullets (*Fig.* 15). However, the facts that the bullets:—

i. Lay superficially in subcutaneous tissue,
ii. Were not associated with any discernible bleeding,

iii. Did not show any rifling on extraction from the bodies and, perhaps most important of all,

iv. Were accompanied by percussion caps and the debris of distorted cartridge cases (*Figs*. 15, 16, 17),

showed that these bullets had not exploded in the breach of a firearm. When identified, the bodies in which these bullets were found, proved to be those of soldiers, members of Mr. Hammarskjöld's bodyguard. They had had magazines of ammunition in their possession and it could only be concluded that it was this ammunition that had exploded in the post-crash fire and 'shot' the partly incinerated cadavers nearby. It was confirmed later, by questioning rescuers, that ammunition was exploding in the still-burning wreckage when they reached the scene 16 hours after the disaster.

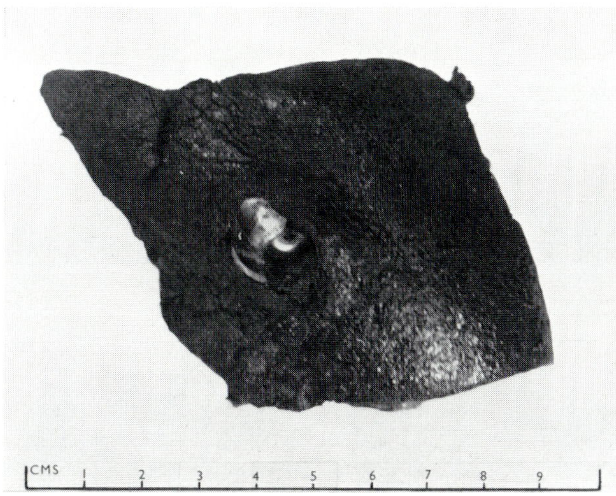


*Fig*. 17.—The cartridge case seen in *Fig*. 16. It has penetrated charred but intact skin, and is seen lodged partly in the underlying subcutaneous tissue.

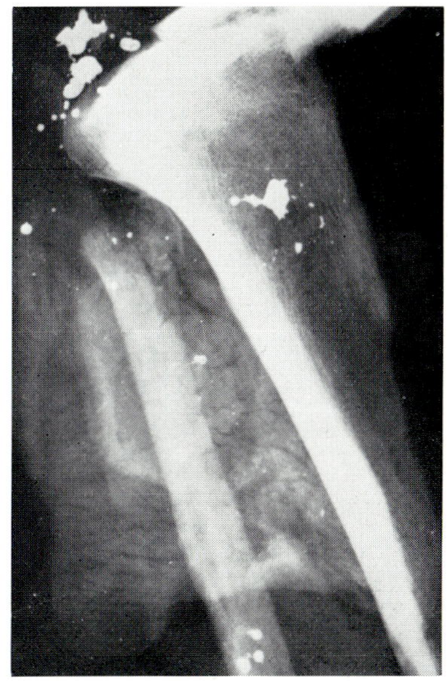

*Fig*. 18.—Radiograph from another victim from accident number 151 showing the characteristic shapes of fused aircraft metal which often contaminates bodies incinerated in a post-crash fire.

The metallic objects in the other radiographs proved to be of no importance. They consisted either of fused pieces of aircraft metal or of fragments of personal property which had become embedded superficially in the charred tissues. The appearances of fused masses of aircraft metal are quite characteristic; they are of irregular shape with smooth outlines and have the variety of 'pseudopodia' that are produced when a mass of molten metal drops and quickly solidifies (*Fig*. 18).

No universally acceptable explanation for this accident was ever discovered. There were two commissions of inquiry into the accident, one appointed by the Federal Rhodesian Authorities and one by the United Nations. The Rhodesian commission concluded, admittedly largely on the basis of the exclusion of other possible causes, that the accident was due to pilot error in that, while making a visual approach to land at night, the pilot inadvertently allowed the aircraft to descend too low during the outward leg and as he turned to line-up with the runway (Federation of Rhodesia and Nyasaland, 1962). The United Nations commission acknowledged that pilot error could not be excluded but that, in the absence of evidence, neither could a number of other hypotheses; in the circumstances they could not conclude that any particular hypothetical cause was more likely than any other (United Nations Organization, 1962a). Both commissions accepted that there was no evidence of sabotage, either in the wreckage which was painstakingly and exhaustively examined by Professor Frei-Sulzer, Chief of the Scientific Department of the Zurich Police, or in thc bodics. Gavshon (1963) reported that there was a conflict of medical evidence on one aspect of the medical investigation only, namely whether or not Mr. Hammarskjöld lived briefly and could have been helped by prompt rescue. It is perhaps understandable that his fellow countrymen were inclined to take the view that his life might have been saved, especially as there was undoubtedly a delay in raising the alarm and organizing search and rescue facilities. However, as one of the three pathologists who performed the post-mortem examination, I hold the opinion that, although there was evidence that cardiovascular function had continued for a brief period (there was bone-marrow and fat embolism of moderate degree and haemorrhage in association with some but not all injuries), the injuries received by Mr. Hammarskjöld were such as to be inevitably and rapidly lethal. In fact, there was very little conflict of medical opinion on the evidence in this accident; in dealing with the question of Mr. Hammarskjöld's brief survival, the Swedish medical report (United Nations Organization, 1962b) contained some unlikely suppositions but then concurred that 'Hammarskjöld's wounds would have been fatal in any case'.

## ACCIDENT NUMBER 241

In this accident the aircraft broke up in the air over mountainous country in apparently perfect weather conditions and the possibility of some form of sabotage had to be entertained. Extremely careful and methodical police mapping and labelling of bodies followed by identification of each individual body enabled plots to be prepared showing the position of each named body in relation to the aircraft wreckage. The aircraft had split into two in the region of the bulkhead between the first-class and economy-class passenger sections of the cabin; the forward section had caught fire and burnt out after falling to the ground. As a seating plan of the occupants in the aircraft was available a number of deductions could be made.

Firstly, the bodies that had been scattered widely over an area of approximately 700 × 300 metres were those of several first-class passengers, the first row of the economy-class passengers and 2 individuals from economy-class seats located several rows further back. The incinerated bodies that had been retained in the forward part of the fuselage were found to be those of the steward who normally would serve in the first-class compartment from the forward galley, the only passenger in the front row of the first-class compartment and 2 female passengers from the rear two rows of the first-class seats (they may have been still strapped into their seats at the time of the accident or possibly in the forward toilets, and in either case thus prevented from falling out when the aircraft broke in two).

Most of the occupants of rows 9 to 15, in the economy-class compartment, immediately behind the break in the fuselage, had been thrown out when this part of the aircraft struck the ground; nearly all these bodies were found around the inner part of the broken-off right wing. Occupants of row 16 and rows aft were in the vicinity of the smashed rear fuselage. A steward and two stewardesses were found near to the wreckage of the rear galley.

Eleven bodies of passengers and cabin crew were found to have areas of skin desquamation. This change, often referred to as 'skin slip' occurs as a normal post-mortem phenomenon (Marshall, 1968) but usually takes several days to develop in temperate or cold climates. I have found on several occasions, since I first observed it

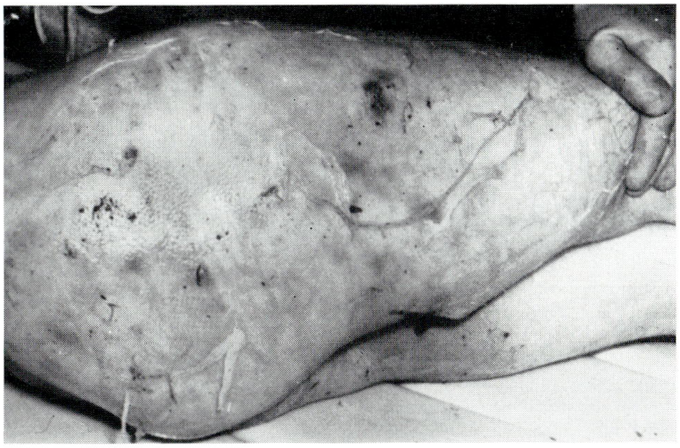

*Fig.* 19.—Skin desquamation typically due to post-mortem soaking of the skin with aviation fuel.

in the body of a military pilot in 1960, that long before the changes of putrefaction are at all advanced, skin desquamation can occur in those areas of a body which have been soaked with aviation fuel (*Fig.* 19). Heat may cause blistering of the skin, of course, and when there has been a fire this cause for skin desquamation must not be overlooked. When due to fuel, the change most often appears on areas covered by intact, fuel-soaked clothing and is observed when there has been no fire.

The passengers from accident number 241 whose bodies showed this change were found all to have occupied seats in rows 9 – 14 with but one exception; he had been in row 16. They were, therefore, immediately behind the break in the fuselage; some were among those flung out when the aircraft broke up and others among those thrown out at ground impact. It is likely that broken fuel lines at the point of fracture would have resulted in spraying of both forward fuselage and central cabin areas, although only the former caught fire. The skin desquamation therefore provided additional indirect evidence about the position of certain passengers at the time the aircraft broke up in the air.

The conclusion that could be drawn from all the above evidence was that all aircraft occupants appeared to have been in their appropriate positions at the time of the catastrophe. There was nothing to suggest that the captain had been out of his cockpit (as for example in Mason's case quoted earlier in this chapter) or that a passenger had been on the flight deck with or without a gun.

The use of a time-bomb or other explosive device is the commonest form of sabotage; it occurred in all but one of the 20 cases listed in *Table IV* that were truly sabotage, i.e., deliberate destruction or attempted destruction. Evidence may be found in the human remains and serve merely to confirm the conclusions reached by the technical investigators from their own investigations, as in *Case* 18 in *Table IV* (Mason and Tarlton, 1969). Alternatively, the pathological examination may provide the prime source of evidence leading to the correct reconstruction of the accident as in *Case* 10 in *Table IV* (Doyle, 1968).

The investigators' examination of the wreckage of the main fuselage and tail in accident number 241 rapidly excluded a bomb having exploded in that part of the aircraft. It was not so easy for them to exclude sabotage from an examination of the forward fuselage which had been largely destroyed by fire. Radiographs of the bodies of the crew failed to reveal any evidence of an explosion in the crew compartment for no films showed any foreign object. Although not conclusive—for negative evidence is never conclusive—the medical and pathological examinations suggested that the accident had not been caused by sabotage. Eventually, the Commission of Inquiry concluded that it had resulted from freak meteorological conditions and the machine encountering 'abnormally severe turbulence . . . which imposed a gust load considerably in excess of the design limit'.

*Chapter 6*

# PATHOLOGICAL EVIDENCE OF EVENTS PRIOR TO AN ACCIDENT

THE fourth amendment (1963) to the Air Navigation Order of 1960 made it mandatory for all jet aircraft over 12,500 lb. in weight and all piston-engined aircraft over 60,000 lb. in weight to carry a flight recorder so constructed and located in the aircraft as to make it likely to withstand the destructive forces encountered in an accident. At the present time this equipment records altitude, air speed, magnetic heading, vertical acceleration ('g') and pitch attitude against a time scale. It is, therefore, likely that a great deal of evidence will be available about what has happened to a modern aircraft during the minutes before a crash.

## ACCIDENT NUMBER 187

Before the introduction of these flight recorders a particular aircraft descended through cloud over mountainous terrain after the captain had declared his intention of staying at a safe altitude to await the expected improvement in local weather conditions. The aircraft struck the side of a mountain and was destroyed and all on board were killed. One of the problems presented to the Commission of Inquiry was to determine whether the descent was deliberate, or the result of sudden loss of control. Had the descent been due to loss of control and accompanied by excessive turbulence within the aircraft at a time when the passengers had not had their seat belts fastened (a likely state of affairs if a landing were not contemplated in the following few minutes) then, in these circumstances, some of the passengers could have been thrown about inside the cabin with consequent non-lethal bony injury. Such injury would have been likely to produce pulmonary fat and bone-marrow embolism; this would have arisen before impact against the mountain side caused immediate lethal injuries with dissolution of their cardiovascular systems. Full histological examination of specimens of lungs from a representative 30 of the 81 passengers and cabin crew, failed to reveal any evidence whatsoever of pulmonary embolic phenomena. This negative evidence was of some value in that it supplemented inconclusive non-medical evidence that the aircraft's descent had been deliberate and not due to sudden loss of control.

## ACCIDENT NUMBER 231

The main feature of medical interest in this accident, which was the subject of a public inquiry, was the possibility of spatial disorientation in the pilot. The aircraft was approaching on the third attempt to land in marginal weather conditions. At an altitude of about 200 ft. a decision was made to abandon the attempt and overshoot; a few seconds later the aircraft dived and crashed onto the runway.

Incapacitation of a pilot from natural disease was discussed in Chapter 3. Incapacitation from disorientation cannot be detected at autopsy with present knowledge, and must be deduced from a reconstruction of events prior to an accident, and, in the modern context, in relation to the evidence provided by a flight recorder; it is therefore appropriate to consider the subject in this chapter.

The tendency for a pilot to become spatially disorientated in flight in various circumstances, and to respond inappropriately to the true situation, has been appreciated for a long time (Vinacke, 1947, 1948; McFarland, 1953; Clark and Nicholson, 1954; Jones, 1957). Benson (1965) quoted Anderson (1919) as reporting in the early days of flying that it had been found that pilots could not maintain a desired attitude or direction of flight when deprived of visual clues to orientation. In early reports this was often referred to as 'aviator's vertigo'. As 'vertigo' implies a sensation of rotation it should be used only when strictly appropriate. It is best to follow Clark and Graybiel (1956), quoted by Benson (1965), and to use the term 'spatial disorientation' for 'all those incidents in which the pilot fails to appreciate correctly, or is uncertain of, the attitude or position, or changes in attitude or position, of himself and his aircraft with respect to the earth's surface'.

What was called the 'dark night take-off phenomenon' was recognized in night-bomber operations during the Second World War and disorientation has been blamed for numerous military and civilian crashes over the years (Newton, 1951; Department of Civil Aviation, Australia, 1958; Nuttall and Sanford, 1959; Dougherty, 1965; Ogden, Jones, and Chappell, 1966; Bryan, 1967). It is by no means a problem related to inexperience (Moser, 1969). The increased speed of acceleration of modern aircraft has enhanced the risk of a pilot becoming disorientated. Buley (1967) discussed disorientation and loss of control in jet transport aircraft and summarized the applied physiological basis for disorientation in these circumstances as follows: 'During flight manœuvres a pilot's apparent gravity vector (the direction of gravity as sensed non-visually) continually changes since it is the result of the true gravity vector and a flight acceleration vector (determined by flight speed and path)'. Quoting Martin and Jones (1965) he continued, 'Illusions of attitude can arise in the absence of visual references if the apparent gravity vector is identified with the true gravity vector'. Jones (1957) illustrated the point as shown in *Fig*. 20.

In accident number 231 an aviation physiologist's conclusions as to the pilot's possible perceived flight path drawn on the basis of the accelerations the pilot experienced (calculated from the flight recorder data) showed that the accident could well have resulted from the pilot believing that his aircraft had begun to climb steeply. If the pilot did suffer such an illusion and was unable to suppress it by concentrating on the evidence of his instruments, or if the information from his instruments had been itself conflicting, he could have pushed the control column forward and the aircraft's nose down believing that he was making the correct response to the circumstances. In this investigation, as in most investigations, the medical evidence could not be evaluated in isolation. Here the medical evidence was based upon circumstantial and technical evidence; the hypothesis conceived required to be judged in the light of all the evidence about the accident before it could be given the appropriate weight by the investigating commissioner.

The contribution of a pathologist in accidents possibly due to disorientation is likely to be very small unless he discovers in the pilot's body evidence of natural disease or a drug, the effects of which could be the impairment of powers of concentration and

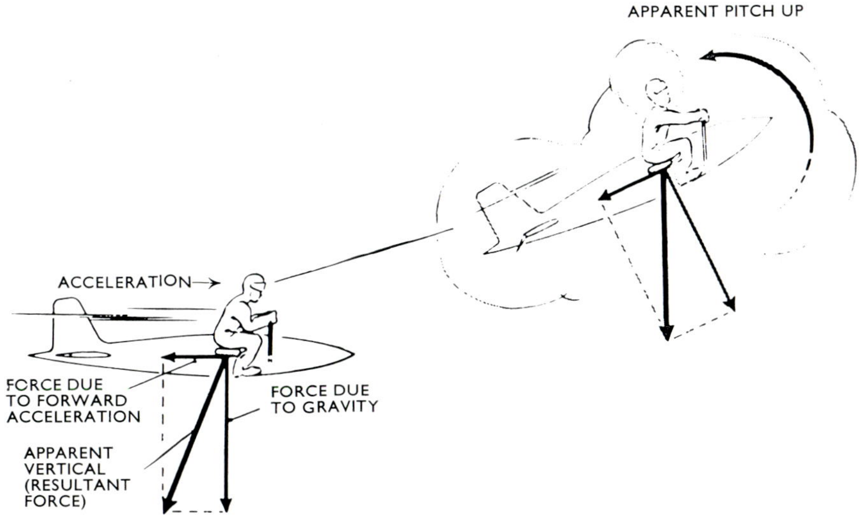


*Fig*. 20.—This diagram from Jones (1957) illustrates simply the illusion of attitude that can result from horizontal acceleration in the absence of visual cues. A pilot senses the resultant of the forces acting upon him as the true vertical and therefore misinterprets his attitude relative to the earth's surface. (*Crown Copyright, reproduced by permission of the Controller of Her Majesty's Stationery Office.*)

therefore increased susceptibility to disorientation. The extent of burning and mechanical injury to the bodies of the crew in the case quoted precluded a full assessment of the state of health of the pilots concerned. As far as was possible, the presence of disease and drugs was excluded. However, light aircraft accident number 244, discussed in Section II, was a possible instance of pilot disorientation and the pathological evidence was of much greater importance on that occasion.

## *Chapter 7*

# RECONSTRUCTION OF EVENTS AT IMPACT AND IMMEDIATELY AFTER AN ACCIDENT

## SURVIVAL AND ESCAPE

ONE of the most important aspects of an accident in which there are both fatalities and survivors is the assessment of whether the outcome could have been influenced by improved design of the aircraft or its escape facilities; the training of its crew; the training of, or equipment available to, local rescue services; or anything else subject to practical remedial action. Following such accidents many questions arise, for example:—

i. Why did those who were killed not escape?

ii. From what did they die? Were they killed outright or did they die in the post-crash fire?

iii. If they died from fire, were they incapacitated by injury or trapped in the wreckage?

iv. How did the survivors escape?

v. Were the emergency exits used, adequate in number and most advantageously sited?

The answers to these questions can only be provided on the basis of full post-mortem examinations to determine the causes of death, the nature of the injuries sustained and the presence of life during the post-crash fire. This evidence must be correlated with the individuals' seating positions, their location as found by rescuers, the position of escape exits, the seat orientation and other factors relative to each person's immediate environment in the aircraft. All this evidence must be interpreted in the light of survivors' evidence about the circumstances of their own escape and the evidence to be derived from a detailed examination of the aircraft wreckage.

### ACCIDENT NUMBER 152

This was an example of an accident in which there were survivors and fatalities. As recorded in Chapter 3 the aircraft stalled on take-off, struck the ground in a flat attitude, broke in two, decelerated over a considerable distance and caught fire. Two views of the wreckage are shown in *Figs*. 21 and 22. Twenty-seven persons (20 passengers and 7 crew) of the 34 on board were killed. Much of what could be discovered from the investigation of this accident is incorporated in *Fig*. 23. This shows the seating positions of the survivors and some of those who were killed, and the positions of a number of seats deduced to have been vacant.

As soon as the first facts about this accident were known it was expected that the survivors would be found to have occupied the rear half of the aircraft as this is generally regarded as being the safest part and it appeared in this case to be the least damaged (*Fig*. 21). However, in this instance the rear of the aircraft did not prove to have been

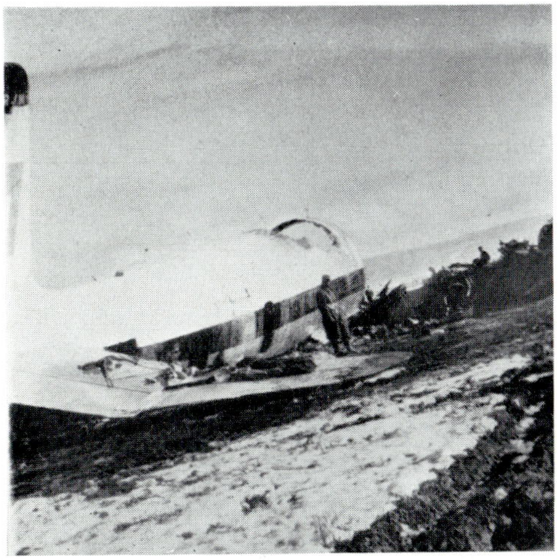

*Fig*. 21.—A view of the wreckage from accident number 152. The rear half appears relatively undamaged and is lying tipped a little to the right. The door shown was blocked and could not be opened by rescuers; a door on the opposite side was found by rescuers to be open and one passenger had escaped through it.

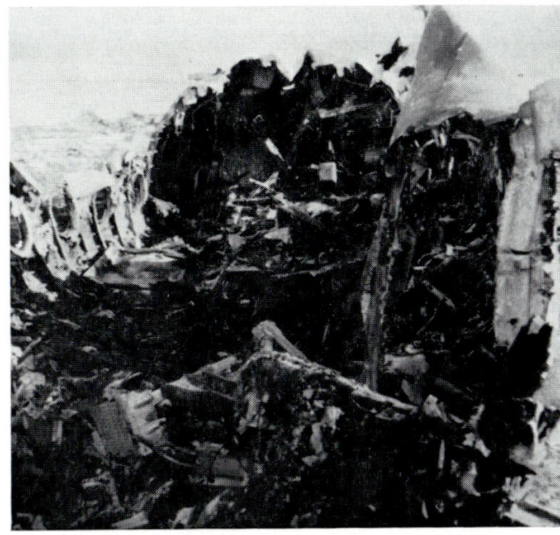

*Fig*. 22.—A view of the forward passenger compartment taken from a position just in front of the break in the fuselage. The whole of this area has been completely burnt out. At the far end the bulkhead between the cockpit and the passenger compartment can be seen. Fire had not extended very much beyond that bulkhead.

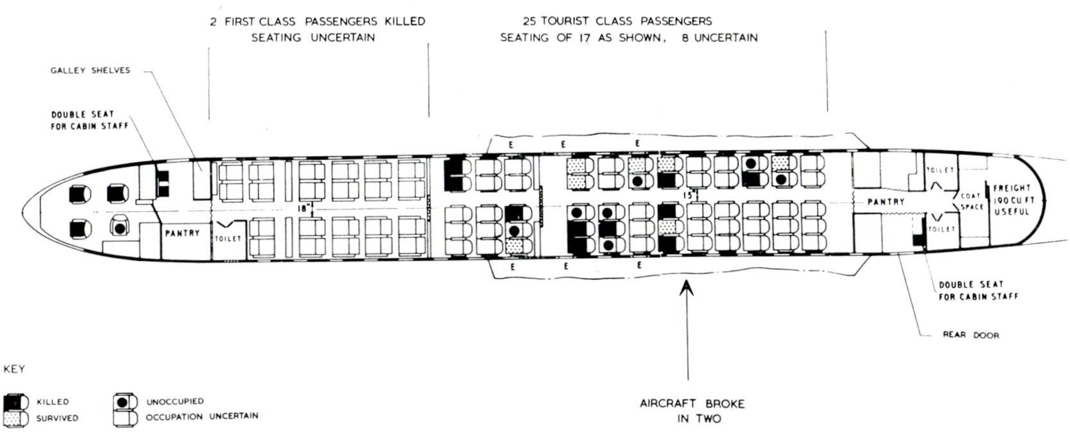


*Fig*. 23.—Plan of the aircraft showing the fate of the occupants relative to their seating positions and other features of their immediate environment (accident number 152). (*Reproduced from Stevens (1968a) by permission of the Editor 'Medicine, Science and the Law'*.)

the safest; all but 1 of the survivors were found to have been seated in the centre section (*Fig*. 22) beneath which were the main fuel tanks; they had been, therefore, in a very vulnerable position in view of the post-crash fire. The positions of the emergency exits as shown in *Fig.* 23 suggested that these may have been important factors in the survivors' escape. This also proved to be incorrect; none of the survivors used an escape exit for it was discovered that the fuselage had broken away on either side of the centre section before the aircraft came to a standstill and sections containing emergency exits were distributed along the wreckage trail. Survivors told how they had recovered from their initial, dazed state and discovered that they could escape from the flames merely by climbing out onto the aircraft's wing and jumping down to the ground.

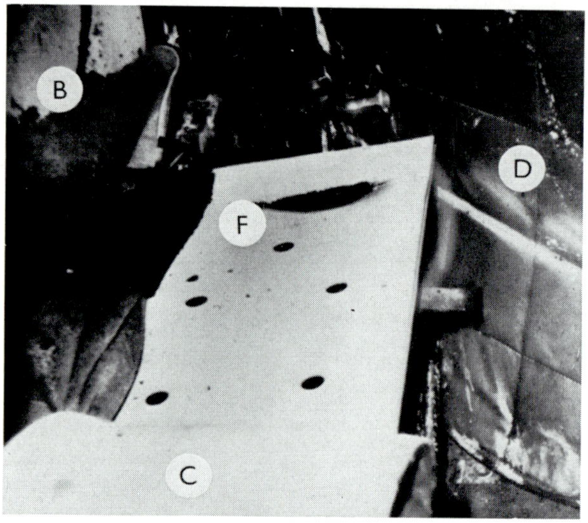


*Fig.* 24.—Double seat for cabin staff at rear of aircraft in accident number 152 (*see also Fig.* 23). The cushion C has been rolled back to show the depressed fracture F of the wooden seat. This damage suggested that it was occupied when considerable vertical deceleration was applied. In normal use the seat had to be folded up against bulkhead B to allow the door D, ajar in this photograph, to be fully opened inwards. (*Reproduced from Stevens (1968a) by permission of the Editor 'Medicine, Science and the Law'.*)

The account of his escape given by the sole survivor in the rear section was of considerable importance in the reconstruction of events in that part of the aircraft. The passenger in question had anticipated the accident; he was himself an ex-pilot and realized that the aircraft was climbing too steeply and that it would probably stall. He bent forward and braced himself in preparation for the crash. He quickly recovered from the jolt of the impact and, through the darkness and smoke, made his way to where he expected to find, and to have to open, the rear exit door. Finding the door already open, he climbed through and reached safety. On direct questioning later, he remembered that someone had brushed past him going forwards as he, himself, made his way to the rear door.

Examination of the wreckage showed that the rear cabin crew's double seat had been occupied by at least one person when the aircraft struck the ground. This seat was of the tip-up variety and it required to be in the 'up' position before the rear door could be opened (*Fig.* 24). The bodies of two stewards were found in the rear half of this aircraft; they were neither injured nor burnt but both had died from asphyxiation due to the inhalation of products of combustion. Rescuers did not recall exactly from where they recovered these two bodies, but it was possible to conclude that at least one of them had been sitting in his correct seat at take-off. Further, it seemed that he had probably worn his restraining seat strap, that he quickly recovered from the immediate effects of the crash and opened the aircraft's rear door before going forward to try to assist passengers. Had he had breathing apparatus readily available he might have saved some passengers and survived himself. Following this investigation a suggestion was made that breathing apparatus be supplied for cabin crew to use in this type of accident but the idea was not followed up. However, several recent examples of death in similar circumstances—in a post-crash fire following a survivable impact—have resulted in the design and preliminary trials of a protective polyimide 'smoke hood' for use by passengers (McFadden, Reynolds, and Funkhouser, 1968). More recently a proposal has been made that the Federal Aviation Administration regulations be amended to require certain aircraft to carry smoke hoods for the use of passengers and crew members in appropriate emergencies (*Aerospace Medicine*, 1969).

*Table V.*—THE CAUSES OF DEATH OF THE PASSENGERS KILLED IN ACCIDENT 152

| | |
|---|---|
| Passengers, total | 27 |
| killed | 20 |
| *Causes of Death:—* | |
| Asphyxiation from fumes due to fire | 15 |
| No autopsy (religious reasons) but probably asphyxiation from fire | 1 |
| Asphyxiation—inhalation of blood | 1 |
| Multiple lethal injuries | 1 |
| Burns (died after some hours) | 1 |
| Cause undetermined | 1 |

Two stewards had occupied the forward cabin crew seats; they too died from asphyxiation with apparently little or no incapacitating injury. One had a bruise on the back of the head, the other a minor fracture of the sternum. The particular seats they had occupied were rearward-facing but of relatively weak construction with insubstantial head rests. They were located opposite the galley shelves which were unguarded by doors. The vertical deceleration of the aircraft had resulted in collapse of the seats; the forward deceleration had resulted in the contents of the galley shelves being pitched forward. It appeared that these loose objects had caused some of the injuries sustained by the two stewards and that it was quite possible that they had lost their lives because of the inadequately stressed and poorly padded seats, complicated by the effects of unguarded pantry equipment storage—both factors readily amenable to improved design.

All three operating crew died. Two of them were killed virtually instantaneously from their head injuries. The other suffered a severe but not essentially lethal head injury and was asphyxiated in the ensuing fire. All three had failed to fasten their shoulder harnesses although they had fastened their seat belts. The cockpit was distorted in the crash and the captain's legs were trapped; there is little doubt that had they correctly fastened their shoulder harnesses they would all have survived the ground impact and the forward deceleration. It is very probable that two of them would have been capable of extricating themselves before they were overcome by the fire, as the cockpit was the part of the aircraft furthest away from, and least affected by the fire; it is even possible that they would have been able to release and rescue the captain.

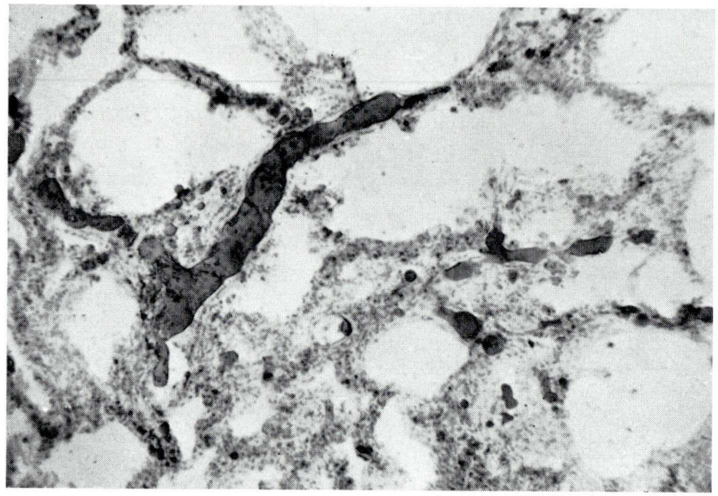

*Fig*. 25.—A section of lung from a victim of accident number 152. Fat emboli are seen in the capillaries. (15 $\mu$ sections.) Oil-red O. ($\times$ 60.)

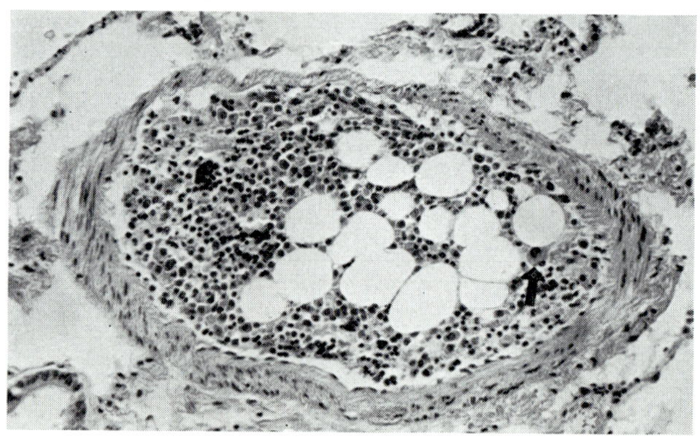

*Fig*. 26.—A megakaryocyte can be identified among the mass of haemopoietic tissue which comprises this bone-marrow embolus in a pulmonary vessel of one of the victims of accident number 152. The spaces contained fat which has been dissolved out in the processing. H. & E. ($\times$ 60.)

The causes of death of the 20 passengers who were killed are shown in *Table V*; of the 16 who were asphyxiated, 6 had bony injuries such as fractures of spine, ribs, sternum, or a long bone, or a combination of such injuries. These 6 all had pulmonary fat embolism and unequivocal pulmonary bone-marrow embolism (*Figs*. 25, 26). Two other asphyxiated passengers had extensive fat and bone-marrow embolism but no evidence of the bony trauma from which the emboli had originated; as both bodies were severely incinerated, it may be accepted that fire had probably obscured the evidence of ante-mortem bony injury. In the other 8 passengers who were asphyxiated there was no microscopic or macroscopic evidence of injury to explain why they failed to escape. Some may have been too far away from breaks in the cabin wall to be able to make their way out through the darkness and smoke before they were overcome by fumes; 1 or 2 appeared to have been as fortuitously favourably placed as some of the survivors, but they had nevertheless died. It is probable that several passengers were temporarily incapacitated by minor concussive injury of which no post-mortem evidence was detectable. Unfortunately rescuers did not record the exact positions in which the bodies were found; it was not known how many were still in their seats and how many collapsed while seeking a means of escape.

As indicated above, the survivors all said they were dazed by the impact when the aircraft crashed. It was not possible to relate this state to minor head injuries, although they may have been a cause; either any such injuries were so minor that they were not clinically evident or they were obscured by the burns to face and scalp which many had received. Vertical deceleration appears to have been of greater importance in this accident than the forward deceleration, although the latter was certainly considerable, at least in the forward part of the aircraft, as was demonstrated by the severe facial and cranial injuries to one of the crew. It was possible that the vertical deceleration experienced by those seated where forward deceleration was minimal had been sufficiently violent to cause transient concussion. It was extremely difficult, therefore, to assess the significance of the universal forward-facing passenger seating in this aircraft; no unequivocal conclusion could be reached. Although rearward-facing seats might not have increased the number of survivors in this particular accident, it was difficult to escape the impression that some of those who failed to escape might have fared better if they had been in rearward-facing seats.

## ACCIDENT NUMBER 158

The evidence from a survivor of accident number 158 indicated that, although his own lap belt was loosely fastened, no order to fasten seat belts had been given and most passengers had almost certainly had no restraint at impact. The pathologists involved in this investigation considered from the general circumstances and from their pathological findings that 'survival would have been the rule rather than the exception had safety harnesses [i.e., belts] been worn'. They did not express an opinion about the relevance of the forward facing seats to death or survival in this accident.

## ACCIDENT NUMBER 255

Except for accident number 212, which a stewardess survived with apparently quite remarkable good fortune, accident number 255 was the only other one in this series from which there were survivors. The aircraft was approaching to land and probably all passengers had their seat belts fastened. As in accident number 152, the evidence in favour of the contention that rearward-facing seats would have resulted in more survivors was equivocal. Again medical investigators thought that there might have been a few more survivors if all the seats had been rearward-facing, but a firm opinion could not be given; the forces in the accident were so great that it was quite fortuitous that there were any survivors at all. It was felt that it would be difficult to refute a claim in this accident that a slight alteration in a survivor's environment—even the provision of a rearward-facing seat—might have reduced his chance of survival and that had this aircraft had rearward-facing seats, different people, not necessarily more, might have survived.

## SAFETY EQUIPMENT

Death may be prevented or injury minimized by bodily restraint during an accident. Moseley and Zeller (1958) found that 'dislodgement of the seat and occupant was the most prevalent injury factor' in passenger aircraft accidents and suggested that the most obvious and easily effected remedy would be the improved structural design of aircraft seats and moorings to withstand deceleration in the fore and aft axis. There are limits to what can thus be achieved, imposed by such considerations as the strength of the air frame itself and the weight penalty of increasing the strength of seats and their attachments; a safe and strong aircraft so heavy that it cannot carry a reasonable payload is not a commercial proposition. With the advent of stronger but lighter materials it may be possible to achieve some improvement without much increase in weight. This problem is largely in the hands of the designers; all the accident investigator can do is draw attention to those cases in which minimal structural damage has occurred to the floor of an aircraft but seats have become detached with consequent severe injury to their occupants. A recent example was the crash survival study of the accident to a Convair 580 aircraft at O'Hare International Airport on 27 December, 1968 (National Transportation Safety Board, U.S.A., 1969b), which showed that 'occupants whose seats and restraint systems remained intact sustained the least overall degree of injury. Conversely, fatalities and most severe injuries were generally associated with failures of the occupant restraint system.'

### Lap Belts

The subject of pilots' safety harness is discussed in Section II, for it is especially relevant to light aircraft aviation. Nevertheless, it is by no means irrelevant to public transport aviation and, as already stated, 3 pilots may have lost their lives in accident number 152 because they failed to use the safety equipment provided for them.

The passengers' lap belt functions in two situations; firstly it serves to prevent injury when an aircraft is flying in turbulent air conditions; on occasions, turbulence can be extreme and unless a passenger is strapped into his seat he may be thrown forcibly around the passenger compartment and consequently injured. Secondly it restrains him in his seat in an accident and prevents injury due to his being propelled against rigid obstacles during the violent deceleration.

The efficacy of a lap belt in the context of a forward-facing seat and fore-aft deceleration is limited. Ruff (1950a) reported a high proportion of head injuries and compression fractures of the lower thoracic or lumbar spine when a lap belt without shoulder straps was used. Moseley and Zeller (1958) found that jack-knifing over a fastened lap belt with flailing of the head was a very common cause of death in transport aircraft accidents. Fryer (1965b) quoted Hawkes (1956) who reported 11 of 22 passengers killed in one accident by penetrating head wounds caused by impact with the backs of the seats in front. Stapp (1953) stated that 88 per cent of persons dependent upon lap belt restraint sustain head injuries in aircraft crashes, and Mason (1962g) concluded that, 'evidence for the relative ineffectiveness of lap belt restraint is so overwhelming, that it must be concluded that its retention in commercial passenger carrying aircraft is based on passenger resistance to additional restraint and the difficulty in fitting such equipment to women and children'.

The subject of the injury potential of lap belts themselves is discussed in connexion with light aircraft accidents for it is, perhaps, more relevant to accidents in which decelerative forces are less than those usually encountered in passenger aircraft accidents. In only one of the accidents in the present study (number 158) did it appear that passengers may have died because they did not have fastened lap belts. In none did it seem that death resulted because lap belts had themselves caused lethal injuries. In only one accident in which there were survivors (again number 158) was it possible to conclude that lap belts were a significant factor in survival of those that escaped.

It is difficult if not impossible to dissociate the question of lap belt restraint in the passenger from that of his seat orientation, certainly from the point of view of one investigating an accident, although differentiation in experimental circumstances is possible.

## The Orientation of Seats

The case for rearward-facing seats has been put by many workers including Gilson, Stewart, and Pekarek (1943); Dudgeon (1947); Moseley (1955); Moseley, Townsend, and Stembridge (1958); Fryer (1958, 1959) and Campbell (1960). In his review of the subject Fryer (1958) discussed the arguments advanced against the adoption of rearward-facing seats and showed that the majority were insubstantial if not completely invalid. The aircraft of the Royal Air Force Air Support Command (formerly Transport Command) have been fitted with rearward-facing seats since 1947 as have all civilian aircraft employed under charter for trooping. The reluctance in the commercial field to equip passenger aircraft with such seats is probably largely economic. It would be extremely costly to convert aircraft already in service; it is not merely a matter of turning existing seats around. Rearward-facing seats require strengthened seat backs and duplicate locks on recline mechanisms and certain other modifications. If they were introduced only in new aircraft it is feared that there might be some adverse reaction among potential passengers who might either think that the newer aircraft were more likely to crash or be reluctant to fly in aircraft continuing in service with forward-facing seats.

Such fears about passenger reaction are probably ill-founded; probably as spurious as the alleged adverse passenger reaction to facing backwards for other reasons (Dudgeon, 1947; 'R.B', 1954; Shaw, 1956; Campbell, 1960). I discussed the subject with a representative of an airline which had at one time had a Government trooping charter; it had several piston-engined aircraft equipped with rearward-facing seats for all passengers. Having lost the contract, it put the aircraft into service on a route flown by several other airlines, all having forward-facing seats. The representative assured me that during the several years this situation existed, his company had had its fair share of passengers and the orientation of their seats had been apparently of no consequence in this regard.

Perhaps of more importance is the undoubted drawback of the discomfort experienced in a rearward-facing seat in the steep take-off of the modern jet conforming to the noise abatement regulations. Probably most important of all is the fact that any particular airline has very few accidents. When accidents do occur injuries are either minimal in any case, or the accident is completely unsurvivable. In any one year the number of lives or serious injuries that might be saved in aircraft accidents by the universal adoption of rearward-facing seats is probably small; with the increase in volume of aviation the number may well increase.

The controversy over rearward-facing seats, therefore, continues. As pointed out by Fryer (1965c), it is important for experienced personnel to continue to make an appraisal of the value of various protective measures during accident investigation, but statistical evidence from aircraft accidents will never be sufficient by itself due to the small numbers involved and the infinite variety of circumstances that influence the outcome in the individual accident; the evidence from accident investigation must supplement a combination of theory and experiment.

*Chapter 8*

# GENERAL CONCLUSIONS

THE pathological findings were of appreciable importance in the investigation of at least 7 of the 18 public transport accidents in this series. In 2 accidents potentially significant natural disease was found in a pilot and in 1, carbon monoxide intoxication of all the operating crew was discovered. In 2 cases pathological evidence helped to exclude the sabotage that at first had been considered highly probable. In 1, some evidence, albeit of a negative nature, was offered to the Commission of Inquiry and supported the non-medical evidence that tended to exclude one possible set of circumstances leading to the aircraft's descent through cloud and collision with a mountain.

In 3 accidents pathological evidence was found and correlated with evidence from other sources to reconstruct the means of escape of a few survivors and explain the failure to escape of those who died. In 1 of these accidents, it was shown that most of the deaths were due not primarily to the mechanical forces experienced in the accident but to the post-crash fire and were, therefore, potentially preventable. The deaths of the operating crew in this same accident had been due to a failure to use the safety equipment provided; two of the cabin crew died probably because of inadequate seating and the lack of doors guarding the pantry storage shelves. It was shown that the actions of at least one member of the cabin crew had been faultless in that immediately after the accident he had opened the escape exit and prepared to assist passengers, ignoring his own personal safety.

The number of crew involved in this small series of accidents is too small to provide a basis for any firm conclusions about the incidence of natural disease or the adequacy of the medical standards of airline pilot selection or surveillance. There is certainly no suggestion from the findings that there is any gross deficiency.

# *SECTION II*

# *LIGHT AIRCRAFT ACCIDENTS*

---

## *Chapter 9*

## INTRODUCTION

### ACCIDENT TRENDS

THE term 'light aircraft' has no precise definition. In the United States of America it is popularly used to cover those aircraft up to 12,500 lb. in weight, and coming under the category of general aviation aircraft. In the United Kingdom the term has been generally used to include aircraft up to 5000 lb. in weight only, and the accidents reviewed in this section are to aircraft thus defined.

Brooks (1966) described the growth of British light aircraft aviation between the two world wars, and showed how the British pioneered the field in the 1920's but lost their leadership to the Americans in the 1930's. During the Second World War, and for the following 15 years, it remained static in the United Kingdom; no new types of British light aircraft were produced and the import of machines built in the U.S.A. was virtually impossible due to strict import licence control. With the relaxation of this restriction in June 1959, in respect of machines of up to 4500 lb. in weight, light aircraft aviation began to increase once more in this country.

Official statistics about light aircraft aviation are not published. This is because there is an absence of information about the hours and miles flown and the numbers of passengers carried; it is difficult, therefore, to compile any accident rates. Vivian (1967) published some statistics derived from the number of registered light aircraft, the number of people holding student and private pilot's licences (S.P.L.s and P.P.L.s), and the number of fatal and non-fatal accidents recorded in the United Kingdom in recent years. *Table VI* was prepared from his data and demonstrates a steady increase both in pilots and aircraft during the period 1961–6. Vivian concluded that total notifiable accidents per 100 pilots had decreased slightly but that there had been an upward trend in fatal accidents and total fatalities, both in absolute numbers and when related to the numbers of pilots licensed and aircraft registered. He further stated that his findings did not seem to be very different from those in other countries and cited the combined figures for the 19 states of the European Civil Aviation Conference. For example, for the years 1962 to 1964 the fatalities per 100 British aircraft averaged 1·43; those for the E.C.A.C. were 1·45.

The impression gained from these figures is that there is an increasing volume of light aircraft aviation apparently without much, if any, improvement in safety. Indeed, the fatal accident and fatality rates, as well as the absolute fatality figures, appear to be increasing rather than decreasing. This suggests that, as with public transport aircraft accidents, all aspects of each fatal accident should be studied in a search for a full explanation and for evidence upon which to base proposals for improving flight safety.

## THE CASE MATERIAL

Forty-two fatal light aircraft accidents on the files of the Department of Aviation Pathology are reviewed in this Section. One accident involved a helicopter, the remainder occurred to fixed-wing machines. Four of the accidents involved university air squadron pilots and one a Service pilot; since these 5 were essentially civilians, it was

*Table VI.*—BRITISH LIGHT AIRCRAFT ACCIDENT DATA: 1961–6 (*after* Vivian, 1967, *reproduced by permission of the Editor, 'Flight Safety Bulletin'*)

| YEAR | NUMBER OF VALID S.P.L.S AND P.P.L.S | NUMBER OF AIRCRAFT | NUMBER OF ACCIDENTS | NUMBER OF FATAL ACCIDENTS | TOTAL FATALITIES | ACCIDENTS PER 100 PILOTS | ACCIDENTS PER 100 AIRCRAFT | FATAL ACCIDENTS PER 100 PILOTS | FATAL ACCIDENTS PER 100 AIRCRAFT | FATALITIES PER 100 PILOTS | FATALITIES PER 100 AIRCRAFT |
|---|---|---|---|---|---|---|---|---|---|---|---|
| 1961 | 10,720 | 965 | 65 | 6 | 10 | 0·61 | 6·73 | 0·06 | 0·62 | 0·09 | 1·04 |
| 1962 | 10,856 | 990 | 64 | 9 | 18 | 0·59 | 6·46 | 0·08 | 0·91 | 0·17 | 1·82 |
| 1963 | 11,032 | 1036 | 60 | 4 | 8 | 0·54 | 5·79 | 0·04 | 0·39 | 0·07 | 0·77 |
| 1964 | 11,842 | 1052 | 75 | 10 | 18 | 0·63 | 7·11 | 0·08 | 0·95 | 0·15 | 1·71 |
| 1965 | 12,600 | 1087 | 73 | 9 | 14 | 0·58 | 6·64 | 0·07 | 0·83 | 0·11 | 1·29 |
| 1966 | (estimated) 13,775 | 1185 | 71 | 13 | 25 | 0·52 | 5·99 | 0·09 | 1·10 | 0·18 | 2·11 |
| | | Totals | 408 | 51 | 93 | | | | | | |

considered appropriate to include them in the series. The fatalities from the 42 accidents totalled 72 persons: 42 pilots-in-charge, 10 second pilots and 20 passengers; there were 5 injured survivors. Two of the pilots had airline transport pilots' (A.L.T.P.) licences and 9 had commercial pilots' licences (C.P.L.); 1 of these professional pilots was killed on a commercial flight but the others while flying light aircraft for private purposes. Thirty-six pilots had private pilots' licences (P.P.L.) and the other 5 were flying under the aegis of the Royal Air Force.

General safety aspects of light aircraft aviation are discussed in Chapter 12; crash safety factors are common to both civilian and military light aircraft, and a further 14 accidents, all involving military pilots flying light aircraft, are analysed in this context with the 42 accidents involving civilian pilots. The helicopter accident was excluded because the crash forces in rotary wing aircraft accidents may differ considerably from those in fixed wing aircraft accidents, although Bezreh (1963) and Keil and Blumberg (1963) reported that the causes of death were similar and occurred in similar proportions in both helicopters and ordinary aircraft.

## THE AIMS OF THE PATHOLOGIST'S INVESTIGATION

The aims of each investigation were exactly as set out in Chapter 2 with respect to public transport accidents. As might be anticipated, there were some differences in emphasis but the search for evidence to explain and reconstruct the accident fully was the basic purpose. The series provided no good example of either clues to a non-medical cause for an accident or evidence of important events in flight prior to an accident, arising from the pathological evidence. Section II does not, therefore, contain the equivalent of Chapters 5 and 6 in Section I; however, it is likely that continued careful routine pathological investigation of light aircraft accidents will result in contributions of this nature from the pathologist in the future.

*Chapter 10*

# NATURAL DISEASE IN THE PILOTS

PRIVATE pilots are required to have periodic medical examinations (every 25 months if they are under 40 years of age and every 13 months if they are over 40 years of age). It is possible that they are less likely to maintain quite such a high standard of fitness as most professional pilots who are subject to more frequent medical examinations (annually for military pilots, every 6 months for commercial and airline pilots). A man whose career depends upon his maintaining a high standard of fitness will be more likely to attempt to do so than a private pilot whose career is not at stake. However, the great majority of diseases are no more likely and no less likely to afflict private pilots than commercial pilots.

As was discussed in Chapter 3, there are many diseases which may cause acute incapacitation and thus precipitate an accident and many others which may so lower a pilot's efficiency as to contribute to an error of skill; any disease is of greater potential seriousness in a pilot who is flying solo or in a machine with only one set of controls than in the public transport aircraft with two or more pilots on board. Coronary artery disease is the most prevalent cause of sudden unexpected death and, although it has been discussed at some length in relation to airline pilots and accidents to public transport aircraft, it merits further consideration in relation to light aircraft accidents and private pilots.

## CORONARY ARTERY DISEASE

What may have been the first fatal flying accident to be attributed to collapse of a pilot in flight from an attack of coronary insufficiency, occurred in 1948; it has not been reported previously in the medical literature and this account of its investigation as given by the accident inspector concerned (Warren, 1967) is of some historical interest.

'A trainee pilot, aged 44 years, took off in an aircraft with an open cockpit for a local flight of approximately 30 minutes' duration. Immediately before this he had had a check flight with an instructor lasting about 10 minutes; during this flight he handled the aircraft competently and made a satisfactory landing. After taking-off solo the pilot flew in the area for approximately 15 minutes. The aircraft was then seen by witnesses on the ground to be approaching from an easterly direction at about 300 feet, one mile north of the aerodrome. It commenced a fairly steep turn to the left and started to lose height. The turn continued and the rate of descent increased until the aircraft struck trees and crashed into a wood. During the latter part of the descent the witnesses were unable to see anyone in either cockpit of the aircraft as they were accustomed to do when aircraft flew low near the aerodrome. One of the witnesses said that the engine appeared to be cutting-out, or was throttled back and popping during the descent. The pilot died shortly after being admitted to hospital. At the time the wind was light and the sky three-quarters covered by cloud at 800 feet; visibility was over 3 miles.

'Although the aircraft was extensively damaged it was salvaged and subjected to a detailed examination. No evidence of any malfunction or structural defect was found in the airframe; the engine was in good mechanical order and revealed nothing to suggest that there had been a loss of power or other failure.

'As no material evidence was found in the wreckage to account for the manœuvres of the aircraft prior to impact, special consideration was given to the possibility of failure in the human element. Suspicions were aroused in this connexion by the fact that witnesses, who did not know whether the aircraft contained one or two occupants,

*Table VII.*—FATAL LIGHT AIRCRAFT ACCIDENTS: PILOTS FOUND TO HAVE NATURAL DISEASE OR ADVERSE MEDICAL HISTORIES

| ACCIDENT NUMBER | TYPE OF LICENCE | DISEASE FOUND OR HISTORY ELICITED | ASSOCIATION WITH CAUSE OF ACCIDENT |
|---|---|---|---|
| 131 | C | Immature personality; accident prone; failed flying training | Highly probable |
| 178 | A | Severe coronary artery disease | Probable |
| 186 | P | Cerebellar arteriovenous aneurysm | Improbable |
| 207 | P | History of attacks of vertigo and recent insomnia; probably under influence of alcohol at time of take-off | Probable |
| 211 | S | Migraine | Improbable |
| 225 | P | Myocarditis; encephalitis | Equivocal |
| 244 | P | Acute U.R.T.I.; patchy pneumonitis; equivocal myocarditis; had taken antihistamines | Highly probable |
| 258 | P | Chronic anxiety state; untreated hypertension; had taken amphetamine | Equivocal |

A = Airline Transport Pilot's Licence. C = Commercial (or Senior Commercial) Pilot's Licence. P = Private Pilot's Licence. S = Student Pilot's Licence.

were unable to see anyone in either cockpit, although they should have been able to see the pilot in the conditions pertaining when they had the aircraft in view. A post-mortem examination of the pilot was ordered by the coroner. The pathologist found severely diseased coronary arteries and stated at the subsequent inquest that in his opinion the accident "may well have been caused by the deceased suffering a cardiac (anginal) attack whilst flying".

'The possibility of malfunction of the engine could not be eliminated entirely, but not only was there no evidence of malfunction but the aircraft was not being manœuvred in a manner to be expected if a forced landing were being attempted. If, on the other hand, the pilot had become seriously ill in some way in flight, he might well have throttled back the engine before losing his faculties. This would account for the witnesses having the impression that the engine was not functioning normally; the fact that the pilot could not be seen in the cockpit when the aircraft was at low height could be explained by his having collapsed in his seat. After consideration of all the evidence I came to the conclusion that there was no structural failure or mechanical defect in the aircraft and that the probable cause of the accident was loss of control following incapacitation of the pilot due to a heart attack.'

As shown in *Table VII* only one of the present series of light aircraft accidents—number 178—seemed likely to have been due to coronary artery disease in the pilot.

## ACCIDENT NUMBER 178

This involved an airline pilot flying a privately owned light aircraft for pleasure purposes. He had stated that he intended to carry out circuits and landings. Two circuits and landings were carried out and the machine took off a third time. About half way around the third circuit the engine was heard to be throttled back to about the power required for a normal approach for landing and the machine appeared to be under control and slowly losing height; it then turned across wind, too low and too near the airfield for a normal landing, with the engine still throttled back. The wings were seen to 'wobble' and then the engine was heard to open up to about full power. At a height of about 100 ft. the machine turned towards a wooded ridge, passed through a gap in the trees but then the undercarriage struck a tree and the starboard wing struck another and the machine plunged into a lake.

At post-mortem the pilot was found to have a moderate degree of myocardial fibrosis and severe coronary artery disease, but without complete occlusion of any coronary artery. No pre-crash failure was demonstrated in the aircraft and no adequate non-medical explanation for the accident was discovered. It was possible, therefore, in view of the extensive coronary artery disease and the myocardial fibrosis that the pilot had suffered an attack of acute coronary insufficiency; the coroner's pathologist reported death to have been due to 'coronary thrombosis' and no inquest was held.

Reals, Davidson, and Karnitschnig (1964) reported a series of 178 persons killed in an unstated number of light aircraft accidents. Eight of the accidents were thought to have been precipitated by natural disease—in each case coronary atherosclerosis. No other pathological conditions were present in the pilots they studied. Siegel and Mohler (1969) claimed that the National Transportation Safety Board's records showed about six cases each year of in-flight incapacitation of the pilot from either a coronary occlusion or a cerebrovascular accident. Dille and Morris (1967) reported 122 fatal general aviation accidents (autopsies were performed on 86 of the pilots) and stated that none was thought to have been caused by natural disease in the pilot; in only 2 pilots was severe narrowing of one or more coronary arteries found.

The findings of Reals and others (1964) are in contrast to the absence of any accident in the present series caused by coronary artery disease in a private pilot (accident number 178 involved a professional pilot, although he was flying a privately owned light aircraft when he was killed). An attempt was made, therefore, to compare the extent of coronary artery disease in the private pilots in this series with that found in several studies of the disease in professional military pilots and controls reported in the literature. Of the 52 pilots, 12 were excluded because they were professional pilots (1 military and 11 civilian) who happened to have been killed flying light aircraft; 3 were excluded because detailed information about the state of their coronary arteries was not available. Of the remaining 37, 18 (49 per cent) had no coronary artery disease beyond slight thickening of the intima, 16 (43 per cent) had Mason's Grade I, and 3 (8 per cent) had Mason's Grade II or Grade III atherosclerosis. These figures are compared in *Table VIII* with those from the various studies collected and reported by Mason (1963b); despite their high average age the civilian light aircraft pilots appear to have been as fit as any of the groups of professional pilots and as fit as most of the groups of controls. Only Enos's soldiers, who were much younger, appear to have been healthier as judged by the state of their coronary arteries.

*Table VIII.*—ASYMPTOMATIC CORONARY ARTERY DISEASE IN AVIATORS AND CONTROLS (OCCURRENCE IN %) (*after* Mason, 1963b, *reproduced by permission of the Editor, 'British Medical Journal'*)

| GRADE OF DISEASE | CATHERMAN AND OTHERS (1962) (AVIATORS) | GLANTZ AND STEMBRIDGE (1959) (AVIATORS) | STEVENS (1961) (AVIATORS) | MASON (1963) | | ENOS AND OTHERS (1953) (SOLDIERS) | RIGAL AND OTHERS (1960) (CONTROLS) | PRESENT SERIES CIVILIAN LIGHT AIRCRAFT PILOTS |
|---|---|---|---|---|---|---|---|---|
| | | | | AVIATORS | CONTROLS | | | |
| 0 | 24 | 30 | 34·5 | 38 | 50 | 58·4 | 36 | 49 |
| 1 | 38 | 49 | 43 | 37 | 33 | 29·3 | 46 | 43 |
| 2 and 3 | 38 | 21 | 22·5 | 25 | 17 | 12·3 | 18 | 8 |
| Average age | 30 | 28 | — | 28·3 | 26·3 | 22·1 | 25 | 32·9 |
| Total in Series | 96 | 222 | 190 | 180 | 90 | 300 | 167 | 37 |

## OTHER CONDITIONS

There was either evidence of natural disease at post-mortem or on subsequent laboratory examination, or an adverse medical history was discovered, in another 7 of the 52 pilots killed in the 42 accidents (*Table VII*). They form a miscellaneous group and their case histories demonstrate how different are the circumstances in each one. Every accident is unique. Were it possible to give a percentage probability figure to the association of the disease in the pilot and the cause of the accident, it would probably differ markedly in each case as a result of several subtle points in the assessment as well as a number of more obvious ones.

### ACCIDENT NUMBER 131

The pilot had failed his flying training in one of the Services following several adverse reports for carelessness, inattention, and poor airmanship. After being grounded he had suffered a car accident and later required psychiatric investigation and treatment. He was discharged from the Service with a reduced medical category and a diagnosis of immature personality. After discharge he was involved in two further motor car accidents and sustained a broken leg. However, he subsequently completed a civilian course of flying training and was granted a commercial pilot's licence.

The accident in which he was killed was his first commercial engagement. The accident inspector's investigation revealed that he had failed to refuel before taking off, despite the fact that he knew that the aircraft had made several flights previously that afternoon. He failed to use the correct techniques for fuel management in flying the particular type of aircraft. During take-off he should have used the main fuel tank which had a gravity feed to the carburettor rather than the auxiliary tank which had a pump feed; this procedure is designed to reduce the chance of engine failure due to fuel starvation at what is a critical phase of flight. When safely airborne, he should have switched over from the main tank, which had a fuel gauge, to the auxiliary fuel tank which had not; this practice is adopted so that in the event of the auxiliary tank becoming empty during flight, the main tank can be used and its fuel gauge provide an accurate indication of the fuel remaining.

In the event, the pilot took off using the main tank and flew the aircraft until that tank was empty. Then, apparently in confusion, he failed to switch to the reserve tank which had, in fact, plenty of fuel in it, although normally it would have been empty if the main tank was empty. Having thus precipitated an emergency, he tried to glide the machine down on to some school playing fields; this he might well have accomplished successfully had he quickly released the advertising trailer he was towing. Apparently he forgot about the trailer until the drag this produced on the aircraft had caused so much loss of flying speed that the aircraft stalled.

In retrospect, it was clear that this man was quite unsuited to be a pilot. He had not revealed his full medical and flying history when he applied for a commercial licence. Had he done so, his Service medical history would have been available on a confidential basis to the licensing authority. The only way that intentional deceit of this nature could be detected would be for the Services to provide the civil licensing authority with a 'black-list' of pilots, student or qualified, grounded or discharged from the Service for either medical or airmanship failure. The undesirable features of such an arrangement are apparent, but so are the dangers to the public of its lack. This aircraft crashed during the rush-hour period only a short distance from a very busy main road of a large city; it was fortunate that an open space was available for the attempted forced landing. Having a commercial licence, this pilot was entitled to carry fare-paying passengers in those aircraft for which his licence was endorsed; in view of his indifferent competence as a pilot, it is probable that he would not have advanced to become an airline transport pilot but nevertheless he could have killed several people in the course of flying even a light aircraft.

## ACCIDENT NUMBER 186

A reserve military pilot was giving air experience to a cadet. During the flight the aircraft was seen to make a climbing turn at the top of which it appeared to stall. It then dived towards the sea, flattened out slightly but struck the water; after floating briefly, it sank. When the machine was raised it was found to contain only the body of the pilot still fully strapped into his seat. The passenger's harness was unfastened and the body missing. At post-mortem the pilot was found to have an arteriovenous aneurysm (*Fig.* 27) approximately 1 cm. in diameter, situated on the anterior margin of the lateral part of the anterior lobe of the cerebellum, just above the right superior cerebellar peduncle. On microscopic examination it appeared that this lesion had not bled acutely although there were numerous haemosiderin-laden macrophages in the adjacent tissue.

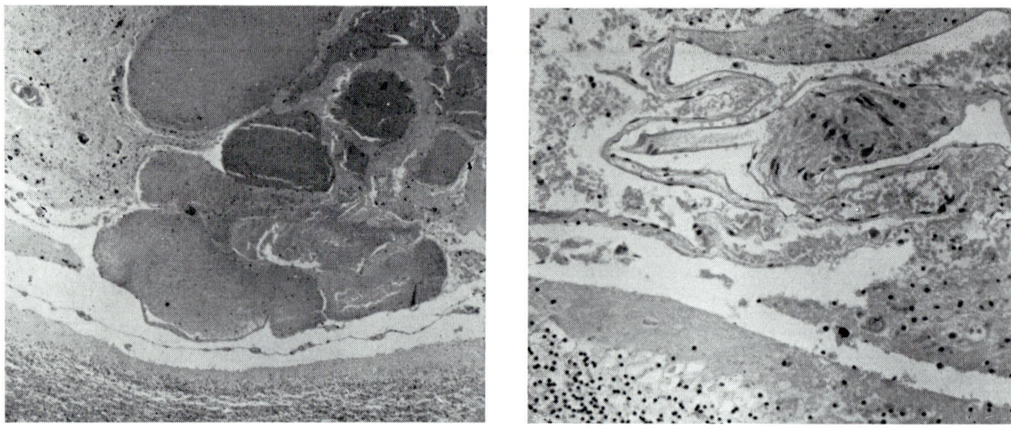

A B

*Fig.* 27.—A, Low power (H. & E., × 16) and, B, High power (× 66) views of an arteriovenous aneurysm of the cerebellum found in the pilot involved in accident number 186. The masses of blood in A are all within vessels; there has been no fresh bleeding around the lesion but the dark granules in the adjacent tissues are deposits of haemosiderin indicating old haemorrhage.

Two main questions arose in the attempt to appraise the significance of this lesion in relation to the cause of the accident. The first was whether the aneurysm had contributed to the accident. Since it had not bled, the only effect it could have had upon the pilot would have been a subtle impairment of his proprioceptive senses; this might have contributed to his error in permitting the aircraft to stall, if he were flying it 'by the seat of his pants' rather than by the use of instruments.

The second question was whether the aneurysm was associated with the pilot's failure to escape. It was inconceivable that the passenger, making his first flight, would not have been fully strapped into the aircraft; since his harness was found undone in the recovered aircraft, it could be presumed only that the passenger was not incapacitated, was able to unfasten the harness and escape from the aircraft but that he was subsequently drowned. Since the aircraft wreckage showed very little damage to the cockpit area, there was no doubt that the pilot had not been trapped by distorted aircraft wreckage. No evidence was found at post-mortem to suggest that he had been incapacitated when the aircraft struck the sea; yet unlike the passenger, he had not made any attempt to escape. There was no satisfactory explanation for this. The possibility that he was unable to unfasten his harness because of incoordination due to the effect of the aneurysm without it having bled acutely seemed sufficiently remote to be dismissed.

## ACCIDENT NUMBER 207

An aircraft carrying an instructor and a pupil took off one afternoon from an airfield on the South Coast; after performing some aerobatics above the airfield it flew out over the English Channel and crashed into the sea in unknown circumstances; a small quantity of wreckage was later recovered. On investigation it was discovered that during the preceding year, the instructor had had a period of 5 months off flying because of attacks of dizziness that were said to have been diagnosed as labyrinthitis. Examination of the hospital notes, however, revealed that his symptoms had been regarded as psychogenic. At one time he had been advised to give up flying but it was later decided that the vertiginous attacks had been due to emotional tension and that, as these stresses were thought to have been resolved, his flying licence should be renewed. Investigation also revealed that 2 or 3 weeks before his death, this pilot had suffered from insomnia. He had sought medical advice and received a prescription for sodium amytal; an empty sodium amytal bottle was found in the boot of his car at the airfield.

The instructor's headless and limbless body was recovered from the sea 12 weeks after the accident; no evidence of natural disease was found in the torso at autopsy and histological examination was of extremely little value due to autolysis. In the circumstances a search for intracranial or middle ear pathology was precluded; the possibility that he had suffered another attack of vertigo and thus precipitated the accident could not be assessed.

This accident is discussed further in Chapter 11, for there were certain aspects of toxicological interest and importance.

## ACCIDENT NUMBER 211

This accident also involved an aircraft carrying two pilots. One, the holder of a student pilot's licence, was known to suffer from migraine; he was accustomed to treat himself for this and found that two codeines were usually sufficient. The aircraft crashed when a forced landing was being attempted, apparently due to bad weather conditions.

A strongly positive test for salicylates was obtained on testing a specimen of urine taken from the student pilot at post-mortem. It was not known for certain which pilot was attempting the forced landing. However, the student had passed all but his ground examinations for a full private pilot's licence and, as a pilot, he was probably equal in ability, if not better than the pilot in command. The machine had dual controls (except for wheel brakes) and the convention is for such aircraft to be flown from the left hand seat; in this case that seat was occupied by the student pilot. It is probable, therefore, that it was he who was attempting the landing. It was he who had taken salicylates and was presumably suffering from or recovering from a migrainous headache. No further evidence could be found to help to determine whether or not his illness had contributed to the accident. The possibility was sufficiently strong for the case to be of value as an example with which to warn pilots of the dangers of flying when not perfectly fit.

## ACCIDENT NUMBER 225

A light helicopter, being flown solo by its owner, crashed a few minutes after take-off for a cross-country flight. At routine post-mortem examination patchy scarring of the myocardium was noted. Microscopy confirmed the presence of myocardial fibrosis (*Fig.* 28); it also revealed a focal myocarditis (*Figs.* 29 and 30) and a

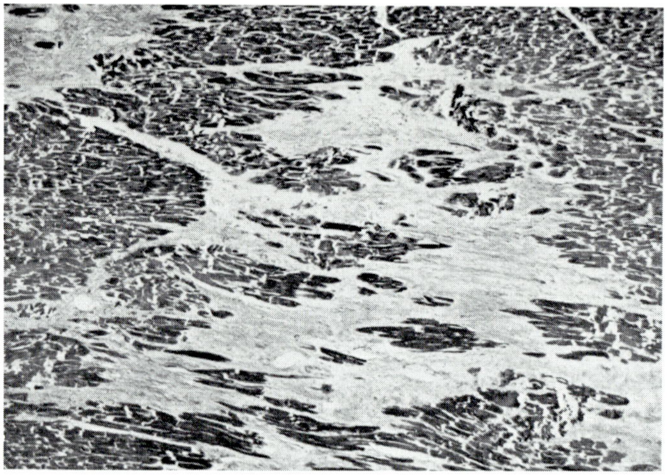

*Fig.* 28.—A low-power view of myocardium from the left ventricular wall of the pilot killed in accident number 225. It shows replacement of much of the muscle by fibrous tissue. P.T.A.H. (× 15.)

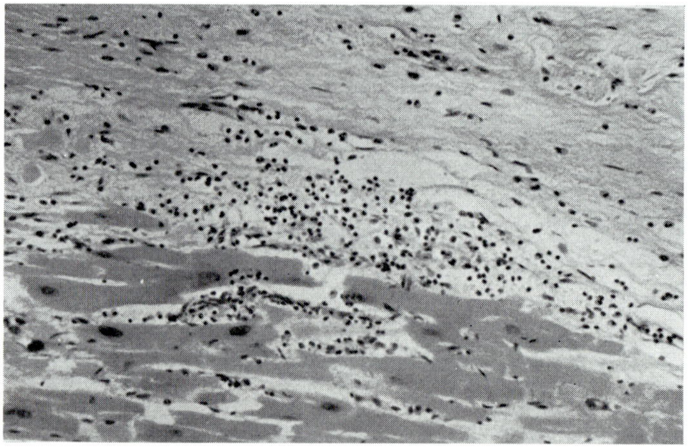

*Fig.* 29.—A higher-power view of the edge of the area of fibrosis shown in *Fig.* 28. There is an inflammatory infiltrate that consists mostly of lymphocytes but there are occasional plasma cells and eosinophils. H. & E. (× 66.)

marked perivascular lymphocytic inflammatory infiltrate in some sections of the cerebral cortex (*Fig.* 31). In other areas of the brain, occasional vessels had a slight lymphocytic cuffing; there were also plasma cells, some with Russell bodies, and macrophages containing granular yellow-brown pigment (*Fig.* 32). Detailed investigation of this man's recent medical history failed to reveal any evidence of clinical illness.

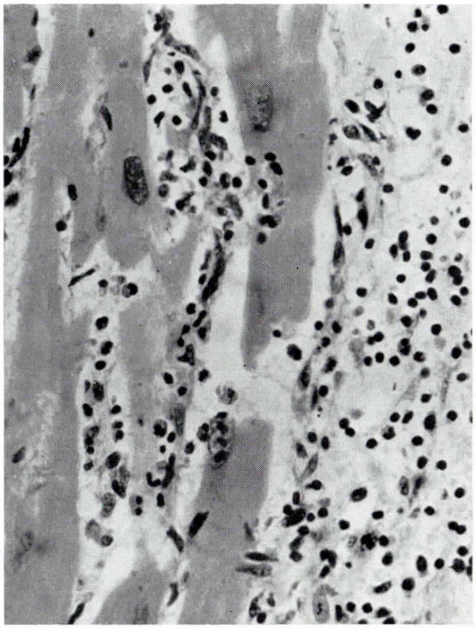

*Fig*. 30.—Higher-power view of part of the field shown in *Fig*. 29. Muscle necrosis is present with interfibrillary cellular infiltration of the damaged muscle-fibres. H. & E. (× 33.)

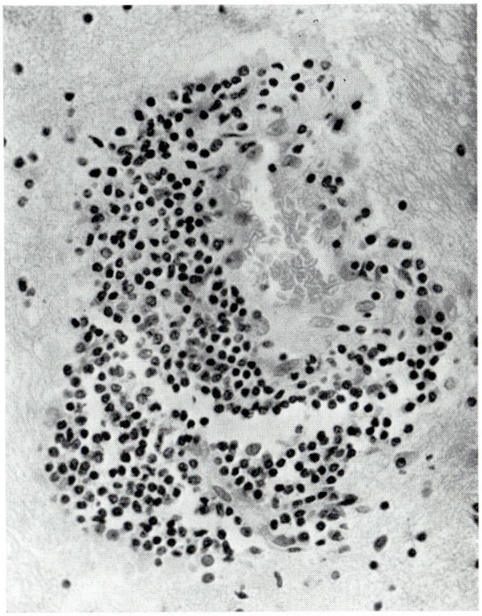

*Fig*. 31.—Section of frontal cerebral cortex of the pilot killed in accident number 225. There is a prominent perivascular cuffing with lymphocytes. H. & E. (× 150.)

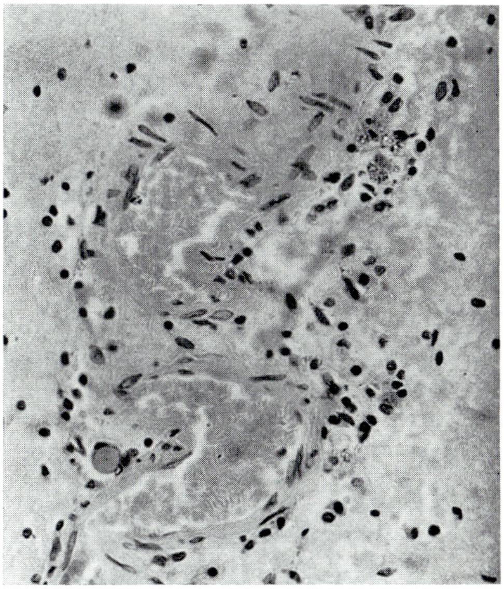

*Fig*. 32.—The same case as *Fig*. 31: another area of cerebral cortex. This shows a capillary with an associated mild lymphocytic and plasma cell infiltrate. One plasma cell contains a Russell body. There are also macrophages containing granular yellow-brown pigment. H. & E. (× 30.)

A V.D.R.L. test was performed on a post-mortem specimen of blood, because of the histological findings in the brain; it was negative. This result was regarded as reliable, although, had it been positive, considerable caution would have been necessary in its interpretation.

There was no evidence of pre-crash failure in this aircraft. Sudden incapacitation of the pilot due to the myocarditis had to be considered, therefore, as a possible cause of the accident. There was little evidence which could be found to support or refute the hypothesis; an equally plausible explanation was pilot incompetence, for he was known to have been extremely casual to the point of being careless in his approach to flying. Furthermore, in this particular helicopter, two control knobs were so placed on the cockpit floor that it would have been difficult for any pilot to see them, whatever his build; the deceased pilot had been unusually obese, for he weighed 240 lb. although he was only 5 ft. 10 in. tall. With such a stature, it would have been quite impossible for him to see the two control knobs in question and he would have had to select the one to operate by touch. Actuation of the wrong control was a very acceptable hypothetical explanation for the accident in the opinion of the accident inspector, having regard to the manner in which the aircraft was seen to crash. Unfortunately this hypothesis was incapable either of proof or disproof; technical examination of the wreckage did not help. A relationship between this man's illness and his accident, therefore, could not be established; but neither could it be dismissed.

## ACCIDENT NUMBER 244

Two pilots and a passenger were on board an aircraft fitted with dual controls, making a cross-country flight. Again, it was not known for certain which pilot was flying the machine, but it seemed most likely that the usual convention would have been followed, and that it would have been flown by the pilot occupying the left hand seat; he was, incidentally, the more experienced of the two.

Meteorological evidence indicated that there were layers of broken stratus cloud at levels between 450 and 8000 ft. at the time the accident occurred. A few minutes after take-off, a message from the aircraft reported that it was being flown in cloud at 2000 ft. Shortly thereafter, it was seen to dive out of cloud and crash into rising ground; eye-witnesses suggested that there was some attempt at recovery. No evidence of pre-crash failure in the aircraft or its engines was found; however, the machine was so badly damaged that the possibility of mechanical defect could not be eliminated entirely.

The medical investigation revealed that the pilot in charge, who was the pilot believed to be flying the aircraft, was suffering from a moderately severe cold. He had, that morning, reported to a doctor and asked for Triominic tablets. These tablets were prescribed by the doctor who did not know of the proposed flight.

Autopsy examinations showed gross mechanical trauma in all three bodies. Fragments of lung were recovered from the partially eviscerated torso of the pilot in charge, and histological examination of these showed that there was a patchy pneumonitis present in some areas (*Fig.* 33). Histological examination of the available fragments of heart showed a very minor degree of focal myocarditis; the foci of lymphocytic infiltrate were so few in number, so small in size and without evidence of myocardial degeneration that the diagnosis of myocarditis was equivocal. The specimens of kidney were subjected to toxicological analysis and traces of the three antihistamines constituting the preparation Triominic were found; there was no doubt, therefore, that this pilot had commenced treatment with the tablets he had requested from his doctor on the day of the fatal flight.

The possible relationship between this pilot's illness and the accident was evaluated as follows: a pilot flying in cloud has no cues about his orientation in space as was discussed in relation to accident number 231 in Chapter 6. In such circumstances, he

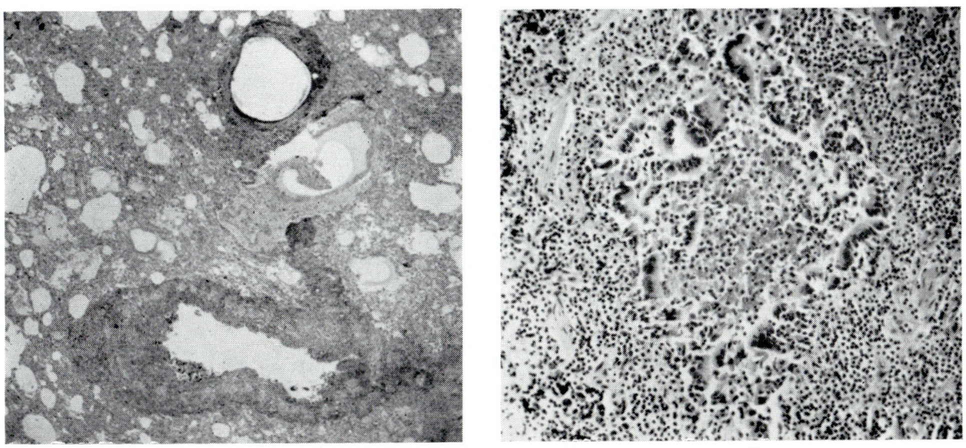

A B

*Fig.* 33.—Microscopic view of two areas of lung from a pilot in accident number 244. There is patchy bronchopneumonia and pneumonitis. A, H. & E. (× 20.) B, H. & E. (× 84.)

has to use instruments which include an artificial horizon; this is normally sufficient for the suppression of false sensations and the pilot is thus able to keep himself correctly orientated. Occasionally, even an experienced pilot may suffer from disorientation despite his instruments, and may find difficulty in suppressing false sensations and re-orientating himself. This is especially liable to occur to a pilot when flying at night or in cloud, or when suffering from a medical condition which disturbs labyrinthine function; it may occur when a pilot is tired or not fully alert or is distracted for some other reason. The Triominic in this case might have produced symptomatic relief of the pilot's upper respiratory tract congestion but it might well also have made him slightly drowsy—a common side effect of antihistamines. Having regard to all the circumstances of the accident, and in particular the lack of a reasonable alternative hypothesis, loss of control due to disorientation was regarded as the most acceptable explanation.

## ACCIDENT NUMBER 258

A schoolmaster who had designed and built an aircraft at his home, was allowed to test fly it within a certain restricted area after it had been checked from the design aspect by the Air Registration Board. A series of successful flights were made over a period of some months. Subsequently, during a flight on which handling tests were being carried out, the aircraft went out of control; some attempt at recovery appeared to have been made according to the evidence of eye-witnesses, but the machine crashed.

No evidence of any significant natural disease was found at post-mortem or on subsequent histology. However, it was discovered that the pilot had had a history of acute psychiatric illness some 6 years before his death, and almost continuously from that time had taken tranquillizers for a chronic anxiety state. The unfixed tissues routinely taken at autopsy were subjected to toxicological analysis. No tranquillizers were found but amphetamine was discovered in the urine in an amount consistent with his having taken a dose of from 5 to 10 mg. a few hours before death. Despite exhaustive enquiries, the source from which the pilot had obtained amphetamine was not discovered. A variety of drugs were found in the medicine cabinet at his home; some belonged to his wife, some had been prescribed for him, but none contained amphetamine. Why he should have taken it on the day of his death, when there was no evidence to suggest that he had ever taken it before, remained a matter for conjecture. One hypothesis was that he had regarded the particular flight as more important than usual; it was being watched by an acquaintance who, it was believed, was considering marketing the aircraft abroad. Possibly the pilot was given the amphetamine by a friend to 'pep him up' for the occasion.

The association between the small dose of amphetamine and the pilot's handling error which apparently caused the accident was also obscure. Although amphetamine is a drug used to stimulate the nervous system, lessen the sense of fatigue and produce a state of well-being, it is known that in excess it can cause nervousness and impair judgement. Repeated doses can cause insomnia and symptoms similar to an anxiety neurosis; larger doses may cause hallucinations. Susceptibility to amphetamine, as with all drugs, varies with individuals; it was considered unlikely, however, that one dose of 5–10 mg. would have caused appreciable deterioration in this pilot's ability to handle his aircraft. Nevertheless, it was just possible that it had induced a state of sufficient well-being that, in combination with his relatively small flying experience and moderate skill, it had caused him to perform a variety of aerobatic manœuvres to test his aircraft at a height which most cautious and experienced pilots would have regarded as too low for safety. Having lost control, there was insufficient height for him to recover completely. A closer association between the drug and the accident could not reasonably be advanced.

## SUICIDE

In Section I the subject of sabotage and attempted sabotage was discussed (Chapter 5); some of the reported cases were due to passengers intent upon suicide. No reports of sabotage to light aircraft have been found in the literature and no case has occurred among the light aircraft accidents my colleagues or I have investigated. However, the possibility of suicide was considered in each one investigated; in the majority, the circumstances were such that suicide could be dismissed as a possibility so remote as to be negligible.

Only in accident number 207, already mentioned in connexion with natural disease in the pilot, alcohol and drugs, was the question of suicide given more careful consideration than usual. No direct evidence of suicide could be adduced but the pilot in question had a history of considerable social and domestic difficulty; he had recently suffered from insomnia and had taken off, apparently under the influence of alcohol, and had commenced his flight with a series of aerobatics, described by eye-witnesses as 'high powered'. In this connexion it is of interest that Gibbons, Plechus, and Mohler (1967) reported 6 cases of accidents to light aircraft apparently caused by pilot's suicidal acts; in 3 the pilots were under the influence of alcohol and in 4 the pilots engaged in aerobatics prior to the accident.

## THE INCIDENCE OF ACCIDENTS CAUSED BY NATURAL DISEASE

The incidence of accidents caused by natural disease in the pilots in the series reported by Reals and others (1964) was probably about 8 per cent (assuming an average of less than two persons involved per accident); in the study by Dille and Morris (1967) the incidence was between 1 and 2 per cent. In the present series there were 8 cases of natural disease from 42 accidents. In only 4, however, was the condition considered to be a probable or highly probable cause for the accident; in only 2 of the 4 was there evidence of organic disease at autopsy or on histology. These figures suggest an incidence for the association between natural disease in pilots and the cause of light aircraft accidents of something between 5 and 10 per cent. It is to be appreciated, however, firstly that the series is small; secondly that the probability of an association between the disease found and the cause of the accident in a given case is a subjective assessment rarely capable of proof; thirdly that the chance of finding evidence of natural disease at autopsy or on subsequent laboratory investigation, or by delving into a pilot's medical history, is very much affected by the motivation and diligence of the pathologist concerned. The only acceptable conclusion is that up to 10 per cent of light aircraft accidents may be caused by illness in the pilot, but the true incidence is probably nearer 5 per cent.

## THE INCIDENCE OF NATURAL DISEASE IN PRIVATE PILOTS

In the present series there were 6 private pilots out of 37 who had evidence of natural disease of potential importance with regard to the safety of their flying; this is an incidence of about 17 per cent which seems unduly high. These cases, however, do not suggest that the present arrangements and standards of medical fitness for private pilot licensing are inadequate. In two instances (accidents numbers 211 and 244) the pilots concerned were suffering from an acute illness; only indoctrination of the pilots themselves in the importance of not flying with acute, though minor, illness can prevent accidents so caused.

In 3 instances (accidents numbers 207, 211, and 258) the pilots' medical histories were known to the medical licensing authority; in 2 of these, very careful assessments of their suitability for renewal of their flying licences were made. In retrospect it may be concluded that those responsible came to the wrong conclusions; it must be accepted from the documentary evidence, however, that their decisions were not made lightly. The pilots killed in accidents numbers 186 and 225 were suffering from conditions unlikely to have been discovered at a clinical examination even immediately prior to take-off on their last flights.

## CONCLUSIONS

It is concluded from this study of natural disease in pilots killed in light aircraft accidents that:—

i. As would be anticipated, occasional accidents occur due to illness in the pilot.

ii. Routine pathological investigation is necessary to detect a large proportion of such cases; even though illness in the pilot be the cause, rarely will the circumstances of the accident be such as to reveal the necessity for a full medical investigation at the outset; when the need is realized, it may be too late.

iii. There is no evidence from this study that the current practice in medical surveillance of private pilots is deficient or less efficient than that of commercial pilots.

iv. There is an indication that some cases where difficulty has been encountered in deciding whether a pilot with an adverse medical history should have his licence renewed, may have been settled too leniently in favour of renewal.

v. It may be that concealment of previous failure of flying training or of medical unfitness to fly is too easy. In practice, however, it is difficult to guard against deliberate deception of this type and it is almost certainly an infrequent occurrence. Apart from those quoted in this chapter, I know of only 2 cases which have ended either in tragedy (the accident at Ardmore discussed in Chapter 3 involving an airline pilot) or a near miss (*Flight Safety*, 1968, involving a private pilot); both these cases occurred in the U.S.A.

## *Chapter 11*

# IMPAIRED EFFICIENCY OF THE PILOT DUE TO INTOXICATION

## ALCOHOL

In only 2 of the 42 accidents has there been the possibility of a close association between the accident and alcoholic intoxication of the pilot.

### ACCIDENT NUMBER 207

Some aspects of this accident were described in the last chapter. As recounted, the aircraft and the two occupants were lost at sea. However, eye-witnesses who saw the instructor on the airfield prior to take-off stated that he had appeared unsteady and had given the impression of having been drinking. The body of the pupil was washed up on the seashore one week after the accident; his urine alcohol was found to be 60 mg. per 100 ml. The instructor's body was not recovered until 12 weeks after the accident; urine alcohol in his case was approximately 30 mg. per 100 ml. and liver alcohol approximately 50 mg. per 100 g.; all estimations were checked by gas chromatography. It was considered, however, that these figures were of little significance as the specimens had been taken so long after death. Putrefactive production of alcohol might have occurred; it has been reported present within a few hours of death in appropriate conditions (Chapter 4); alternatively a high ante-mortem level could have been greatly reduced during the several weeks of immersion in the sea. The importance of alcohol was, therefore, yet another aspect of this case which could not be appraised satisfactorily.

### ACCIDENT NUMBER 243

An aircraft took-off from a private airfield at the conclusion of a public flying display. On board were a pilot, an unlicensed student pilot, and two passengers. It was intended that after a short trip one of the passengers would be returned to the airfield prior to the aircraft being flown back to its base. According to eye-witnesses, the take-off was normal; after a brief initial climb at a normal angle, the aircraft began to climb very steeply to a height of about 250 ft. Then it appeared to stall, one wing dropped and the machine turned, fell, and crashed into an area occupied by spectators and motor cars. The pilot and 2 spectators were killed; the other 3 occupants of the aircraft and 3 spectators were all seriously injured.

No natural disease was discovered at autopsy in the pilot. Blood was taken five hours after death and the level of blood alcohol found to be 161 mg. per 100 ml. It was discovered, thereafter, that the pilot, who had not been involved in the air display, had been drinking brandy and beer at various times during the day, both in the refreshment tent on the airfield and in a public house nearby. Some of the drinking had been in the company of the intended passengers, one of whom reported that the pilot had said, on leaving the refreshment tent for the aircraft 'we will now go and give the Cessna a thrashing'; but he stated at the subsequent inquest that he considered there was nothing in the pilot's speech or manner to indicate that he was under the influence of alcohol.

There was inadequate evidence to decide whether the pilot himself had been at the controls and had made the dangerously steep climb resulting in a stall, or whether he had allowed the inexperienced pupil/passenger (who had often handled the controls under his supervision) either to take-off or to take over control at too low a height. In either event, it was impossible not to associate the raised blood alcohol in the pilot and his lack of skill and/or judgement. Aksnes (1954) showed that levels of alcohol considerably below 150 mg. per 100 ml. seriously affected flying skills and 'there can be very few persons in whom impairment of the ability to drive' (or fly) 'properly and increased risk of being involved in accidents are not present to a significant extent at blood-alcohol concentrations in excess of 80 mg. per 100 ml.' (British Medical Association, 1965b). Harper and Albers (1964) stated that from the work of Aksnes (1954) and Drew, Colquoun, and Long (1958) it appeared 'that flying skills were measurably decreased by one-fourth the amount of alcohol necessary to produce measurable decrease in driving skills'. Although individual tolerance to alcohol varies considerably (Newman, 1947), Borkenstein, Crowther, Shumate, Ziel, and Zylman (1964) showed that car drivers with blood-alcohol levels of 150 mg. per 100 ml. are 25 times more likely to have an accident than drivers having levels of less than 10 mg. per 100 ml.

## DISCUSSION

Analyses for alcohol were performed on specimens from 46 persons (35 pilots and 11 passengers) from 29 of the 42 accidents investigated. Twenty-six of the pilots and all 11 passengers had values defined as negative by Harper and Albers (1964), that is, less than 15 mg. per 100 ml. of blood. In a further 5 pilots, levels of between 15 and 20 mg. per 100 ml. were found and it appeared unlikely that these had any bearing upon the causes of the accidents concerned. One pilot had a level of 53 mg. per 100 ml. of blood; the specimen was taken several days post-mortem and the result was considered unreliable. In only the one accident described earlier (number 243) was alcohol considered a definite main causal factor, and only in one other accident (number 207) was it considered a possible causal factor.

The figures from this series, therefore, give a maximum of 2 out of 29 accidents associated with alcohol, or 3 out of 36 pilots with raised blood alcohol; this suggests an incidence of alcohol-associated fatal light aircraft accidents of about 7 per cent, and just over 8 per cent for alcohol intoxication in pilots killed in light aircraft accidents. Reals and his colleagues (1964) did not state the incidence of raised blood alcohol in their series, but their report implied that it was about 6 per cent; they did not record in how many casualties the search for alcohol was undertaken, and it is possible that the incidence in their series was rather higher. Dille and Morris (1967) stated that 17 of 83 pilots from their 122 fatal accidents had levels of blood alcohol in excess of 30 mg. per 100 ml.;

5 were in excess of 250 mg. per 100 ml. Their findings gave an incidence of alcohol-associated fatal light aviation accidents of 20·5 per cent. This is considerably higher than that found in the present series, or that found by Reals and his associates (1964); all three reports, however, contrast markedly with the dramatic figures of Harper and Albers (1964) who found 56 accidents out of 158 to be associated with alcohol (an incidence of 35·4 per cent), and even those of Gibbons, Ellis, and Plechus (1966) who found 36 cases out of 117 (30·8 per cent) to be associated with measurable levels of blood alcohol—in 33 (28 per cent) of these the level was over 50 mg. per 100 ml. Due account, however, must be taken of the fact that Harper and Albers (1964) did not state how many of their pilots had levels between 15 and 30 mg. per 100 ml. Had they done so, it would have been possible to make a more adequate comparison between their findings, those of 2 of the other 3 studies quoted and the present series.

Mohler, Berner, and Goldbaum (1968) reported that in 1967 74 per cent of fatal general aviation accidents in the U.S.A. had toxicological examinations performed on post-mortem tissues from the pilots; 23 per cent were found to have levels in excess of 150 mg. per 100 ml. and Siegel and Mohler (1969) observed that, though a number of these 'may be "false" positives due to putrefaction, contamination, or other factors, many are substantiated by a history of pilot consumption of alcohol immediately prior to the fatal flight'.

It is probably fair to conclude that alcohol is not an important cause of light aircraft accidents in Britain but it may well be in the U.S.A. This is likely to be due to the fact that private light aircraft are used much more widely in the U.S.A. for pleasure and social purposes when a car would be used in this country. Even with the increasing number of private light aircraft in Britain, it is considered the 'don't drink and drive campaign' will have its effect in controlling any tendency to a marked increase in flying accidents due to alcohol.

## DRUGS

There are at present no facilities for the routine screening of a dead pilot's tissues for any drug of possible importance as discussed in Chapter 4. However, it has become possible recently for analyses for drugs to be undertaken at the combined Home Office/R.A.F. toxicological facility at Aldermaston in selected cases when the presence of particular drugs is suspected. In two cases drugs were found but the pilots both had natural disease and for this reason the accidents were described in Chapter 10.

Haddaway (1963) reported the death in a flying accident of a pilot who had taken barbiturates, thyroid extract, and amphetamine; he referred to several other flying accidents in bad weather where the pilots had taken drugs and he emphasized the importance of toxicological analyses as a routine part of an aircraft accident investigation. Reals and others (1964) reported that drugs were detected in the tissues of only 2 pilots in their series; in 1 instance it was chloroquine and in the other a low level of barbiturate. In neither case was it considered that the drug was relevant to the cause of the accident. Dille and Morris (1967) reported that barbiturate was discovered in 2 pilots from 122 accidents (but they did not state in how many an analysis was performed); that in 2 further accidents the pilots had with them a variety of medicaments but in neither instance did toxicological examination of tissues produce evidence that the drugs had been ingested. Dille and Mohler (1969) discussed the potential danger of flying while taking a wide variety of drugs but quoted only 9 fatal accidents (including our accident number 244) in which the pilots were found to have ingested various drugs; in several of these a doubtful causal relationship existed with the accidents concerned.

From these reports it would appear that there is not a frequent association of fatal light aircraft accidents and the presence of drugs in the pilots. This is probably a valid conclusion but it must be accepted with some reserve until routine and comprehensive screening has been carried out on a large series of pilots involved in accidents, both fatal and non-fatal, and a control series of pilots who have not had accidents; this is a research project that it is envisaged will be undertaken in the Department of Aviation Pathology in due course.

## CARBON MONOXIDE INTOXICATION

In no pilot or passenger from this series of 42 accidents was a raised carboxyhaemoglobin level found that did not appear to have resulted from survival in a post-crash fire. Reals and his colleagues (1964) did not report any accident in which carbon monoxide intoxication appeared to have been a significant causal factor; but Dille and Morris (1967) reported 1 such case among their 122; a father and son were found to have levels of 27·4 and 40 per cent carboxyhaemoglobin respectively and 'the direct and distractive effects' of this 'were felt to have caused this accident which was fatal to both occupants'. Siegel and Mohler (1969) recorded the case of a pilot who could not account for an hour of his two-hour flight, made a gear-up landing, and was found mumbling incoherently when helped from the aircraft; this was thought to be a 'near-miss' due to carbon monoxide contamination of cockpit atmosphere.

Carbon monoxide contamination of light aircraft cockpits may arise in a number of ways. In certain circumstances, while an aircraft is taxying or waiting for a long time for take-off with the engine running, exhaust fumes may enter the cockpit in considerable quantity. After take-off it is likely that the level of contamination will fall and that ventilation will be such that any levels achieved in the occupant's blood will be lowered—but only slowly. Carboxyhaemoglobin levels fall by about 50 per cent in four hours when the subject breathes air (Roughton and Root, 1945). Defects in exhaust systems can result in continuing cockpit contamination in flight.

An interesting relevant case is recorded in the A.I.B. files (Ministry of Civil Aviation, 1953). An Auster aircraft had been used for aerial photography one afternoon; as it approached the airfield on its return it suddenly dived to the ground from a low altitude. The aircraft had been modified to take two cameras but on the fatal flight only an oblique camera was fitted. The aperture at which a vertical camera was usually located in the floor of the aircraft, was covered by a metal disk held in place by a somewhat crude expedient—a breeze block! There were eye-witnesses who reported they had seen the aircraft land on a rough field near to the factory being photographed; after a few minutes it had taken off again. The possibility was raised several days after the accident that the aperture for the vertical camera might have become uncovered during that landing and take-off and that carbon monoxide from the engine's exhaust might have thus contaminated the cockpit.

The Coroner had not ordered a post-mortem examination on the pilot and no estimation of carboxyhaemoglobin in the pilot's blood had been made. By the time it had occurred to the investigators that carbon monoxide intoxication might have been the cause of this accident, it was too late to secure appropriate medical evidence. In an effort to test the hypothesis to some extent, trials were conducted in another aircraft with a similar defect in the floor and it did appear that carbon monoxide contamination might have occurred as suggested. A routine autopsy and routine toxicological investigations would have settled the issue; indeed, they might have provided the first clue to the true cause of the accident as in accident number 261 described in Chapter 4.

*Chapter 12*

# RECONSTRUCTION OF EVENTS AT IMPACT

THIS aspect of the pathological investigation of a fatal light aircraft accident is confined to an assessment of the survivability of the crash and an evaluation of the safety equipment provided; this includes an appraisal of the use or abuse of the equipment, its efficiency or malfunction. Two accidents are described below to exemplify the problems that arise.

## SAFETY AND SURVIVAL

### ACCIDENT NUMBER 245

A pilot and 2 passengers on board a light aircraft were approaching to land on an island. After a run across the airfield, the aircraft headed out to sea and appeared to be making a turn for the final approach; during the turn it stalled and crashed into the

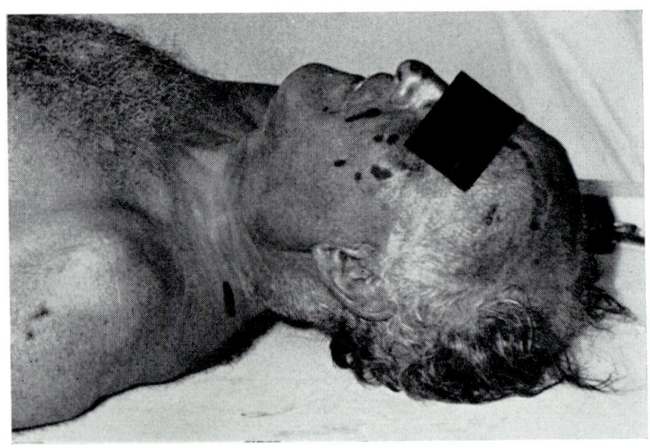

*Fig*. 34.—A victim of accident number 245. In common with his two companions he received superficial abrasions of the face and forehead but there was no fracture of the skull or intracranial injury. The only other injury sustained was a crush fracture of the lumbar spine. Death was due to drowning. (*Reproduced from Stevens (1968b) by permission of the Editor 'Aerospace Medicine'*.)

water, floated briefly, and then sank. Divers recovered the bodies several hours later; all 3 were found in their seats with fastened lap belts. Post-mortem examinations showed that death was due to drowning in each case, and that none had sustained a potentially lethal injury, although 2 had compression fractures of the lumbar spine; all 3 had minor abrasions on or about the forehead (*Fig*. 34) but none had a fracture of the skull or evidence of intracranial injury.

Examination of the cockpit showed relatively little distortion. It appeared that this accident should have been survivable, but there had been no attempt by any occupant to escape; none had even unfastened his lap belt. It was concluded that the spinal fracture and the minor blows to the head had resulted in each case from a combination of vertical deceleration and forward deceleration, with jack-knifing over the fastened seat belt; the resulting concussion was doubtless the main cause for there being no attempt to escape. Restraint by a full harness would have reduced or prevented the injuries in each case; the use of protective helmets would have provided added protection.

## ACCIDENT NUMBER 243

The circumstances of this accident have been outlined already (Chapter 11). The pilot was intoxicated and allowed the aircraft to climb too steeply; it stalled and crashed into a car park coming to rest upside down (*Fig*. 35). He was the only one of

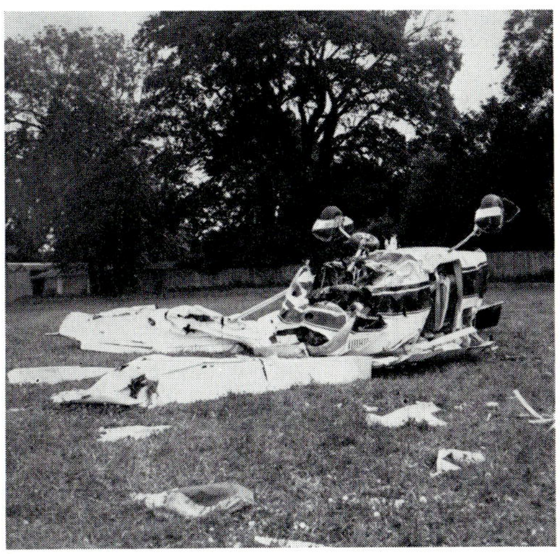

*Fig*. 35.—General view of the aircraft wreckage from accident number 243.

the 4 occupants to be killed; death was due to severe multiple lethal injuries. A student pilot (better, perhaps, called a 'passenger' as he was unlicensed) was in the right-hand front seat and suffered only minor injuries; 2 passengers in the rear seats sustained severe internal injuries that required surgery. The only safety equipment available was lap belts; the passengers at the rear were known to have had theirs fastened when the aircraft taxied from dispersal but at that time the pilot and the front passenger had not fastened theirs.

Examination of the aircraft wreckage showed that the pilot's seat had become detached from the floor during the accident; it is seen to be missing in *Fig*. 36. The floor attachments of the other seats were partially broken, but their anchorages had not failed completely. The lap belts in the type of aircraft involved are bolted to the aircraft's frame independently of the seats as can be seen in *Fig*. 36. It is probable that it was the fastened seat belts that provided sufficient restraint and 'tie-down' effect upon the 3 passengers to prevent their seats from breaking away completely. Moseley and Zeller (1958) were quoted in Chapter 7 as stating that failure of seat attachments at impact was a main cause for injury and death in public transport aircraft; this accident would suggest that it may also be an important factor in light aircraft accidents.

The pilot's lethal injuries were at two sites. His sternum had been fractured and there were ruptures of the interatrial septum, the pulmonary artery and the aorta. It seemed probable that these injuries were caused by a fairly circumscribed object such as the control column; that on the left-hand side (the machine had dual controls) had been broken in the accident (*Fig.* 36) possibly from impact with the pilot's body. If

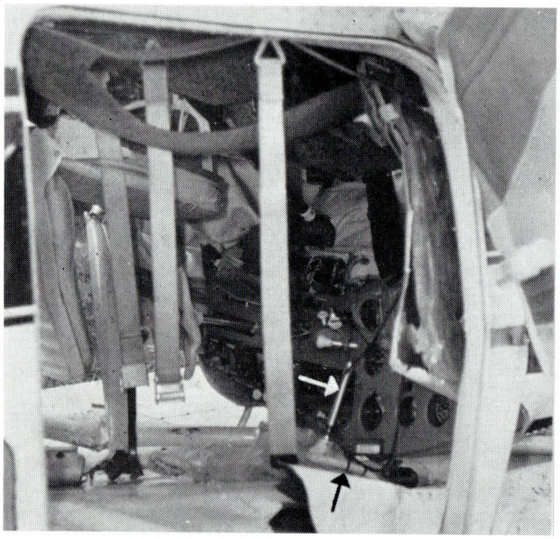

*Fig.* 36.—A view of the left-hand side of the inverted cockpit of the wreckage shown in *Fig.* 35. The left-hand seat is missing having become detached from the floor during the accident. The broken control column is arrowed. It may well have been this object that caused the pilot's thoracic injuries.

the pilot had had a fastened lap belt his seat might have been retained in position; he might or might not have been spared his chest injuries, however, since he would undoubtedly have jack-knifed over the belt. A fastened full harness would almost certainly have prevented him striking his chest on the control column for the engine and instrument panel had been pushed backwards into the cockpit only a relatively slight distance.

His other lethal injuries resulted from a blow on the head that had fractured his skull and lacerated the brain. A fastened lap belt might have minimized these head injuries; two of the passengers with fastened lap belts were concussed only, the third had no head injury. Had the pilot worn a full harness and a protective helmet, it is very likely that he would not have received any lethal injury.

Considerable caution must always be exercised in drawing conclusions such as these. One serious injury received by the pilot was a horizontal laceration above the thyroid cartilage; this was apparently caused by the leading edge of the right-hand wing which had broken forwards and sliced round in a scything action to cut into the roof of the cockpit as the aircraft struck the ground. It is very difficult to be sure that, had the pilot's seat been retained in the aircraft, and had he been wearing a full harness and a protective helmet, he would have been protected from this particular injury; it is possible that, being held in a more or less erect (though inverted) position, he would have sustained just as severe, if not worse injuries from the starboard wing.

Two of the 3 passengers were concussed; they lost their memories for the events immediately prior to the accident. Protective helmets would undoubtedly have lessened the severity of their injuries and possibly prevented them altogether. The passenger in the right-hand front seat was one of those concussed; if, as was thought, his seat belt was fastened (the evidence of rescuers was equivocal on this point) it was surprising that

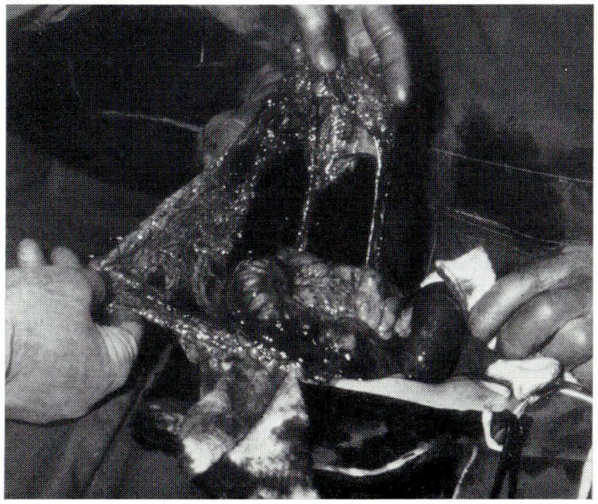

*Fig.* 37.—A view of the lacerated mesentery found at laparotomy on a passenger from accident number 243. This undoubtedly resulted from forced flexion over a fastened—probably loosely fastened—seat belt. (*Reproduced by permission of Mr. G. R. C. Peatfield, Bedford General Hospital.*)

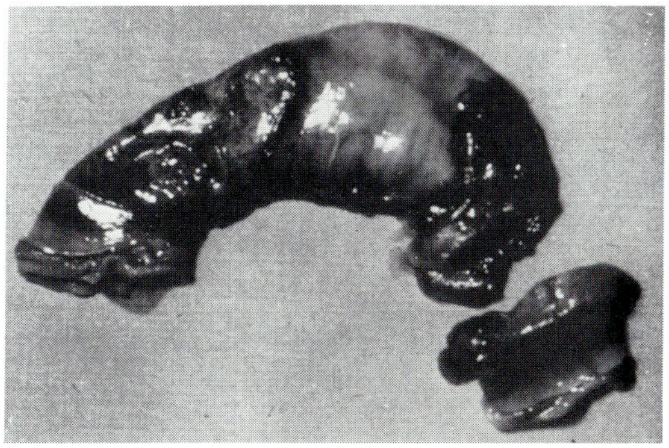

*Fig.* 38.—The surgical specimen from laparotomy on another passenger from accident number 243. There was a rupture of the small bowel and a segment on either side of the injury was resected. This also was an injury sustained from forced flexion over a lap belt. (*Reproduced by permission of Mr. G. R. C. Peatfield, Bedford General Hospital.*)

he did not also receive severe forward decelerative injuries to his chest from jack-knifing. Although his seat was retained in the aircraft, there was considerable distortion of the cockpit in the vicinity, and the lack of chest injury can only be regarded as fortuitous; the control column on his side was quite badly distorted suggesting that his body may have come into contact with it but, presumably, with insufficient force to cause him harm.

The 2 rear passengers both sustained ruptures of the intestines. The surgeon in charge noted bruising of the lower abdominal walls and, despite relatively little clinical evidence of an abdominal emergency, decided upon laparotomy in each case; 1 proved to have a lacerated mesentery (*Fig.* 37) and 1 a ruptured small bowel (*Fig.* 38); Peatfield (1966) attributed these injuries to the lap belts.

### The Injury Potential of Lap Belts

The aircraft in the years following the First World War had open cockpits and were usually fitted with safety belts designed to prevent the occupant from falling out. Human nature being what it is, it is not surprising to find in the A.I.B. records that this equipment was not always used; in 2 of the 4 fatal accidents in 1920, neither pilot nor passenger had fastened their safety belts. In 1926 a passenger fell from an aircraft during a stall turn; he had not been strapped in and neither had the pilot. Two years later a pilot fell out of his aircraft while performing aerobatics; his misfortune occurred because his safety belt broke under stress.

With the advent of the closed cockpit there was no need to strap people into an aircraft to stop them falling out. However, lap belts were retained to provide restraint during turbulence and because it came to be appreciated that some form of restraint in the event of a crash was an advantage—a fact that has been much publicized in recent years in connexion with the automobile.

Although it would seem that forceful jack-knifing over a lap belt in an accident is potentially dangerous due not only to the possibility of striking the head upon an obstruction but also to the chance of an intra-abdominal injury, there are relatively few reports of such injury either in motor cars or in aircraft. Teare (1951) was the first to incriminate seat belts as a cause of injury. He attributed several cases of rupture of the aorta in an aircraft accident to the snubbing action of the belt with forced flexion of the torso over the belt. DuBois (1952), however, strongly criticized Teare's conclusions. Ruff (1950b) reported injuries to kidney, stomach, intestines, and liver in casualties from gliding accidents in which the aircraft were only slightly damaged; he believed the injuries were caused by restraining belts. De Haven, Tourin, and Macri (1953) studied the injury potential of seat belts in light aircraft accidents, and concluded that this equipment was a rare cause of injury and any injuries sustained were rarely dangerous; that injuries apparently caused by seat belts usually resulted from other causes such as vertical deceleration, and that any danger from their use was far outweighed by the protection they afforded in an accident.

Williams, Lies, and Hale (1966) found in the literature only 10 cases of intra-abdominal injury resulting from the wearing of a seat belt, and they reported 4 further cases. All 14 occurred in car accidents. They concluded that the small bowel and its mesentery were the intra-abdominal organs most vulnerable to this type of injury which could occur from direct violence, sheering, torsion or 'entrapment', or by a combination of these mechanisms. They reported that the injuries were initially often unsuspected and that the resulting delay in treatment was associated with a high morbidity and mortality. Porter and Green (1968) further emphasized these points, reviewed the literature and reported 3 more cases of intra-abdominal injury due to seat belts sustained in car accidents.

Fish and Wright (1965) reported seat belt injury in 4 of 18 passengers in military transport aircraft; Gerritsen, Frobese, and Pezzi (1966) reported 2 more cases in car accidents and concluded that loosely fastened seat belts were especially likely to cause injury; 2 cases of lumbar spine injury similarly caused were recorded by Carroll and Gruber (1968).

To return briefly to accident number 243; it can be summarized as one which was survivable; 3 of the 4 occupants survived. The fatality was probably the only one whose body was completely unrestrained and whose seat completely broke away at impact. It was an accident in which the 3 survivors received injuries that would almost certainly have been much less severe, if not completely avoided, had they had a better restraint system such as full harness and some head protection.

The two accidents described above strongly suggest that the safety equipment available was less than adequate. As I have already pointed out, unequivocal conclusions cannot be drawn from individual or small numbers of accidents. It might be argued, for example, that had the passenger in the right-hand front seat in accident 243 been wearing a full harness, and thus been held in a near erect position, he might have suffered more severe injuries when the aircraft crashed nose down and inverted, than in fact he did. Reliable conclusions about safety equipment are likely to result from an evaluation of a number of accidents.

*Table IX*.—INJURIES TO VICTIMS OF FATAL LIGHT AIRCRAFT ACCIDENTS: FINDINGS IN THE PRESENT SERIES COMPARED WITH THOSE OF REALS AND OTHERS (1964)

| TRAUMA | REALS AND OTHERS | | PRESENT SERIES | |
|---|---|---|---|---|
| *Fractures:* | *No.* | % | *No.* | % |
| Skull | 104 | 70 | 63 | 67 |
| Facial Bones | — | — | 45 | 48 |
| Cervical spine | 19 | 13 | 11 | 12 |
| Dorsal spine | 18 | 12 | 21 | 23 |
| Lumbar spine | 15 | 10 | 17 | 18 |
| Ribs | 83 | 56 | 59 | 63 |
| Arms | 94 | 63 | 52 | 56 |
| Pelvis | 35 | 24 | 25 | 27 |
| Legs | 110 | 74 | 68 | 73 |
| *Laceration or Rupture:* | | | | |
| Brain | 78 | 53 | 52 | 56 |
| Lungs | 50 | 34 | 33 | 36 |
| Heart | 51 | 34 | 33 | 35 |
| Aorta | 34 | 23 | 36 | 39 |
| Liver | 72 | 49 | 33 | 35 |
| Spleen | 61 | 41 | 32 | 34 |
| Kidneys | 28 | 19 | 21 | 23 |
| *Penetrating Wounds:* | | | | |
| Chest | — | — | 8 (4*) | 8·5 |
| Abdomen | — | — | 16 (5*) | 17 |
| *Burns* | 51 | 34 | 39 | 42 |

* These numbers indicate cases possibly due solely to fire. Fire can burn away part of the abdominal or thoracic walls and produce appearances suggestive of mechanical injury; it may be difficult in some cases to decide whether there has been a penetrating wound followed by incineration or whether fire has been entirely responsible for the damage found on post-mortem examination.

## ANALYSIS OF SURVIVAL ASPECTS

I have reported previously upon the survival and safety equipment features of 55 fatal light aircraft accidents (Stevens, 1968b). These 55 accidents included 40 of the 42 accidents presently reviewed in this section, and 15 military light aircraft accidents. The latter were included as it was considered that the safety aspects of light aircraft accidents were not affected by the status of the pilot or the ownership of the aircraft, except in so far as ownership might influence the question of the safety equipment provided.

The injuries received by the 92 individuals killed in the 55 accidents, were compared with those reported in light aircraft accidents by Reals and others (1964) (*Table IX*). This did little but confirm that the two series of accidents produced essentially similar injuries and in approximately the same frequency.

The 92 individuals killed in the 55 accidents, were categorized on the basis of whether they had been involved in unsurvivable or potentially survivable accidents. This was a subjective classification and was determined by the extent of the damage to the cockpit in the vicinity of the casualty, the nature of the injuries sustained and their apparent cause; any bias was towards putting doubtful cases into the survivable category. These individuals were further grouped on the basis of their having worn a fastened shoulder harness or lap belt, or their having used no restraint at all, and, further, on the basis of their having used, or not having used, protective helmets (*Table X*).

*Table X*.—THE ASSOCIATION BETWEEN THE LACK OF SAFETY EQUIPMENT AND DEATH IN LIGHT AIRCRAFT ACCIDENTS

| FATALITIES IN UNSURVIVABLE ACCIDENTS | SAFETY EQUIPMENT USED | | | FATALITIES IN SURVIVABLE ACCIDENTS |
|---|---|---|---|---|
| | *Shoulder harness* | *Seat belt* | *Protective helmet* | |
| 12 (13%) | + | | + | 1 (1%) |
| 26 (28%) | + | | − | 5 (5%) |
| 16 (18%) | | + | − | 9 (10%) |
| 13* (14%) | ? | ? | ? | 10† (11%) |
| 67 (73%) | | | | 25 (27%) |

* In several the probability is that a safety harness was used, in several a lap belt only was available.

† In 6 it is probable that only a lap belt was available and no protective helmet was worn; in a further 2 cases it is known that the shoulder harness available was not fastened.

Shoulder harnesses and protective helmets can only be expected to protect from lethal injury in the potentially survivable accident. If they are truly effective in this function, one would expect that relatively few wearing such equipment would die in survivable accidents; most of those killed while wearing such equipment would be expected to die in essentially unsurvivable accidents. The figures in *Table X* show that this was indeed so. The ratio of unsurvivable to survivable accidents was less than 3:1; yet, only 1 of 13 individuals known to be wearing both a full shoulder harness and a protective helmet died in a survivable accident and only 5 of 31 individuals known to be wearing a full shoulder harness but no protective helmet, died in a survivable accident. In contrast, 9 out of 25 individuals having only a lap belt died in potentially survivable accidents. These figures emphasize, therefore, the importance of these items of safety equipment in the appropriate circumstances.

The causes of death of the 19 individuals without shoulder harness restraint or protective helmet and killed in survivable accidents, were: drowning (3 cases), burning without evidence of incapacitating injury (8 cases), a single lethal injury to the thorax (5 cases), and a single lethal injury to the head (3 cases). It seemed probable that some of those drowned or burned to death might well have failed to escape because they had received minor concussive blows to the head that had resulted in temporary incapacitation for vital seconds; several might have escaped with their lives if they had had the advantages of full harnesses and protective helmets.

Five people died in survivable accidents despite fastened shoulder harnesses; 2 of these died from head injuries and 1 drowned. It is quite possible that protective helmets, in addition to full harnesses, would have saved these 3 also.

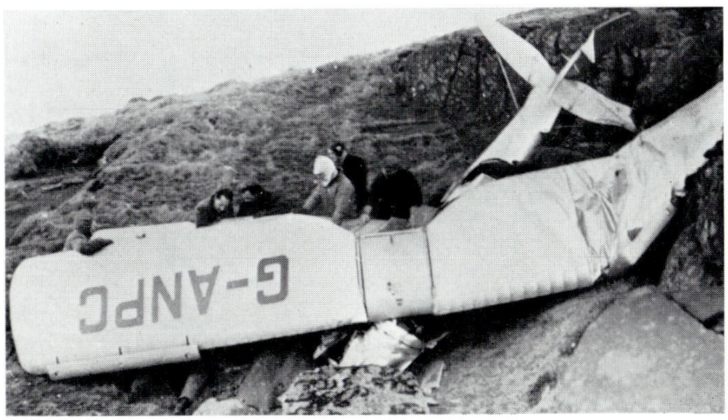


*Fig*. 39.—Wreckage of a light aircraft from which the pilot, who had worn a fastened shoulder harness and a protective helmet, stepped unharmed. (*Reproduced by permission of Mr. W. Lawson, Scottish Gliding Union, Ltd.*)

The role of the Royal Air Force Aviation Pathology Department has not included the investigation of non-fatal accidents. However, over the last few years a number of accidents is known to have occurred in which the pilot of a light aircraft has worn a shoulder harness and a protective helmet, has stepped from the wreckage with little or no injury and has attributed his good fortune to the fact that he had worn a protective helmet in addition to shoulder harness; the smashed aircraft from such an instance is shown in *Fig*. 39. On the other hand, a certain military pilot suffered a traumatic pituitary insufficiency that resulted from a fractured base of skull (*Fig*. 40) received in a light aircraft accident (*Fig*. 41); he had not worn his protective helmet although his shoulder harness had been fastened.

Fifty-five aircraft accidents comprise a relatively small series and the categorization of these accidents as survivable or non-survivable was, as explained, largely based upon subjective criteria. It might be contended, therefore, that any conclusions drawn are of doubtful validity. However, it happens that the conclusions drawn are essentially those of numerous authors whose papers on the subject of safety equipment in light aircraft have been published during the last 20 years. De Haven and Hasbrook (1952),

Reals and others (1964), Hasbrook and Dille (1964), and many others have forcefully argued the need for protection of the upper torso and head by a comfortable full

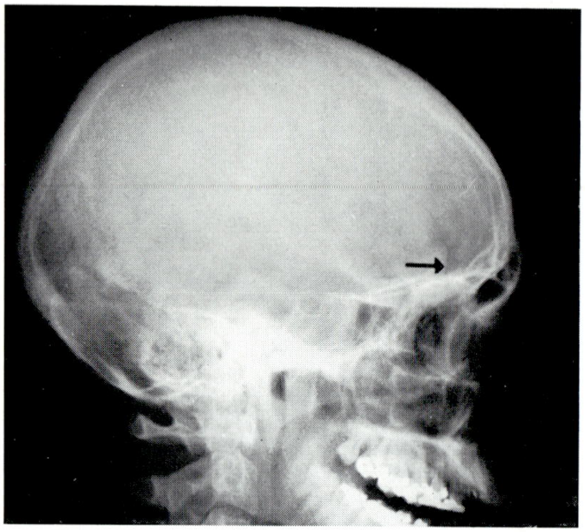

*Fig.* 40.—Radiograph of the skull of the pilot of the light aircraft shown in *Fig.* 41. This man survived but he had not worn a protective helmet. The fracture he sustained (arrowed) passed back along the floor of the anterior fossa and involved the sella turcica and resulted in damage to the pituitary.

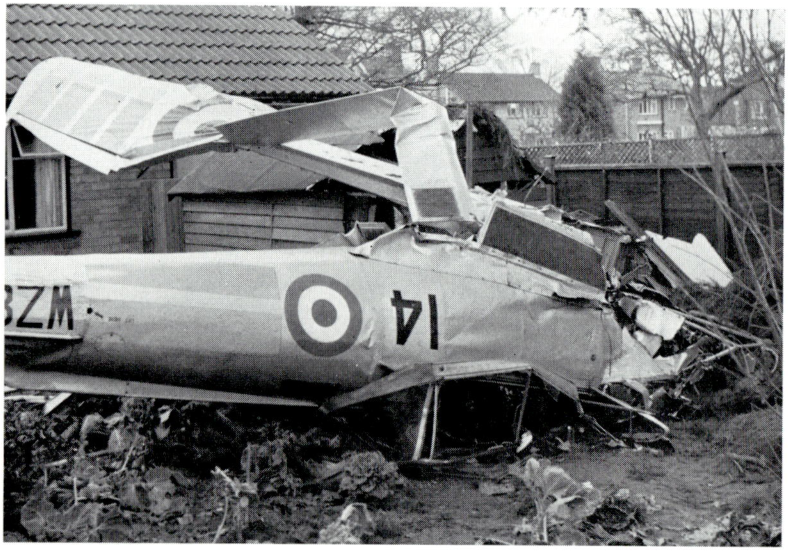


*Fig.* 41.—Wreckage of a light aircraft the pilot of which had not worn his protective helmet. He sustained a serious fracture of the skull (*Fig.* 40) which would almost certainly have been prevented by a protective helmet. (*Reproduced by permission of the Controller of her Majesty's Stationery Office.*)

harness and protective helmet in those flying light aircraft. Mason (1962g), citing several other workers, concluded 'the evidence of the relative ineffectiveness of a lap belt is overwhelming'. Pearson (1961, 1962a,b, 1963) published the results of far larger and more detailed analyses than has been accomplished in the present study, and showed clearly the use of protective helmet and shoulder harness to be essential if the chance of receiving critical injury to the head and upper torso in a light aircraft accident were to be minimized. Haley, Turnbow, Macri, and Walhout (1966) reported that 358 of 701 people involved in civilian light aircraft accidents and not wearing shoulder harnesses, sustained some degree of cerebral concussion associated with fractures of the skull or lesser injuries; over three-quarters of the 358 sustained some period of unconsciousness.

The findings, therefore, in my series of British light aircraft accidents do no more than support the conclusions of many other workers, namely, that shoulder harness is an essential piece of equipment for each person in a light aircraft, and that a protective helmet for each occupant is nearly, if not equally important. It is appropriate, therefore, to consider the present position with regard to the availability of such equipment in light aircraft.

## Protective Helmets

Until recently, the desirability and the probability of success of a propaganda campaign to persuade light aircraft aviators to wear protective helmets was doubtful. Many of the helmets available for purchase by private pilots were not readily adaptable to fit any head; they were relatively heavy and somewhat uncomfortable. Perhaps of greater importance, there was the difficulty associated with the fact that light aircraft pilots have very varied preferences in communications equipment and, therefore, very varied design requirements in a protective helmet. Some pilots favour a hand microphone attached to the instrument fascia and a loudspeaker in the roof of the cockpit; helmets worn by such pilots are useless if they cause attenuation of external sound. Other pilots use a head set and throat microphone; such pilots wearing protective helmets need integral earphones with appropriate connexions for a throat microphone or a boom microphone (a boom microphone is one held in front of the mouth by an arm attached to the helmet). These varied requirements have made manufacturers hesitant about marketing helmets likely to appeal to a small section of a limited potential market.

A helmet has recently been produced in the United Kingdom based on a design conceived at the Royal Air Force Institute of Aviation Medicine, Farnborough (*Fig.* 42). It is hoped that it will be on the general market in the near future. This helmet weighs only 4 lb.; it is instantly adjustable to any head without loss of efficiency and it is usable by those requiring integral communications equipment with external noise attenuation and adaptable for those who require no noise attenuation. The helmet, as illustrated, has earphones in the ear-pieces and connexions for a microphone, in this case a throat microphone—a minor modification only is necessary for a boom microphone. The adjustable ear-pieces are essential for head fitting purposes but they can be provided (at reduced cost) with ventilated cushions. When thus modified, the helmet may be used with the two soft side panels of the helmet raised, and it is then possible to have full head protection without noise attenuation. Such a helmet, without communications equipment, is ideal for a passenger.

Even with a suitable all-purpose protective helmet available for all light aircraft users, both pilots and passengers, there remains one major problem; it is that of how to influence peoples' behaviour. I have already commented on human frailty and the tendency for people not to use equipment provided for their safety. Fifteen to 20 years ago, few motor cyclists in Britain wore protective helmets; propaganda campaigns had resulted in 60 per cent of male motor cyclists wearing helmets by 1958 (Moore, 1962)

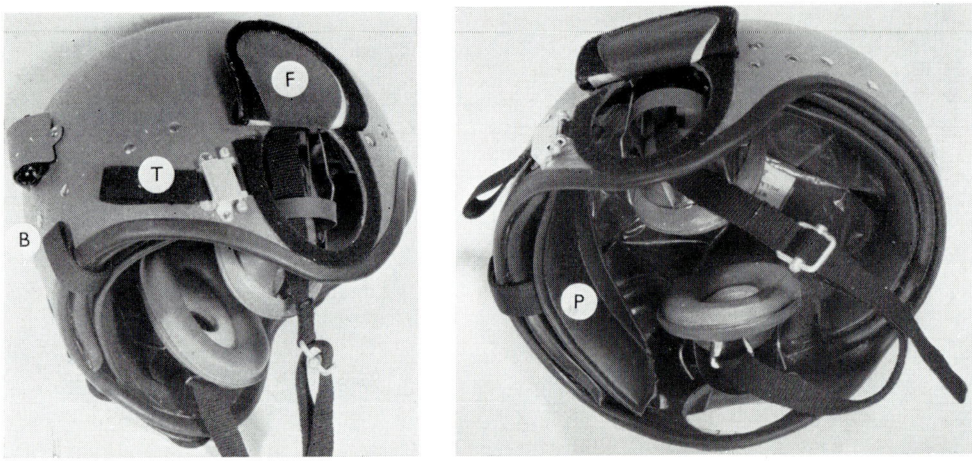


*Fig.* 42.—Two views of the Amplivox/Stadium universal-fitting protective helmet. It is suitable for all light aircraft pilots as it can be provided with or without integral communications equipment. The helmet is put on by opening the side flaps F, using the thumbs to pull the ear pieces outwards and the helmet is then easily slipped onto the head. The springs automatically cause the ear pieces to adjust to the sides of the head. Tab B is unfastened and Tab T is pulled gently to tension the pad P and make the helmet fit snugly in the anteroposterior axis. The flaps F can be replaced to complete the external noise attenuation if desired. If integral communications equipment is not incorporated, the ear pieces have perforations and, with the flaps up, the pilot has full head protection but he can hear external sounds without difficulty.

and by 1964 the proportion was almost 70 per cent (Road Research Laboratory, 1965). I believe that as soon as these inexpensive and generally satisfactory helmets, simply adaptable to nearly all light aircraft aviators' needs, become generally available, appropriate propaganda could be as successful in making it the fashion for light aircraft pilots and their passengers to wear them. If this fashion could be established, there is little doubt that lives would be saved and injuries minimized in those light aircraft crashes that inevitably will continue to occur.

### Shoulder Harness

The present situation with regard to the provision of full harnesses in light aircraft is as follows: the United States of America is the main supplier of this type of aircraft to the western world. What the American Federal Aviation Agency considers sufficient for the granting of a certificate of airworthiness to an aircraft, countries such as the United Kingdom, who import American aircraft, accept on the basis of reciprocal agreement. It is necessary, therefore, to look to the United States of America for a lead in this matter. Young (1966) stated in a Federal Aviation Agency report that 'the use of inadequate or incomplete body restraint systems is a major factor in the current trend of increasing serious and fatal injuries reported from general aviation accidents'. The report proceeded to give advice as to suitable locations for full harness attachment points in five particular types of light aircraft. There has been no annoucement, so far as I can trace, of any intent by the Federal Aviation Agency to do other than try to influence owners and users of aircraft by persuasion and education to fit full harnesses.

I submit that this is not enough but that there should be a further move towards making it mandatory for manufacturers to design and fit harnesses in all new light aircraft. It has been known for long enough that a full harness is a basic piece of safety equipment that ought to be available for every seat in every light aircraft; it is not just an additional luxury to be bought and installed by owners and users at considerable extra cost. It is a matter for considerable concern that it is possible still to buy a new light aircraft, not only without fitted full harnesses but even without provision of adequate attachment points. I believe that at some time in the future it will be made mandatory for manufacturers to supply properly designed safety harnesses as basic equipment; the question is how long it will be for this inevitable decision to be taken. The longer it is delayed unnecessarily, the more deaths and injuries will occur unnecessarily.

The cost of supplying full harnesses in an aircraft will be minimal if these are installed in the first place. Further, if only all new aircraft had this safety equipment fitted, this in itself would be an extra encouragement to owners and users of existing machines to convert theirs. Until the subject is seen by all to be so important as to have been made the subject of regulation, it will be difficult to persuade owners and users that it is a really serious matter. Again it is a question of how best to influence peoples' behaviour patterns for their own good. As soon as a comfortable and properly designed harness becomes a normal piece of equipment in every light aircraft, most people will wear it most of the time and most of the unnecessary preventable injuries will be prevented. The problem is entirely analagous to that which exists in the motor car industry but regulations have already been made to require both British and American manufacturers to fit seat belts in new cars. Although some of my colleagues express reservations, I have no doubt at all of the importance of proper safety harnesses in cars. Surely no one can deny that safety harnesses are even more important in light aircraft and that their provision should similarly be the subject of regulation.

The Australian Government (Department of Civil Aviation) announced in March, 1968, that it would require all new aircraft types introduced onto the Australian Civil Register after July 1967 to have approved safety harnesses fitted for pilots and other occupants of front seats. Certain exemptions were to be permitted, however, in particular where the design of the aircraft was such that 'it would be unreasonable to insist on compliance'. This was clearly a step in the right direction but the provisos were such as to enable manufacturers to ignore the importance of designing new aircraft with harnesses fitted *ab initio*.

# *Chapter 13*

## GENERAL CONCLUSIONS

THE analysis by Vivian (1967) of his 51 fatal accidents did not include a statement about the number of cases in which significant medical findings were present in the pilots. His 51 accidents included 34 of the 42 accidents reviewed in this book and 4 of the 8 cases listed in *Table VII.* Martin (1967) made an examination of the records of the balance of Vivian's cases and found them to include 1 in which alcohol may have been a factor and 1 in which carbon monoxide intoxication, due to cockpit atmosphere contamination, may have been a factor.

It would seem, therefore, from the experience of Reals and others (1964) from Vivian's study (1967), from Dille and Morris's series (1967), and from the present one, that by far the majority of light aircraft accidents are not caused by natural disease in the pilot or intoxication by carbon monoxide, alcohol, or drugs. There is little indication of a particular disease or condition occurring as a frequent causative factor in these accidents. This is not to deny the principle that every accident must be fully investigated and that as a part of this investigation there should be a comprehensive search for a medical main or contributory cause. It does make it clear, however, that one cannot look to improved medical selection or to closer medical supervision of pilots of light aircraft for a dramatic improvement in safety figures in this type of flying. However, a study of the survival and safety equipment aspects of light aircraft accidents strongly suggests that energetic action to ensure the provision of a full harness for each occupant in a light aircraft, and to initiate propaganda concerning the importance of light aircraft aviators wearing protective helmets, would considerably reduce the numbers of dead and injured in light aircraft accidents.

*SECTION III*

# *GLIDER ACCIDENTS*

## *Chapter 14*

## INTRODUCTION

### HISTORY OF THE SPORT OF GLIDING

OTTO LILIENTHAL was the first man to 'mount magnificently into the air' and 'fly properly in gliders' (Gibbs-Smith, 1967). Between 1891 and 1896 he made several 'hang-gliders', from which he was suspended by his arms during flight, and over which he exercised a degree of flight-control by swinging his torso and legs. He perished in a flying accident but his contributions 'directly inspired the next generation of pioneers to master mechanical flight'. Most, if not all glider activity in the following years was directed to the solution of powered flight and culminated, as is generally known, in the Wright Brothers' historic achievements; in their 'Flier I' they made the world's first powered, sustained, controlled flights in an aeroplane in 1903, and their 'Flier III', built in 1905, was the world's first fully practical powered aircraft. From then until the First World War the story of aviation is that of powered flight.

Interest in gliders re-awakened after the War; Klemin, Sayre, and Raspet (1963) and Gibbs-Smith (1967) described how the Germans, whose construction of powered aircraft was strictly limited for a time by the Versailles Peace Treaty, made notable advances in the design and operation of gliders. Gliding as a sport developed in Britain more slowly. At a *Daily Mail* Contest in 1922, 35 gliders assembled at Itford on the South Downs but many of the rather wild contraptions failed to become airborne; the world record for duration of a glider flight had been 6 minutes until this contest which was won for a flight of 3 hours and 21 minutes by a glider with two identical wings and a pilot's seat slung between them. In 1929 the British Gliding Association (B.G.A.) was formed to run the affairs of the sport in Britain and in 1933 it took over a paper *The Sailplane and Glider* first published by the journal *Aeroplane* four years earlier; the paper, now *Sailplane and Gliding* has been the official magazine of the B.G.A. ever since.

During the 1930's gliding was confined to a few enthusiasts, operating mainly from the London Gliding Club on Dunstable Downs, and with the advent of the Second World War, gliding as a peaceful pursuit ceased altogether in this country. Between 1939 and 1945 the only British gliders flown were of the troop-carrying variety, towed by a powered aircraft and used for the invasion of Sicily in 1943 and later of occupied Europe; a few conventional machines were flown off the South Coast during certain radar experiments (Wills, 1966).

After the Second World War gliding recommenced and, for the first time, the sport expanded rapidly in Britain. From the early 1950's there was increasing success in international competitions for British machines and pilots. The B.G.A. grew steadily and by 1967 had at least 65 member clubs with a further 18 Armed Services' clubs affiliated through their parent bodies, namely, the Army Gliding Club and the Gliding and Soaring Associations of the Royal Air Force (R.A.F.G.S.A.) and the Royal Navy (R.N.G.S.A.). With the steadily increasing volume of gliding activity, the sport earned and maintained a reputation for being a particularly safe form of flying. The B.G.A.'s safety panel has reported in considerable detail upon total accident rates among its civilian members from time to time (British Gliding Association—Paul, 1959, 1960; Neaves, 1968) but there have been no published figures for total fatal glider accidents in relation to total gliding activity in this country; such figures would provide a basis for the calculation of fatal accident rates and show whether gliding has become more or less safe in recent years.

## GLIDER ACCIDENT TRENDS

Only 2 fatal gliding accidents are to be found in the A.I.B. files of the inter-World War period; but as stated, little gliding took place during those years. The first was in 1931 when a new launching gear was being tested; the glider dived to the ground from a height of 40 ft. but few details appeared in the report. The second was in 1935; a structural failure occurred during the application of negative 'g' and the pilot failed to escape although he had a parachute. In neither case, apparently, were possible medical aspects investigated.

In the post war years from 1946 to 1949, 3 fatal accidents occurred. The first involved an in-flight structural failure; no mention of any medical aspects appeared in the report. An uncomplicated launch and a short period of normal flight preceded a dive to the ground in each of the other two accidents. In one of these a medical investigation was carried out but apparently it consisted only of an autopsy at which nothing abnormal was found.

*Table XI* shows the magnitude of the increase in gliding in Britain since 1950, the rise in the numbers of fatal accidents and fatal accident rates calculated for quinquennia in terms both of hours flown and of launches made. The figures are calculated for quinquennial periods because so few fatal accidents occurred in any single year that wide fluctuations in annual fatal accident rates tend to result solely from chance. The statistics presented were collected from published and unpublished records of the various British gliding communities' activities; the full details are recorded in the Appendix. I believe the totals for fatal accidents to be completely accurate; in some years one or two clubs failed to report their operational statistics to the B.G.A. but the consequent inaccuracies are undoubtedly insignificant for the reasons given in the Appendix.

The volume of gliding in Britain increased steadily over the whole period. There were approximately three times as many launches made in the mid-1960's as compared with the early 1950's; the increase was nearer four-fold in terms of hours flown. The absolute numbers of fatal accidents varied little throughout the 1950's; only in more recent years has a sustained rise occurred to a level of approximately three times that at the beginning of the period. These facts are reflected in the fatal accident rates which both show a trend toward improved safety during the 1950's, but a reversal of that trend since then. These figures suggest, as does the analysis of non-fatal civilian gliding accidents in 1967 published by the B.G.A.'s safety panel (Neaves, 1968), that the gliding fraternity must not take the reputed safety of gliding for granted. The panel concluded that most accidents that had happened could have been avoided. Our experience has shown that a full medical and pathological investigation of each fatal accident is necessary if all possible causes are to be fully assessed and no measure for the avoidance of similar accidents overlooked.

*Table XI.*—British Fatal Glider Accident Data: 1950–68

| Quinquennium | Total Hours Flown | Total Launches Made | Total Fatal Accidents | Fatal Accident Rates | |
|---|---|---|---|---|---|
| | | | | *per* 10,000 *hours* | *per* 100,000 *launches* |
| 1950–4 | 81,354 | 767,304 | 7 | 0·86 | 0·91 |
| 1951–5 | 87,023 | 808,322 | 5 | 0·57 | 0·62 |
| 1952–6 | 94,061 | 833,970 | 5 | 0·53 | 0·60 |
| 1953–7 | 105,205 | 870,028 | 3 | 0·29 | 0·34 |
| 1954–8 | 113,285 | 917,880 | 4 | 0·35 | 0·44 |
| 1955–9 | 131,342 | 1,014,870 | 5 | 0·38 | 0·49 |
| 1956–60 | 144,779 | 1,109,062 | 5 | 0·35 | 0·45 |
| 1957–61 | 167,258 | 1,275,884 | 6 | 0·36 | 0·47 |
| 1958–62 | 192,630 | 1,450,734 | 8 | 0·42 | 0·56 |
| 1959–63 | 213,302 | 1,587,949 | 8 | 0·38 | 0·51 |
| 1960–4 | 237,954 | 1,747,737 | 11 | 0·46 | 0·63 |
| 1961–5 | 264,445 | 1,895,654 | 14 | 0·53 | 0·74 |
| 1962–6 | 286,671 | 2,022,963 | 15 | 0·52 | 0·74 |
| 1963–7 | 310,546 | 2,113,695 | 18 | 0·58 | 0·85 |
| 1964–8 | 351,213 | 2,273,197 | 22 | 0·63 | 0·79 |

## CASE MATERIAL

Fourteen of the 23 fatal gliding accidents that occurred between 1960 and 1967 are included in the files of the Royal Air Force Department of Aviation Pathology. There were 17 fatalities, 1 seriously injured survivor and 1 uninjured survivor from these accidents.

Five of the 14 accidents occurred to aircraft operated by one of the Armed Services' clubs or the Air Cadets; the remainder involved machines belonging to civilian organizations as did, incidentally, 8 of the 9 accidents which were not investigated by a Royal Air Force pathologist.

Limited toxicological analyses were carried out following 8 of the 14 accidents. No evidence was found that a pilot had taken drugs or that any pilot had had his efficiency impaired by alcohol (in accident number 119, the pilot should have been taking drugs for his illness, may have been taking drugs but probably was not! But this was one of the cases in which toxicological analyses were not carried out—*see* Chapter 15); there is, therefore, no chapter in this section equivalent to Chapter 4 in Section I or Chapter 11 in Section II.

## *Chapter 15*

# NATURAL DISEASE IN GLIDER PILOTS

No less than 7 of the 14 gliding accidents were associated with, although not necessarily caused by, natural disease in the pilots (*Table XII*).

*Table XII.*—FATAL GLIDER ACCIDENTS: PILOTS FOUND TO HAVE NATURAL DISEASE OR ADVERSE MEDICAL HISTORIES

| ACCIDENT NUMBER | DISEASE FOUND OR HISTORY ELICITED | ASSOCIATION WITH CAUSE OF ACCIDENT |
|---|---|---|
| 119 | Epilepsy, pulmonary tuberculosis (instructor). | Highly probable |
| | Bilateral pneumothoraces (pupil) | None |
| 161 | Coronary artery disease (instructor) | Probable |
| | None (pupil—survived) | |
| 185 | Coronary artery disease | Probable |
| 213 | Obesity, fatty liver, coronary artery disease | Improbable |
| 246 | Coronary artery disease, recent blackouts | Equivocal |
| 257 | Coronary artery disease | Probable |
| 260 | Mild focal myocarditis | Improbable |

## ACCIDENT NUMBER 161

A tandem two-seater glider was being flown with a cadet pupil in the front seat and an extremely experienced instructor, aged 43, in the rear. As the machine was turning at a height of about 300–400 ft. it was seen to go into a spin that continued until it struck the side of a hut. The cadet escaped unhurt; the instructor was found dead on the roof of the hut. At autopsy a gross open injury to the chest was found, the heart was badly lacerated and indeed the left ventricle was avulsed and recovered from outside the body. A detailed examination of the coronary arteries was possible, however, and showed moderately severe atherosclerotic changes at many levels; in the left anterior descending artery the degree of occlusion was 70 per cent in several places. The right coronary artery showed an adventitial haemorrhage at its origin; on further sectioning haemorrhage was found in the intima and, in one section, an intravascular fragment of thrombus was present. Two inches from the origin of this artery the lumen appeared almost completely blocked by atheroma peeled off by haemorrhage.

It was not possible to conclude at the post-mortem examination or on subsequent histology whether or not the haemorrhage into the atheromatous plaque of the right coronary artery had been ante-mortem, had occurred during flight, had resulted in an acute myocardial insufficiency in the instructor and had, therefore, precipitated the accident. The possibility that loss of control had occurred for some quite different reason, and that the haemorrhage and blockage of the right coronary artery was cum-mortem and had resulted from the trauma sustained at impact, could not be excluded. However, the combination of all the circumstances of the accident, the instructor's very considerable experience, the relative competence of the pupil cadet and the lack of any acceptable alternative explanation for the loss of control, led to the conclusion that the instructor had very probably suffered an acute coronary insufficiency in flight at a low altitude which had caused the accident.

## ACCIDENT NUMBER 185

A 41-year-old service officer was flying a glider at an altitude of about 1000 ft.; a wing broke and the machine crashed to the ground. At post-mortem examination, the pilot's coronary arteries were found to be severely diseased; in particular, over a length of 1 cm. commencing about 2 cm. from its origin, the right coronary artery showed gross stenosis (*Fig.* 43). No thrombus was present and there was no evidence of

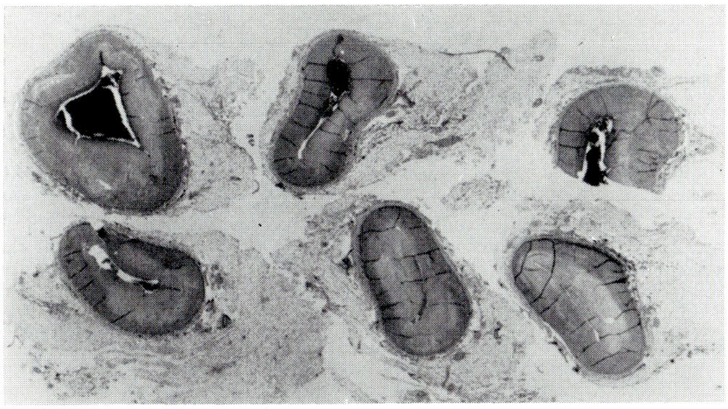

*Fig.* 43.—Sections of the right main coronary artery of the pilot killed in accident number 185. They show stenosis with reduction of the lumen at its narrowest point to about five per cent of its original size. These sections were stained by H. & E. and photographed directly, without the use of a microscope. (*Reproduced from Stevens (1966a) by permission of the Editor 'Zentbl. Verk.-Med. Verk.-Psychol'.*)

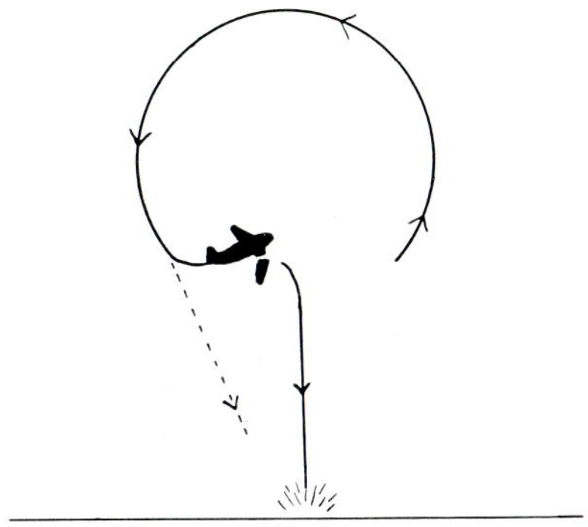

*Fig.* 44.—Diagram illustrating the circumstances of accident number 185. The wing appeared to break off the glider as it completed a loop and flattened out rather suddenly. (*Reproduced from Stevens (1966a) by permission of the Editor 'Zentbl. Verk.-Med. Verk.-Psychol'.*)

ischaemic fibrosis in any of the sections of myocardium. No possible connexion between the coronary artery disease and the in-flight structural failure of the glider was at first apparent. Inquiries of eye-witnesses elicited the fact that immediately before the accident the glider was making a loop. It had apparently flattened out unexpectedly quickly from the downward leg of the loop (*Fig.* 44); to some observers it had seemed as though a second loop were to be attempted—but then the wing snapped.

The pilot was reasonably experienced; it seemed inconceivable that he could, through sheer incompetence, overstress and break the aircraft. His already poor coronary circulation could well have been embarrassed still further by the 'g' imposed during the loop. In this event, he may have had a 'heart attack' as the glider came over the top of the loop and began to dive. Collapse with death or unconsciousness at that stage in the manœuvre was not a tenable hypothesis, however; had either occurred, the pilot would certainly have allowed the control column to go forward, and the machine would have dived straight into the ground. If the pilot had suffered no more than a very severe angina, the sequence of events that did occur could be explained. Chest pain of sufficient severity might well cause even a competent pilot to pull back the control column relatively forcefully in order to get his aircraft straight and level as quickly as possible; such an emergency might easily trap him into overstressing the glider. For this hypothesis to be tenable, it was necessary to show whether a man suffering from an acute angina pectoris would have the strength to pull back the control column with sufficient force to overstress the glider. Technical evidence did show that the type of glider concerned was particularly light on the controls; relatively little pull on the 'stick' would have been required to produce destructive overstressing; but more force than an experienced pilot would be likely to apply in the ordinary course of events. Investigation of this pilot's medical history failed to reveal any recent symptoms such as 'indigestion' that might have been due to coronary artery disease.

## ACCIDENT NUMBER 213

This accident occurred when a single-seater glider was being flown straight and level at an altitude of about 1500–2000 ft. A structural failure occurred; one wing broke and folded back along the fuselage. Expert examination of the wreckage revealed evidence of the wing having been damaged sometime before the fatal flight and as there was a good deal of air turbulence at the time the accident occurred, it was concluded that this had probably caused the defective wing to collapse.

Routine post-mortem examination revealed that the pilot, aged 25 and only 5 ft. 6 in. tall, had weighed 245 lb. His very fatty liver weighed 3000 g.—rather more than one and a half times the average normal weight of that organ. Sections of myocardium taken from the interventricular septum and both ventricular walls showed a minor degree of focal myocardial fibrosis. Sections of left circumflex and left descending coronary arteries showed a moderate degree of coronary artery disease, although at no point was the lumen of either vessel occluded by more than 50 per cent. The right coronary artery, however, showed more severe disease; several sections taken over a 2-cm. length showed reduction of the lumen by up to 80–90 per cent; but there was no thrombus present.

In the circumstances it did not seem possible to invoke partial or complete incapacitation of the pilot from his natural disease as a precipitating factor in this accident. It seemed unlikely that his collapse or death could have resulted in any inadvertent movement of the control column sufficient to produce overstressing of the aircraft without eye-witnesses observing abnormal behaviour of the machine. All the cases in which natural disease has been found in the pilots have raised the question of medical standards for glider pilots; the obesity of this particular man and the associated pathology drew attention to the subject particularly forcefully; it is discussed in some detail in Chapter 18.

## ACCIDENT NUMBER 246

The pilot killed in this accident was attending a gliding course. On the day he died he made two flights with an instructor in a dual-control machine before making three solo flights in another glider. His first two solo flights were less than perfect although they appeared reasonably safe. Following further advice from the instructor, the student began a third solo flight. During the auto-tow launch, the car driver found that the pilot failed to keep the right angle of climb; after making a series of pitching movements in an erratic manner, the glider over-ran the tow-rope which released backwards automatically. The glider continued to make a number of pitching and diving movements, then turned into line with an adjacent runway, dived and struck the runway in a 20° nose-down attitude, bounced 100–150 ft. in the air and finally dived vertically into the ground.

At the post-mortem examination, the only natural disease discovered was gross coronary artery disease. An atherosclerotic plaque was obstructing the lumen of the left descending artery by about 80 per cent at one level; there was obstruction of the right main artery by about 95 per cent. No thrombus was found in the residual lumen in either vessel nor evidence of recent haemorrhage into an atherosclerotic area.

Investigation of the pilot's recent medical history revealed that he had had a series of fainting attacks some months before his death. He had been investigated at a hospital as an out-patient; all tests of his nervous system had been negative. His symptoms were diagnosed as psychogenic and he was treated with phenobarbitone for some weeks. He should have been reviewed at hospital about four months before his death but he failed to keep the appointment. Despite the fact that he was given to recounting his experiences as a war-time bomber pilot, it transpired that his Service had been confined to a short period in a non-aircrew capacity and that he had been discharged on medical grounds with a diagnosis of anxiety neurosis. His total flying experience consisted of some 50 launches in gliders.

Having regard to all the circumstances, it was considered no more than an even chance that the coronary artery disease had contributed to the accident. Had this pilot been truly experienced, his natural disease might have been held to have been the most likely cause of the accident. As he was relatively inexperienced, and as his emotional and psychological stability, as judged by his medical history, was not of the highest order, it seemed more probable that he had made a handling error on take-off or had experienced some difficulty in controlling the machine; that he had lost confidence, panicked and lost control of the aircraft completely.

## ACCIDENT NUMBER 260

This dual-control glider crashed on landing; both the instructor and pupil were killed. The accident history led the inspector of accidents to consider lack of skill and mishandling of the machine as the probable cause of the accident. At post-mortem examinations no natural disease was discovered in either victim but microscopic examination of the instructor's myocardium revealed a focal myocarditis. The inflammatory changes were not extensive in that the foci of inflammation were widely scattered and most were quite small; nevertheless, occasional areas of inflammation could be found in sections from several blocks from each ventricular wall and from the interventricular septum and some were of moderate size (*Fig*. 45).

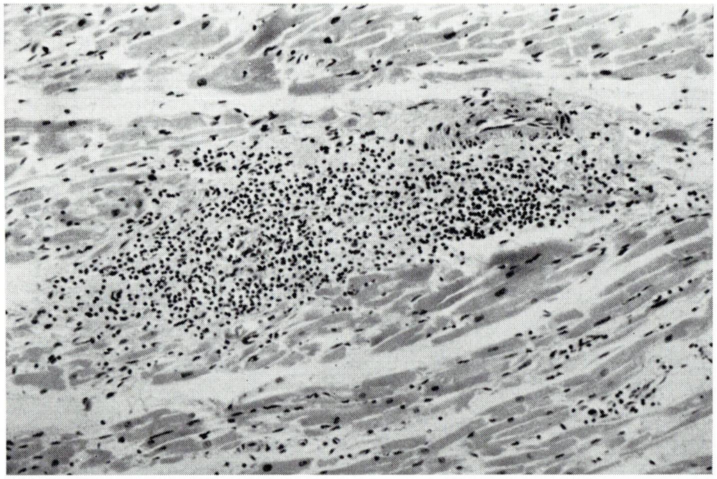

*Fig*. 45.—A view of one of the larger foci of myocardial inflammation from the wall of the right ventricle of the pilot killed in accident number 260. H. & E. (× 60.)

The problem of the significance to be attached to focal myocarditis found in a pilot killed in an accident has been mentioned in Chapter 3 in connexion with two public transport aircraft accidents. I believe that a minor degree of isolated or focal myocarditis is a transient condition, present in a proportion of apparently normal healthy people, that it may rarely cause sudden collapse and death, but that much more frequently its presence is asymptomatic and undetected and it resolves spontaneously. I reported that the natural disease discovered in this instance was a possible but unlikely cause for the accident.

## ACCIDENT NUMBER 257

Two very experienced glider pilots were being launched in a tandem two-seater machine. The man in the front seat had not previously flown this particular machine; he was flying the aircraft and being checked out as a routine by an instructor. The inspector of accident's investigation revealed that the launch was a little slow; the front pilot had indicated this by the accepted procedure of 'waggling the wings' (causing the aircraft to make alternating lateral rotational movements). The tow-rope was released at a height of about 500 ft.—a completely safe height from which to make a circuit and landing. Immediately after release of the tow-rope the glider commenced a right-hand turn; suddenly a right-hand spin developed and persisted until the aircraft hit the ground. Impact was in a slightly nose-down attitude and the marks in the ground showed that the machine had been still spinning to the right as it struck. The pilot in the front cockpit was found dead when reached by rescuers within a minute of the crash; the instructor in the rear cockpit survived despite severe injuries; he suffered retrograde amnesia and could not contribute in any way to an explanation of the accident.

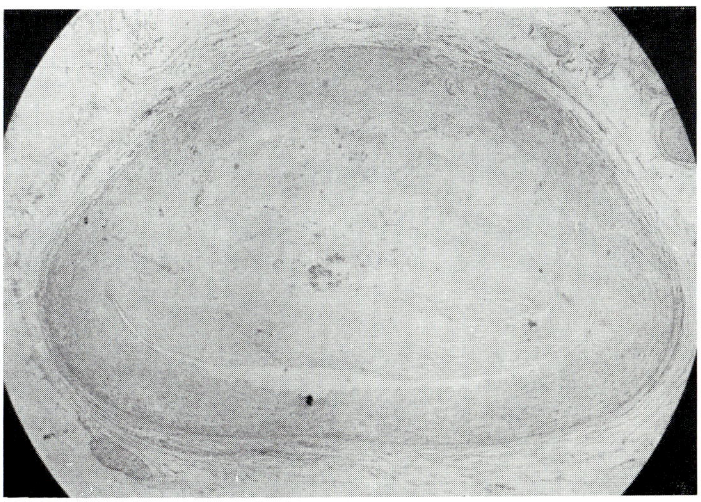

*Fig*. 46.—A section near the origin of the left descending coronary artery of the pilot killed in accident number 257. The large atherosclerotic plaque had caused narrowing of the lumen to about five per cent of its original size. This man may well have had an attack of coronary artery insufficiency in flight. H. &. E. (× 7·5.)

The dead pilot was found to have a large atherosclerotic plaque near the origin of the left descending coronary artery; microscopically the obstruction appeared to be about 95 per cent (*Fig*. 46). The left circumflex coronary artery and the right main coronary artery also showed atherosclerosis but at no point was the lumen occluded to more than 50 per cent in these vessels. An investigation into the dead pilot's history revealed that he had been suffering for some eighteen months to two years from increasingly severe symptoms, almost certainly due to the coronary artery disease; as is so often the case, these symptoms had been misdiagnosed as dyspepsia. Only a few days before the accident he had suffered an attack of pain which had caused him to 'collapse'; he had felt nauseated but had not vomited; he had retired to bed in pain and had felt unable to take anything to drink in an attempt to obtain relief.

This man was nearing his thirty-sixth birthday; his father had died at the age of 36 years from a heart attack. From his medical history it was clear that this pilot had believed that he himself would die a similar death; unfortunately his doctor had considered his symptoms to be psychogenic and had made a diagnosis of cardiophobia.

The technical evidence was especially important in the evaluation of the possible relationship between the pilot's coronary artery disease and the accident. It was shown experimentally following the accident that the type of glider concerned was one which did not spin easily. To initiate a spin it was necessary to pull the control column back and to push one rudder pedal bar forward; unless such action was maintained the aircraft would tend to come out of the spin. The technical investigators felt that since the glider which crashed had continued to spin all the way to the ground and was still spinning when it struck the ground, an explanation had to be found for the control column being held back and a rudder pedal pushed fully forward. One hypothesis advanced was that the pilot had inadvertently allowed his foot to slip off the rudder pedal and had caught it behind one pedal and in front of the other; the two pedals are very close together in this, as in most, types of glider. Paint resembling that on the rudder pedals was found on the side of the pilot's shoe and tended to support the hypothesis. Examination of the wreckage, however, suggested that the two rudder pedals had been in a neutral position and had been equally loaded by a foot on each when the machine struck the ground; both pedals had failed by bending forwards and laterally to a similar degree. Further, the pilot was found to have sustained a fracture-dislocation of each ankle with inversion deformities of the feet; this was consistent with the evidence in the rudder pedals but not with the suggestion that one foot had been caught between the pedals.

It was extremely difficult to decide whether there was any association between the pilot's coronary artery disease and the accident. The front seat of this particular glider was in a semi-reclined position. Had the pilot suffered a complete incapacitation from a heart attack, it is difficult to understand how this would have caused the accident. It is unlikely that he would have forcefully stretched out one leg and it is unlikely that he would have pulled the control column back and held it firmly while the machine continued to spin to the ground. The effect of an attack of myocardial insufficiency is a severe anginal pain or complete collapse with death or unconsciousness. I have been unable to find any report of agonal spasm of skeletal muscle in sudden death from coronary artery disease; only such spasm could explain an inadvertent pull on the control column with sufficient force to prevent the instructor in the rear cockpit from using his column to regain control. Even if the front pilot had had an acute anginal pain as he was executing a right-hand turn, and had this distracted him sufficiently to cause him to depress the rudder pedal too much and at the same time pull the stick back as he clutched his chest, it is difficult to believe that he would not immediately have relaxed and allowed the instructor in the back seat to take over, either because he himself had lapsed into unconsciousness or because he would have been able to react to the instructor's certain order to allow him to take over.

I believe that this accident must have been precipitated by the front pilot suffering a heart attack, although the precise mechanism by which a spinning type of loss of control occurred and was maintained until the machine crashed, could not be explained; but the loss of control could not be explained satisfactorily by any other theory or hypothesis advanced by any other investigator.

## ACCIDENT NUMBER 119

This was the first glider accident that I investigated; it was perhaps the most dramatic of those cases in which natural disease was present in the pilots. There were features of this investigation which serve to introduce the topic of medical evidence as an aid to the reconstruction of events prior to an accident, discussed in the next chapter; it is convenient, therefore, to describe this case as the last in the present group.

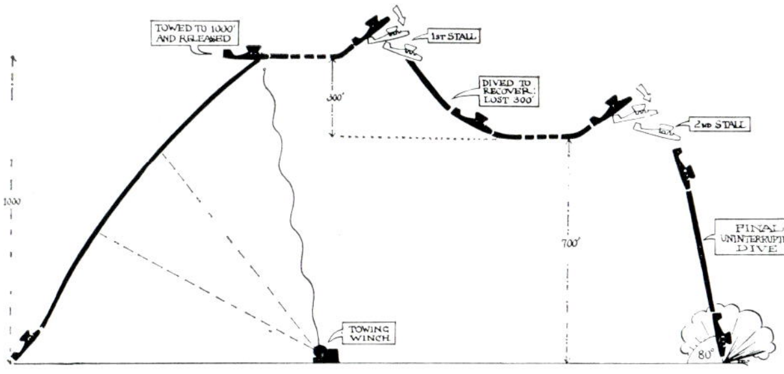


*Fig*. 47.—A diagram depicting the circumstances of accident number 119. While practising stalls and recoveries the glider dived steeply to the ground. (*Reproduced from Stevens* (*1963*) *by permission of the Editor* '*Aerospace Medicine*'.)

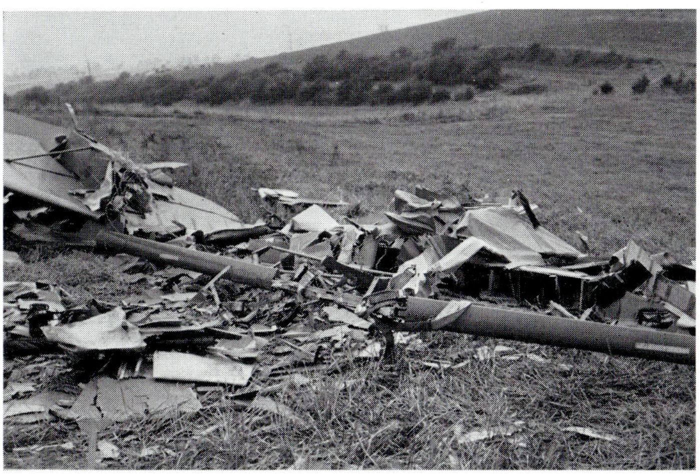

*Fig*. 48.—The disintegrated glider which crashed in the circumstances shown in *Fig*. 47.

*Fig*. 47 depicts the circumstances of the accident. The side-by-side dual-control glider was winch-launched to about 1000 ft. in the normal fashion. It was being flown by an experienced instructor and an inexperienced student who, on his fourth day of a week's residential gliding course, was being taken for a demonstration of the stall and recovery. Shortly after the release of the tow-rope, the machine was seen to stall and recover normally losing about 350 ft. of altitude in the process. Following a second stall, the glider went into a very steep dive; this was maintained until it crashed into the ground and disintegrated (*Fig*. 48). At autopsy both men were found to have died from gross multiple injuries; the only natural disease found in the instructor was an area of active tuberculosis at the apex of one lung. No evidence of natural disease was found in the pupil although, as was discovered later, he had a history of bilateral, but not contemporaneous, spontaneous pneumothoraces within the previous 12 months.

The day following the post-mortem examination, the possibility was raised that the pupil may have precipitated the accident if, through apprehension, he had flexed his knees as the aircraft began its dive to recover from the second stall and if he had inadvertently wedged a foot between the control column and the seat bulkhead. In such a position his foot would have prevented the control column from being pulled

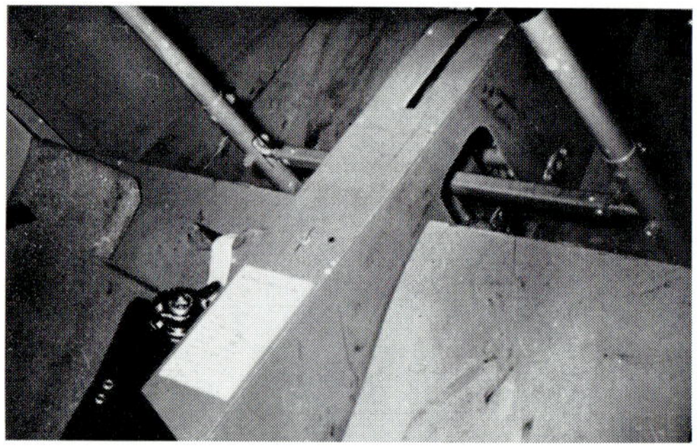

*Fig*. 49.—A view of the inside of the cockpit of the type of glider which was involved in accident number 119. There are linked dual-control columns for the two pilots who sit side-by-side. It can be seen that there is very little space between the control column and the seat bulkhead. An object of moderate size trapped in this position could prevent the control column from being pulled sufficiently far back to bring the aircraft out of a dive. (*Reproduced from Stevens* (*1966a*) *by permission of the Editor 'Zentbl. Verk.-Med. Verk.-Psychol'*.)

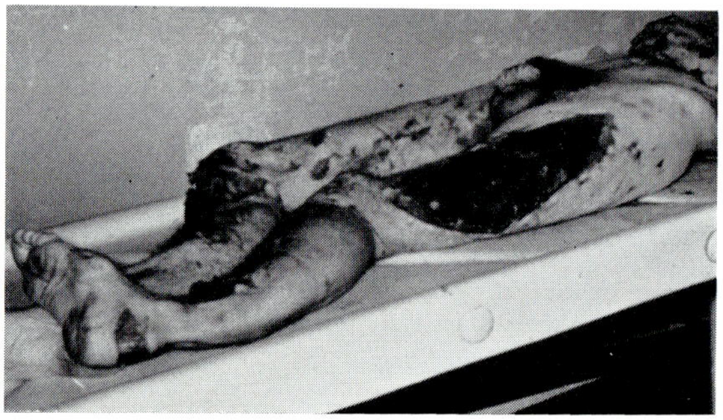

*Fig*. 50.—The injuries to the pupil included unusual damage to the left heel. There was a horizontal laceration around the heel and a horizontal fracture of the calcaneum. (*Reproduced from Stevens* (*1966a*) *by permission of the Editor 'Zentbl. Verk.-Med. Verk.-Psychol'*.)

back far enough by either man to allow recovery from the dive (*Fig*. 49). This hypothesis was advanced on the basis of an accident which had occurred sometime previously at another gliding club; a pupil's camera had swung into the position between the control column and the bulkhead on that occasion, but the instructor had realized the trouble, and, with great presence of mind and very swift action, he had pushed the control column forward to steepen the dive, pushed the obstructing camera away and an accident was averted (Gordon-Burge, 1960).

Our practice of taking numerous photographs of accident victims, their clothing and equipment, has frequently proved its value and did so in this instance. *Fig*. 50 shows that the pupil had an unusual injury to his heel; beneath the horizontal laceration was a fracture of the calcaneum. The police had undressed the casualties prior to the pathologist's examination; this happens all too frequently, but the clothing and, in particular, the pupil's Wellington boots were later recovered from the police station; the left boot had sustained damage that coincided with the injury to the heel.

On examining an intact glider of the type that had crashed, I found that it would have been physically possible for a man of average to large stature as was this pupil, sitting in the right-hand seat, to get his right foot between the control column and the seat bulkhead, although only with considerable difficulty; it would have been impossible for him to get his left foot up over the connecting bar seen in *Fig.* 49 and then into the suggested position. The evidence of several eye-witnesses confirmed that the pupil had sat in the right-hand seat as he should have done; the unusual injury was to the left heel and it was the left boot that was damaged. Examination of the fragments of the seat bulkhead and the control column found in the wreckage showed no traces of the black marks which would have undoubtedly been there had a Wellington boot been trapped

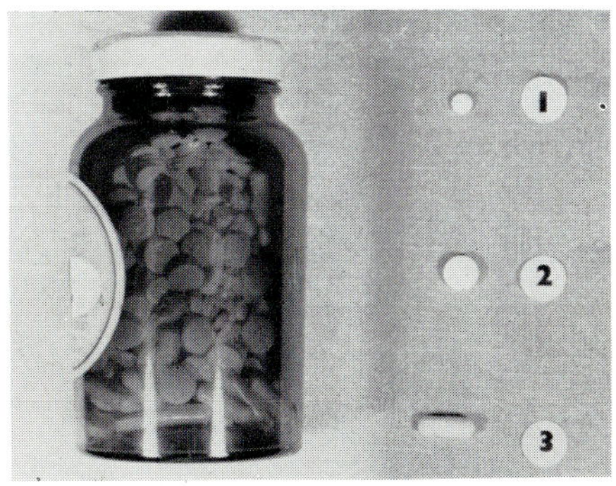


*Fig.* 51.—A bottle of drugs found in the pilot's medicine cabinet. The bottle contained: 1, phenobarbitone, 2, mysoline, and 3, epanutin.

between them at ground impact. It was possible, therefore, to dismiss the hypothesis that the pupil had precipitated the accident in the way suggested; at first it had seemed that there was some supporting medical evidence but when fully evaluated, not only was there no acceptable supporting evidence, there was actually evidence against the hypothesis.

The next step in the investigation was an examination of the instructor's room; he was resident at the club. His medicine chest contained a variety of medicines and tablets; the most significant discovery was the bottle shown in *Fig.* 51; it contained phenobarbitone, mysoline, and epanutin! It transpired that the instructor had been a known epileptic for many years on fairly large doses of suppressive drugs. He had been advised not to drive a car and, indeed, had never attempted to obtain a driver's licence so far as could be discovered. He had had, however, a passion to fly; he had concealed his disability and had joined a gliding club. After some years he had become an assistant gliding instructor and finally the resident instructor. His family doctor in his home town which was far from the gliding club, understood that he was a teacher—he did not know that his subject was gliding! Periodically this pilot had visited his doctor for fresh supplies of the drugs. Fifty-one days before his death he had been given 60 days' supply of each drug; the bottle discovered in his room contained 65 days' supply of phenobarbitone, 100 days' supply of mysoline and 21 days' supply of epanutin. Even if one allows for the inevitable accumulation of tablets or capsules over a period of treatment, the quantities found suggested that at the very least, he had not been meticulous in taking the drugs regularly; it seemed that during the days or weeks before his death he might have been intentionally or unintentionally not taking his treatment. There was the possibility, also, that his active pulmonary tuberculosis might have increased his susceptibility to fits.

The discovery that the instructor was an undisclosed epileptic seemed to offer a probable explanation for the accident; if he had had an attack about the time that the second dive commenced, he could well have held the control column during the tonic phase of a fit for the 7–10 sec. it would take the aircraft to dive to the ground. Initially there was little evidence to support this hypothesis. Nothing found at autopsy had suggested the possibility of an epileptic fit; there was no froth around the mouth, no bitten tongue and no evidence of incontinence. It was considered worth while, however, to interview the police who had removed the bodies from the wreckage and who had undressed them, and to question the mortuary attendant who had prepared the bodies prior to the pathologist's examination.

Indirect questioning of the police sergeant produced evidence that the instructor had had much blood-stained froth around the mouth when he was found in the wreckage; further, his trousers had been soaked around the crutch and thighs with what was obviously urine. The mortuary attendant also had noticed the blood-stained froth but had cleaned this away from both inside and around the mouth in preparing the body for examination. The actions of the police and mortuary attendant had, therefore, destroyed the evidence which could have been the only clues to the cause of this accident. The pilot's personal possessions, including the contents of his medicine chest, could have been removed by his relatives before we, the accident inspector and I, had had an opportunity to examine them; as a matter of fact this very nearly happened. It might well have been impossible to locate this man's doctor had he attended one privately and had he not been a National Health Service patient.

Having regard to all the evidence there was, in my opinion, very little doubt that the accident was caused by the instructor pilot having an epileptic fit.

*Chapter 16*

# RECONSTRUCTION OF EVENTS DURING AN ACCIDENT

## THE CAUSE OF A STRUCTURAL FAILURE

### ACCIDENT NUMBER 134

A PILOT was flying in a glider that had been launched by an aircraft tug to 2500 ft.; he was attempting a 10,000-ft. climb following launch in order to qualify for a Gold C rating. After being airborne for about $2\frac{1}{4}$ hours the glider was seen to perform a rolling manœuvre and to break up at an estimated altitude of 2500 ft. The pilot apparently either succeeded in getting out of the cockpit or fell out—but only at a low altitude;

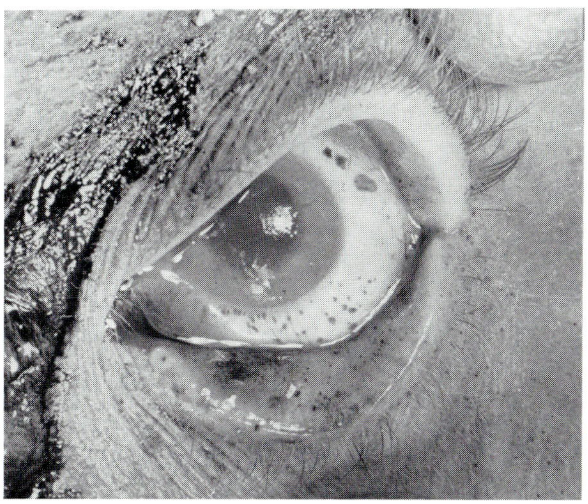

*Fig.* 52.—Subconjunctival petechial haemorrhages probably caused by the pilot's being subjected to negative 'g' at some point during the sequence of accident number 134. (*Reproduced by permission of Dr. G. A. Gresham, Addenbrooke's Hospital, Cambridge.*)

there was sufficient time for his parachute to stream but not to deploy and he died from the multiple lethal injuries he received at ground impact. There was no evidence of pre-existing natural disease at autopsy and the circumstances strongly suggested a structural failure of the glider; but no mechanical pre-crash defect was discovered by the technical investigators.

There was one important clue at post-mortem that helped in the reconstruction of the accident; there were marked bilateral subconjunctival petechial haemorrhages (*Fig.* 52). Possible causes of subconjunctival haemorrhages found in victims of flying accidents are: (1) excessive negative 'g' forces, (2) tumbling in a free fall at high altitude, (3) the effects of ram pressure after jettison of a canopy at high speed, or (4) asphyxia due to strangulation with, for example, parachute rigging lines. In the accident in question only negative 'g' seemed a possible explanation. Subconjunctival haemorrhages result from about — 3 to — $3\frac{1}{2}$ 'g' sustained for a few seconds or from higher forces over shorter periods (Howard, 1965). The glider was built to withstand stresses of the order of — $3\frac{1}{2}$ 'g'; thus, if any manœuvre resulted in a greater stress being placed upon the structure it would be liable to break.

The medical evidence, therefore, indicated that for reasons unknown the man and machine had been subjected to a force of about — $3\frac{1}{2}$ 'g' or more and that this had caused the disintegration of the glider. Forces of about — 4 'g' usually produce unconsciousness; thus there was also here a possible explanation for the pilot's failure to escape from the glider in time to parachute safely.

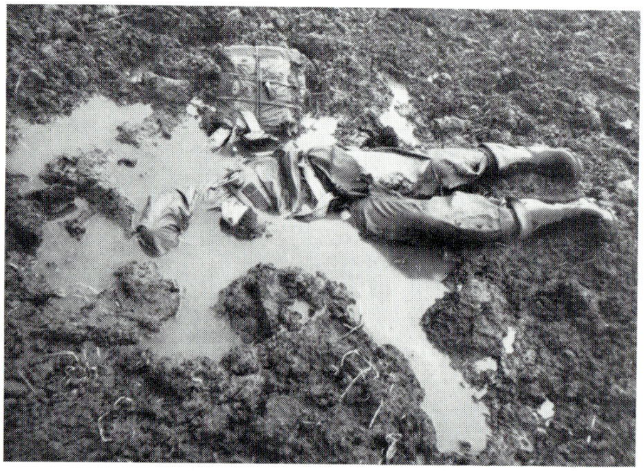

*Fig*. 53.—The body of a pilot who fell into a ploughed field after his glider had been struck by lightning and had disintegrated. He had not apparently attempted to use his parachute. There is damage to his trouser leg and a wound of the left thigh. This wound was approximately 12 cm. long, gaped some 6 cm. and was about 5 cm. in depth.

## A FAILED ATTEMPT TO ESCAPE IN FLIGHT

### ACCIDENT NUMBER 237

The pilot of this glider was also attempting to soar to altitude having been aero-towed and released at about 2500 ft. early one afternoon. The weather was generally fine although there were scattered areas of cumulo-nimbus (thunder clouds). The pilot was in radio communication with an associate on the ground and reported being at a height of 4000 ft. at about 4.30 p.m. Eye-witnesses saw the debris of a disintegrated glider falling out of a thunder cloud at about 4.40 p.m.; the body of the pilot was found to have fallen free from the aircraft wreckage and to have landed in a ploughed field without his parachute having opened (*Fig*. 53). The technical evidence showed that the glider had been struck by lightning; the medical interest in the accident, therefore, centred upon an explanation for the pilot's failure to use his parachute and make a successful escape.

There was no evidence of any pre-existing disease which could have played a contributory part in causing the accident or its fatal outcome. The pilot had died from multiple lethal injuries, clearly received at ground impact. Particular attention was given to a search for injuries which might have been sustained in the air and which could have explained his failure to use his parachute. Only one injury was present which could not be explained readily as having occurred at ground impact; this was the moderately extensive laceration of the left thigh seen in *Fig*. 53. There were no burns on the skin to suggest that he had been struck by lightning and thereby incapacitated. Air in the vicinity of a lightning flash rapidly expands due to the increase in temperature and can produce explosive blast effects; it can thus produce lethal or temporarily incapacitating effects without burning (Mant, 1966). The aircraft's disintegration probably resulted from the excessive turbulence thus caused and in the process the pilot may have banged his head on some part of the glider and suffered from concussion; evidence of in-flight injury to the head would have been obscured by the severe head injuries received on striking the ground.

The excessive turbulence might have caused the pilot to have been thrown out of the glider through the canopy if he had not been strapped in. His seat harness was found intact and unfastened; it was known that he had strapped himself in before take-off and the glider cockpit is such a confined space that it is difficult to imagine what circumstances would have induced him to unfasten his harness while in the air other than to make a deliberate attempt to escape; it seemed most probable, therefore, that he had not been rendered unconscious when the aircraft was struck by lightning, that he had unfastened his harness himself after the strike and that an alternative explanation for his failure to use his parachute was needed.

The possibility that he had become disorientated after leaving the aircraft and unable to locate the 'D' ring with which to open his parachute, had to be considered; this was not, however, a very acceptable hypothesis for there was no evidence from the eye-witnesses or the impact marks on the ground that he had been spinning during the descent. Another possibility was that the parachute itself had been defective but a thorough technical examination failed to reveal any supporting evidence.

It is advocated by many safety officers in the gliding associations that if an escape from a glider has to be made in cumulo-nimbus, a pilot should refrain from opening his parachute until he has fallen free from cloud. This is because of the danger of his being caught in an up-current of air and being carried to quite high altitudes where cold and hypoxia might endanger life. This is not only a theoretical hazard; a number of parachutists have reported the phenomenon. In the light of all the evidence, the following reconstruction was proposed.

The aircraft was struck by lightning in the thunder cloud and became uncontrollable. The pilot was not incapacitated and succeeded in releasing himself and escaping from the machine. According to the parachute manufacturers, it could be assumed that, wearing a back-type parachute, he would probably assume a stabilized attitude of fall as depicted in *Fig*. 54 unless he had actively attempted to adopt some other attitude. His hips may have been rather more flexed than shown by the model for he was wearing Wellington boots, not shoes. Acting on the advice to fall free from thunder cloud before opening his parachute, this pilot would have had to fall a considerable distance, for the cloud base at the time was about 500 ft. It was conjectured that, after falling for some time, he had become concerned and had tried to look over his shoulder to see how near the ground he was. Such an action could have caused a

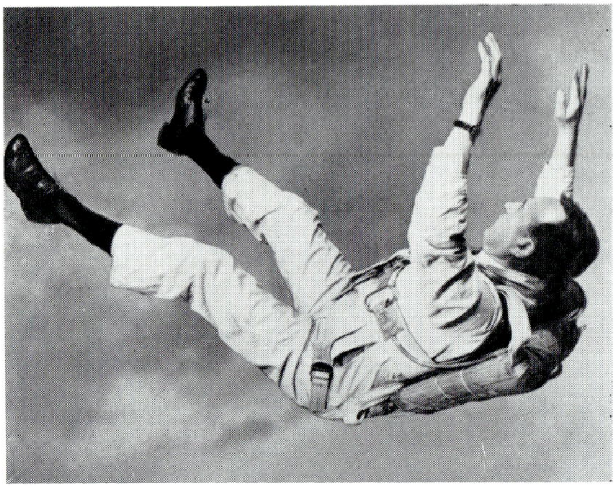

*Fig*. 54.—The stabilized attitude of fall that the pilot involved in accident number 237 may have taken up—though probably not intentionally.

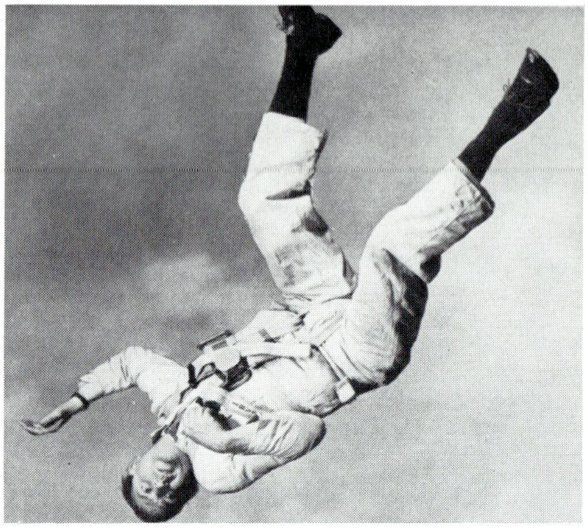

*Fig*. 55.—The possible change in attitude that might occur in a pilot who, in the position shown in *Fig*. 54, attempted to look over his shoulder to see how near he was to the ground. Note the position of the harness box in this type of parachute.

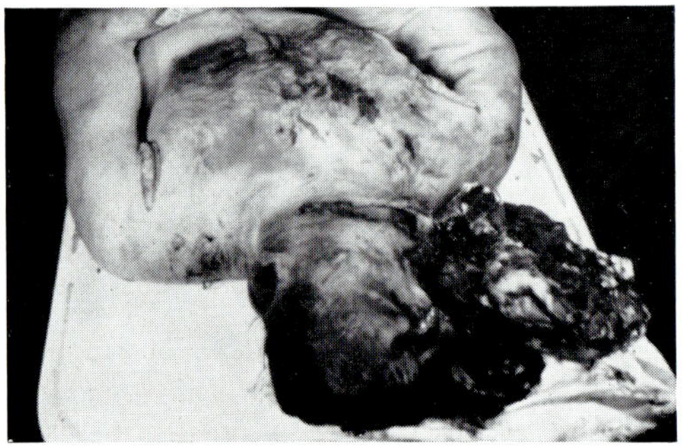

*Fig*. 56.—Severe head injuries which indicate a head first impact with the ground. (*Reproduced by permission of Dr. G. A. C. Summers and Dr. D. MacKinnon, York County Hospital.*)

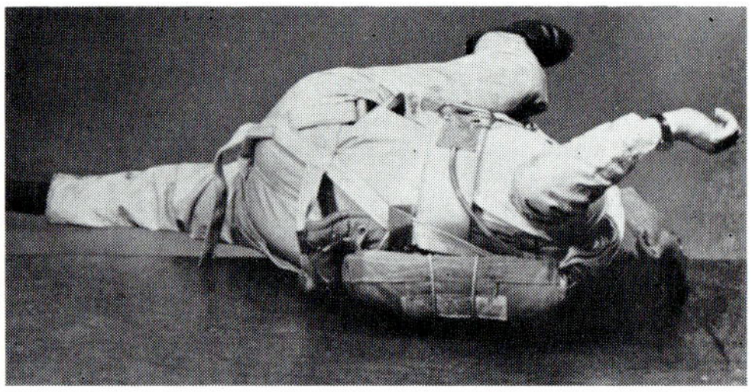

*Fig*. 57.—Reconstruction of the flailing of the limbs that would have occurred when a body in the attitude shown in *Fig*. 55 struck the ground. The left anterior thigh would have come into contact with the parachute harness box and the parachute harness would have been squeezed out to the left and torn away at ground impact, to be discovered as shown in *Fig*. 53.

shoulder to drop and change in attitude to one similar to that shown in *Fig*. 55. If he had struck the ground almost immediately thereafter, the majority if not all the findings at the accident site and at post-mortem examination were explicable.

Firstly the gross head injuries would fit the head-first impact (*Fig*. 56); secondly the way the parachute and harness had become partially torn off to the left of the body as seen in *Fig*. 53, would follow, as the torso, slightly turned to the right, had pivoted on the head and violently smote the ground (*Fig*. 57). Finally, the injury to the left thigh could be understood. On striking the ground in the attitude suggested, an acute flexion of the left hip would have occurred; the thigh would have come into contact

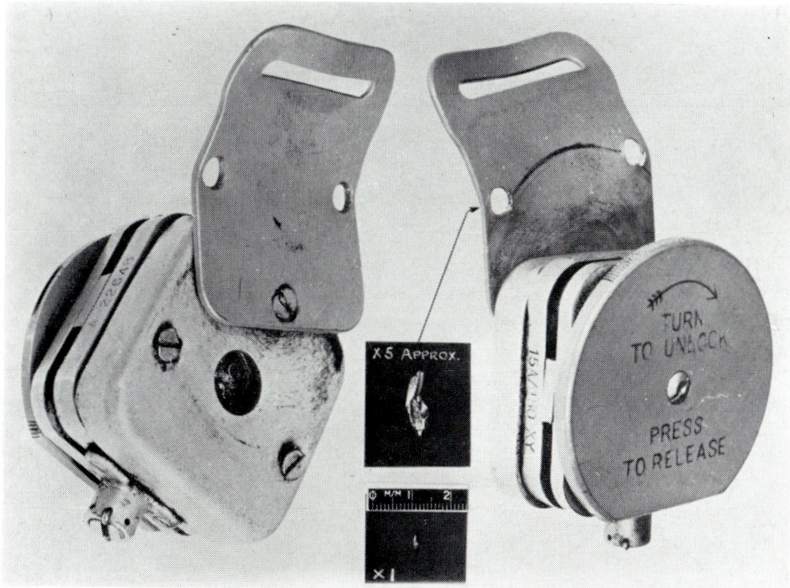


*Fig*. 58.—Views of the parachute harness box from accident number 237. The tiny spicule of metal found deep in the thigh wound (*Fig*. 53) can be seen to have come from the edge of the screw hole in the back plate of the box, as the plate was forced away from the box.

with the parachute harness quick release box which, in this particular type of harness, is located fairly high up (*Fig*. 55). If the thigh struck that box just at the moment that it was being twisted and broken as the parachute was being squeezed out to the left between the body and the ground (*Fig*. 57), the laceration would have resulted. Further, some metallic debris could have contaminated the wound.

A fragment of metal was found in the wound at post-mortem; its origin had been obscure at the time but, on the general principal that no trace evidence of possible significance should be discarded during the investigation of a flying accident, it was saved and given to the engineers for expert examination. As shown in *Fig*. 58, it proved to have come from the edge of the screw hole in the back plate of the quick release box; it had been gouged out as the back plate was forced off the box.

This case is a particularly good example of the value of the correlation of evidence from many sources. A full reconstruction of this failed attempt to escape in flight, was possible only from the sum of the circumstantial evidence, the engineering evidence, the findings in the safety equipment, the parachute manufacturer's evidence and a careful pathological examination of the victim.

## *Chapter 17*

# SURVIVAL AND SAFETY EQUIPMENT

A GLIDER is the most insubstantial of flying machines and there is little to protect the occupant or occupants from injury when an accident occurs. Escape in flight by parachute is possible; when a machine is to be flown higher than a few hundred feet, such a piece of equipment is obviously highly desirable.

The only pieces of protective equipment available for those who crash in their gliders are harnesses and protective helmets. In 12 of the 14 gliding accidents investigated the occupants were in the glider when it crashed and 15 of the 17 people involved were killed. Fourteen of the 15 had had their harnesses fully fastened as had the 2 who survived. One only appeared not to have fastened the shoulder straps of his harness but the lap belt had been fastened. The evidence in the wreckage did not suggest that a fully fastened harness would have saved his life although, in fact, this was accident number 161 in which a pupil survived. The effectiveness of a harness is limited by the strength of the structures to which it can be attached; in a glider this is very low.

None of the 19 people involved in the 14 gliding accidents described wore a protective helmet. The pathological evidence suggested that only 1 of those killed might have lived had he worn a protective helmet; the survivor in accident number 257 would have sustained less severe injuries had he worn a protective helmet and, incidentally, he would probably not have suffered from amnesia and would have been able to help considerably in explaining the accident.

This series of accidents, therefore, has produced no evidence upon which to criticize the harness provided in gliders nor the use of this equipment by those who glide. It does suggest that there is a case for advising the use of a protective helmet. Ellis (1969), however, expressed the view that the wearing of certain types of helmet could cause more injuries than it prevented by causing more accidents. He pointed out that gliders are flown much closer to the stall than powered aircraft and that every glider pilot uses his hearing to detect small changes of speed to a much greater extent than does the pilot of a powered aircraft, any restriction of his hearing by a helmet being, therefore, dangerous. Further, gliders often soar in close proximity to other gliders, perhaps circling in the same thermal current; careful look-out is essential and may be impeded by a bulky helmet in a confined glider cockpit. The majority of glider pilots might be well suited by the simple helmet described in Chapter 12 without the fitted communications equipment; it certainly merits evaluation as a potentially valuable item of safety equipment in this field of aviation.

I have found only one report on the subject of gliding accidents in the medical literature. Wick (1965) reported 117 accidents of which 12 were fatal; he made no observations on safety equipment.

## *Chapter 18*

# GENERAL DISCUSSION

THE 5 fatal gliding accidents in this series that have not been described in detail did not prove to have medical or pathological aspects of particular interest. The group as a whole, considered with the gliding safety figures quoted in Chapter 14, suggest that, although a routine pathological and medical investigation of each fatal accident is amply justified in the interests of a complete explanation and reconstruction, the only general subject that arises is the medical fitness of those who engage in the sport.

As recorded in Chapter 15 half of the pilots in this series were found to have potentially serious natural disease. However, in the instance of the epileptic pilot there had been successful concealment of disability despite medical examination for a P.P.L. In 4 cases the disease was coronary atherosclerosis; this is a condition which is often not detectable at routine medical examination even though it be present to a potentially serious degree. In any case 2 of these 4 pilots were under medical supervision and had been reassured that they were fit. One pilot had mild focal myocarditis—a condition even more difficult to detect clinically. One pilot only may not have passed a medical examination for fitness to glide but it is almost certain that his accident had nothing to do with his state of health (accident number 213).

## MEDICAL STANDARDS FOR GLIDER PILOTS

Before 1960, most but not all civilian gliding clubs required their flying members to complete a declaration of physical fitness. Following the fatal accident in 1960 (accident number 119) I urged that all glider pilots should sign a certificate of physical fitness to be countersigned by their family doctors. In due course, the B.G.A. added to its operational regulations the following:—

'1. All persons joining an affiliated club shall, before flying solo, sign a declaration of physical fitness.

'2. All pilots shall, before starting to give instruction in gliders, have their certificate of fitness endorsed by their own doctor. If it is not possible to obtain the endorsed certificate, a medical check will be required by a doctor, sufficient to enable him to endorse a certificate.'

Pilots holding civil aeroplane pilots' licences or Air Cadets or Service personnel holding appropriate Service medical certificates were exempted from the regulation. The suggested declaration required of a glider pilot was as follows:—

'I hereby declare that I do not suffer from epilepsy, or from sudden attacks of disabling fainting or giddiness, or from any other disability, mental or physical, which would be likely to result in the flying of a glider by me being a source of danger to myself and others.

I understand that it is my responsibility to inform the club of any changes occurring which would affect this declaration.'

Individual clubs were allowed to modify the wording of this declaration if they saw fit. Clubs which had not previously asked their members to sign declarations of fitness were required to incorporate such a declaration in their membership renewal forms so that within the following 12 months all those engaged in gliding in B.G.A affiliated clubs would have signed a declaration.

The doctors' endorsement, mandatory for instructors' certificates, was as follows:—

'From my knowledge of the above named, extending over . . . years, I certify to the best of my knowledge and belief the information vouched is correct.'

### B.G.A. MEDICAL STANDARDS

**PART ONE**

*To be signed before starting to fly as pupil or solo pilot*

I hereby declare that, I have never suffered from any of the following, which I understand may create, or lead to, a dangerous situation in flight.

Epilepsy, Fits, Severe Head Injury. Unusually High Blood Pressure. Recurrent Fainting, Giddiness or Blackouts. A Previous Coronary. I am not regularly taking Insulin for the control of Diabetes.

I further declare that, in the event of my contracting, or suspecting, any of the above conditions in the future, I will cease to fly until I have obtained medical opinion.

Signed .......................... (Name [caps] .................................... ) Date .........

If you cannot sign the above declaration, you must, before flying, obtain the signature of your *regular* G.P., OR that of an approved Board of Trade P.P.L. Examiner, below:

I am the regular G.P. of the applicant<br>I am a B. of T. P.P.L. Medical Examiner } Delete as appropriate.

I understand that the applicant wishes to fly in sporting gliders, but has been unable to sign the above declaration. In my opinion, it is safe for him/her so to fly.

Signed ...................................... Date ..................................

Name/Address .................................... Applicant's name ........................

................................................ ........................................

The following conditions may cause you difficulty while flying. If you suffer, or have suffered, from any of these, you are advised to take medical opinion:

Chronic Bronchitis.
Severe Asthma.
Chronic Sinus Disease.
Chronic Ear Disease.
Eye Trouble (e.g. Inability to read a car number plate at 25 yards—corrective glasses may be used)
Regular, Severe, Migraine.
Diabetes in any form.
Rheumatic Fever.
Kidney Stones.
Psychiatric Disorders.
Severe Motion or Travel Sickness. Any condition requiring the regular use of drugs (Includes any medication whatsoever).

You are further advised that:

(*a*) If you normallly wear spectacles, you should always carry a readily accessible spare pair.

(*b*) Minor illnesses, drugs, and the donation of blood, will probably make you temporarily unfit to fly.

*Fig.* 59A.— Front page of B.G.A. declaration and certificate of fitness to fly gliders (1969).

The B.G.A. advised that the medical endorsement of a certificate of fitness should be applied to all solo pilots and not only to instructors; but a final decision on this point was left to the discretion of each club. Periodic renewal of a certificate of fitness was not required.

In Annex I to the Convention on International Civil Aviation (I.C.A.O., 1962), it is recommended that a member state requires the same medical standards of its glider pilots as of its private pilots of powered aircraft. The express implication of this recommendation was that each government should arrange an initial and periodical medical examination and a licensing system for glider pilots. As Wills (1966) pointed out, gliding in Britain is the only flying movement in the world which controls its own certificates of airworthiness for its aircraft, a standard for its instructors' and pilots'

**B.G.A. MEDICAL STANDARDS**

**PART TWO**

*Passenger Carriers or Instructors (Excluding Professionals)*

Before commencing to carry passengers, or instruct, in sporting gliders, the certificate below must be signed in addition to the signature required at PART ONE. The certification must be renewed as indicated.

Doctors may use the conditions listed in PART ONE as a guide to the requirements.

I am the regular G.P. of the applicant }
I am a B. of T. P.P.L. Medical Examiner } Delete as appropriate.

I understand that the applicant wishes to carry passengers, or instruct, in sporting gliders. In my opinion, he/she is not suffering from any medical condition which might make him/her unfit so to do.

Initial/Renewal Certificate (Delete as appropriate)

Signed ................................ Date ..............................

Name/Address .......................... Applicant's Name ...................

........................................ .....................................

(For Club Use) Valid Until...................................

**Professional Instructors** (Defined, for this purpose only, as any person receiving wages/salary, excluding expenses, for instructing in gliders for any consecutive employment period of 12 calendar weeks or more).

Evidence must be provided, before commencing to instruct in a professional capacity, that the normal P.P.L. Medical Examination has been passed.

**Renewals**

The PART TWO Medical Certificate (or P.P.L. Medical for Professionals) must be renewed as follows:

1. Up to and including age 40—Every Five Years.
2. Age 41 to 50—Every Three Years.
3. Over 50—Annually.

Clubs should calculate the renewal date, using the relevant periods, to the nearest next date of the B.G.A. Annual Return.

**NOTES**

1. In all cases, possession of a *valid* P.P.L., C.P.L. or equivalent Service document, will override the B.G.A. requirements.
2. Foreign certificates may be accepted, provided there is proof that the standard is at least that of the B.G.A.
3. Clubs may demand a *higher* standard, for any of their members, at their own discretion.
4. In the case of defective vision, hearing or physical disability, a club waiver of demonstrated ability may be operated.
5. When a signature is required at PART TWO, PART ONE must also be presented, signed, to the relevant doctor, for his information.
6. In cases of doubt, or non signature of the certificates, the applicant should be referred to the B.G.A. for final arbitration.

*Fig.* 59B.— Reverse of B.G.A. declaration and certificate of fitness to fly gliders (1969).

qualifications, its inspectors and inspection procedure. The B.G.A. is understandably reluctant to have an outside body take over the control of the medical standards of its flying members. Nevertheless, it is concerned that all reasonable measures should be taken to maintain the safety of gliding; to improve its medical standards still further, the Association amended its operational regulations again on 1 January, 1968. The effect of the new regulations was to recommend strongly that a B.G.A. physical fitness declaration should be used by all clubs for all members; to ensure that not only gliding instructors but also glider pilots taking up passengers, should use the particular form of declaration promulgated and should have a doctor's endorsement completed. The form of declaration and certification was again revised in 1969 and is reproduced by permission of the B.G.A. in *Figs*. 59A and B.

Wick (1965) reported that in only 2 of 12 fatal gliding accidents in the United States was a post-mortem examination carried out on a pilot and in neither instance was there any evidence of physical incapacitation which could have explained the accident. He pointed out that many pilots who fly gliders are medically certified for other forms of aviation and, studying 105 non-fatal accidents, he found that pilots possessing such medical certificates appeared to have more accidents than those without! He pointed out that this conclusion was quite possibly invalid as no account had been taken of the 'exposure' to accidents of the two groups but concluded that at least there was no evidence to suggest that an elaborate system of medical certification and licensing of glider pilots would lower the accident rate.

In my opinion, the latest regulations on medical standards imposed by the B.G.A. are likely to result in an acceptable level of medical fitness among those who glide in this country; medical investigation of 14 of the 23 fatal gliding accidents that have occurred in the last 8 years, has not provided any evidence to show that a system of licensing and medical examination of glider pilots would materially increase the safety of the sport.

*Addendum*. The 3 fatal gliding accidents investigated by members of the Aviation Pathology Department at Halton between October 1967 and June 1969 do not include any example of a pilot having pre-existing disease detectable at an ordinary medical examination and which would have called into question his fitness to glide (Mason, 1969).

*SECTION IV*

# *THE FATAL AIRLINER ACCIDENT AS AN EXAMPLE OF MASS DISASTER: MEDICOLEGAL ASPECTS AND THE ORGANIZATION OF THE INVESTIGATION*

---

*Chapter 19*

## INTRODUCTION

### THE MAJOR AIRCRAFT ACCIDENT IN PERSPECTIVE

If a mass disaster is defined arbitrarily as one in which 10 persons or more are killed, then an average of approximately 120 mass disasters occurred each year since 1962 in various parts of the world (*Britannica Books of the Year*, 1963–9); between one-fifth and one-sixth of these were aircraft accidents. Mass catastrophies due to natural hazards such as earthquakes, floods, avalanches, or hurricanes often result in hundreds or thousands of casualties. In those disasters which are so immense as to wipe out whole communities, little can be done to recover and identify the bodies of the dead. In catastrophies of lesser magnitude such as the earthquake at Skopje, Jugoslavia, in 1963, in which just over 1000 people died (Milčinski, 1965), it may be possible to recover and identify the bodies of those killed.

About two-thirds of the disasters each year are associated with man's activities; they include mining accidents, fires, explosions, and accidents during transportation by rail, road, sea, or air; the lives lost in each of these accidents are usually numbered in tens, rarely in hundreds. The worst train disaster in Britain—it occurred at Quintinshill as long ago as May 1915—killed 226 persons (Hamilton, 1967b); the worst air disaster to date in Britain caused 80 deaths and in the biggest accident to a British registered aircraft abroad, 124 persons perished; indeed, the death toll in the greatest single slaughter the worlds' airlines have yet known, the mid-air collision of two airliners over New York in 1960, resulted in only 136 deaths—129 aircrew and passengers and 7 persons on the ground. Provided, therefore, that disintegration of the bodies is not extreme, their detailed examination following an aircraft accident is a practicable proposition. Furthermore, in an aircraft accident more than in any other mass disaster, such detailed examinations should be an integral part of the investigation of the accident itself, as has been demonstrated in Section I.

In other respects also the large aircraft accident tends to differ from other disasters. It is one that often involves people of several nationalities; it often occurs outside the confines of the victims' own countries and often to a machine owned and operated by a country other than that in which the accident occurs. An aircraft accident is one that is especially likely to occur in a remote place, far from the facilities needed for a major medical and pathological investigation. It is a disaster in which the mechanical trauma of the accident itself and the effects of fire in the post-accident phase are especially likely to hamper the task of those handling and examining the human remains.

Any major operation such as the clearing up and investigation of a disaster is more easily and efficiently carried out if there has been some pre-planning and organization by those responsible. In no mass disaster is a pre-conceived plan more important than in an aircraft accident, if the full potential of a medical and pathological contribution to the accident investigation is to be realized. But the complications are many and are particularly evident when an aircraft registered in one country crashes on the territory of another. When this happens many groups of people and organizations are involved either directly or indirectly and they include:—

1. The International Civil Aviation Organization.
2. The commission appointed to inquire into the accident by the state in which the accident has occurred.
3. The local legal authority within whose jurisdiction the accident has occurred.
4. The local police and rescue organizations.
5. The local doctors or pathologists appointed to examine the human remains.
6. The relatives of the deceased.
7. The airline whose aircraft has crashed.

The efficiency, extent, and success of the investigations depends on several of these groups of people; their roles and some of their problems and limitations are discussed in the next Chapter.

*Chapter 20*

# THE VARIOUS AUTHORITIES, OFFICIAL BODIES, AND GROUPS CONCERNED WITH THE INVESTIGATION OF AN ACCIDENT

## THE INTERNATIONAL CIVIL AVIATION ORGANIZATION

AT the invitation of the United States, representatives of 54 nations met at Chicago on 1 November, 1944, for the purpose of reaching agreement to provide control of international aviation and to foster its development. As a result of this convention, the International Civil Aviation Organization (I.C.A.O.) came into being in April 1947.

I.C.A.O. is responsible for co-ordinating all aspects of international civil aviation. Under Article 26 of the Chicago Convention 'in the event of an accident to an aircraft of a contracting state occurring in the territory of another contracting state and involving death or serious injury or indicating serious technical defect in the aircraft or air navigation facilities, the state in which the accident occurs will institute an inquiry into the circumstances of the accident in accordance, so far as its laws permit, with the procedure which may be recommended by the I.C.A.O. The state in which the aircraft is registered shall be given the opportunity to appoint observers to be present at the inquiry and the state holding the inquiry shall report the findings to that state.'

Under Articles 37 and 38 of the Chicago Convention, I.C.A.O. was made responsible for establishing and periodically reviewing standards for air transportation on a world-wide basis. Over the years standards and recommended practices covering a wide variety of matters have been adopted by the Council of I.C.A.O. as annexes to the Chicago Convention. In 1951 standards and recommended practices for aircraft accident inquiries were adopted as Annex 13; in 1966 certain amendments to this annex were agreed. The material in an annex does not have the same legal status as the treaty agreement embodied in the original convention; it is possible for a contracting state to file a notice of departure from the international standards. However, in general, all the contracting states do adhere to the provisions of the original Annex 13 and its amendments.

The original Annex 13 repeated the provisions of Article 26 of the convention whereby the responsibility for the investigation of an accident rested with the state where the accident occurred. It provided further that if the aircraft were registered in another state, then the state of registry should be allowed to appoint firstly 'an accredited representative' to participate in the investigation and secondly advisers to assist the accredited representative to play his full part in the inquiry. According to the original Article 26, the status of an accredited representative was to be that of 'an observer' although the term was not defined. The amendments to Annex 13 passed in 1966 recommended that accredited representatives and their advisers should be allowed specifically—

'1. to visit the scene of the accident,
'2. to examine the wreckage,
'3. to question witnesses,
'4. to have full access to all relevant evidence,
'5. to be provided with copies of all pertinent documents,
'6. to make submissions in respect of various elements of the inquiry.'

These recommendations were made subject to the normal procedures of the state conducting the inquiry. Although no specific mention was made in the annex of medical or pathological advisers to the accredited representative, authority for the inclusion of such advisers would appear to be implicit in its provisions.

I.C.A.O. endeavoured further to promote a high standard of aircraft accident investigation by the publication of a *Manual of Aircraft Accident Investigation;* the third edition appeared in 1959—the fourth is in course of preparation. The manual was not concerned with the form an inquiry might take and was prepared so as not to conflict with the laws of any state. It had no standing whatsoever as an instrument of international law or agreement. It was intended solely to assist those in any country charged with the responsibility of the investigation of an aircraft accident should they wish to use it. The greater part of the manual dealt with the examination of the accident in general and with the examination of the aircraft wreckage in particular. Chapter 9 discussed somewhat briefly the potential value of medical evidence in aircraft accident investigation but put the case for autopsies upon the victims no more strongly than 'in the case of death of any of the operating crew members on flight duty at the time of the accident, particularly where the aircraft crashed out of control and when sudden incapacity in flight was suspected, a post-mortem examination of the crew members concerned should be made and, whenever practicable, an autopsy performed'.

In Chapter 10 of the *Manual* the identification and care of aircraft accident victims was discussed, recommendations of the international criminal police organization were quoted, and a brief account given of the various procedures that may be of value in identification. My experience of major aircraft accident investigation in general supports much of the advice given in Chapters 9 and 10 of the *Manual;* with a number of points I do not entirely agree and in certain other respects the advice offered, in my opinion, could be very much improved; the particular points in question will be raised in the pages that follow.

Most countries now belong to I.C.A.O.; the only notable exceptions are Russia and Communist China. It would seem, therefore, that all reasonable preparations have been made by international agreement and action to ensure a proper investigation in the event of an accident to an aircraft either on an internal or an international flight. However, international agreements made on behalf of governments, do not necessarily result in detailed briefing of those who are locally legally responsible.

It is necessary, therefore, to consider briefly the position and aims of a commission appointed by the civil aviation department of a government under the terms of the I.C.A.O. Convention to inquire into an accident, and also the position and aims of a local legal authority within whose jurisdiction the accident has occurred.

## THE NATIONAL COMMISSION OF INQUIRY

### In the United Kingdom

In Britain the Chief Inspector of Accidents is charged with the responsibility of investigating flying accidents (The Civil Aviation Investigation of Accidents Regulations, 1969). He investigates each accident through one or more of his inspectors and investigating officers. His report is made to the Board of Trade and it is invariably published in due course. Exceptionally a public inquiry is held when a commissioner and a number of assessors hear in open court the evidence of the accident inspectors, the investigating officers, and other witnesses and subsequently report to the Board; this report too is usually published.

The Chief Inspector and his inspectors have statutory powers to carry out their investigations under the Regulations. They may subpoena any witness, expert or otherwise, to appear before them and give evidence provided there are grounds for believing that the witness concerned is able to contribute to the inquiry. Accident inspectors and investigating officers have the right of access to the aircraft wreckage and of its removal to a suitable place for examination. The aims of the Chief Inspector and his officers are to establish in detail the cause of an accident and to assess safety and survivability factors.

The importance of routine comprehensive pathological investigations into fatal flying accidents is fully appreciated by those responsible for the inquiries in the United Kingdom; as was explained in the introduction to this monograph, it has been the practice for several years for the Chief Inspector of Accidents in Britain to ask a Royal Air Force pathologist to act as an adviser to the inspector in charge of an investigation if it has been in this country, or to act as an adviser to the inspector appointed as the British accredited representative when a British aircraft has crashed overseas.

### Abroad

A permanent aircraft accident investigation organization comparable to that in Britain exists in only a few other countries. In most an *ad hoc* commission of inquiry is appointed from people with experience in aviation.

As indicated in the General Introduction, few other countries have pathologists experienced in aircraft accident investigation who routinely assist their accident investigation branches where they exist, or who can be appointed to an *ad hoc* commission of inquiry. Except in Britain, the United States of America, Canada, Australia, Germany and perhaps one or two other states, if any pathological contribution to an accident inquiry is made it comes from those doctors who happen to be appointed by the local legal authority to examine the remains.

## THE LOCAL LEGAL AUTHORITY'S INQUIRY

In Britain as in most other countries the national accident investigation runs concurrently with, but is distinct from, the local legal inquiry which takes place if the accident has been fatal; the latter inquiry is in the hands of one of H.M. Coroners in

England and Wales or a Procurator-fiscal in Scotland. In other countries a magistrate, a local chief of police, or other similar official performs a function roughly equivalent to that of a British Coroner.

### England and Wales

The Coroner's function differs from that of the official accident investigator. The Coroner within whose jurisdiction bodies lie must hold an inquest with a jury into deaths caused by 'accident, poisoning or disease, notice of which is required to be given to a Government Department. . . .' Aircraft accidents come under this heading (The Civil Aviation Investigation of Accidents Regulations, 1969). The Coroner and his jury are concerned to establish who is dead, where, when, and by what means they met their death and to arrive at a verdict. The list of other situations in which the Coroner must summon a jury includes 'death occurring in circumstances continuance or possible recurrence of which is prejudicial to the health or safety of the public or any section of the public'. The Coroner's role in the prevention of accidents is, therefore, established; he can 'mark the importance or gravity of any particular case or circumstances of death arising from the same or similar causes by placing the facts before . . . a jury' (Purchase and Wollaston, 1957a).

Nevertheless, neither the Coroner nor his jury have the knowledge, experience, or skill to conduct a detailed technical inquiry into such a complicated matter as an aircraft accident. As there is a national official inquiry held into the aircraft accident, it is the practice for Coroners to adjourn an inquest until the results of this other inquiry are available. In doing this, a Coroner is expected to keep in mind that the object of his inquest is 'to enable interested persons to ascertain in general terms the cause of the accident . . . . The evidence at the inquest should be sufficient to enable the jury . . . to reach a conclusion . . . as to which is the appropriate verdict to return' (Purchase and Wollaston, 1957b). Possible verdicts are that death was due to accident, misadventure, manslaughter (implying a gross degree of negligence on the part of some person or persons), murder, or suicide, or, failing evidence to support adequately one of these, an open verdict. The technical minutiae of the cause of the accident or, indeed, whether the accident resulted from a pilot's collapse (short of death) in the cockpit, need not of necessity concern the Coroner unless the points bear upon the verdict.

Havard (1960) reported that up to 1953 the use the Coroners made of post-mortem examinations to assist in the determination of the causes of death in the cases reported to them varied very greatly over the country but was generally too low for an acceptable level of efficiency and accuracy. As might be expected, those cases least likely to be autopsied were those in which the causes of death were apparently all too obvious, for example, multiple injuries received in an accident. Nevertheless, it has become general practice in recent years for Coroners to order full post-mortem examinations on the bodies of those killed in aircraft accidents. This has resulted largely from the experience gained by the Royal Air Force pathologists from Halton, and the general appreciation that post-mortem examinations in these circumstances may provide a considerable amount of evidence of importance in the accident inquiry apart from merely confirming the obvious cause of death (Purchase and Wollaston, 1957c).

Coroners, therefore, will now normally call for evidence to be presented at the inquest by pathologists about the causes of death of those killed in the accident, and evidence concerning the presence or absence of pre-existing disease in the operating crew members. Whenever aircraft accidents have occurred in England and Wales my colleagues and I have found that our presence in the A.I.B.'s investigating team has been welcomed both by Coroners and their pathologists.

### Scotland

In Scotland it is a Procurator-fiscal who carries out an initial inquiry into a fatal accident. He then 'presents a petition to the Sheriff, craving him to hold a public inquiry in regard to the cause of death and the circumstances of an accident' (Glaister, 1962) if he considers this desirable. In conducting his initial inquiry the Procurator-fiscal 'precognosces' a medical witness 'who reports on the cause of death, without a post-mortem examination when the cause of death can be so ascertained, otherwise after a post-mortem dissection'. It is the general practice for a Procurator-fiscal to accept 'multiple injuries' as the cause of death deduced solely from an external examination of the body in the case of a victim of an aircraft accident; it is rare for him to petition the Sheriff to issue a warrant for a full post-mortem examination. My colleagues and I have frequently (but not always) found it difficult to persuade a Procurator-fiscal of the need for full autopsies following military and light aircraft accidents; it has frequently been suggested that those believing such examinations to be important should seek permission from the relatives. Whether or not the Procurator-fiscal would be prepared to act in accordance with the recommendations of I.C.A.O. if a public transport aircraft crashed within his jurisdiction is not certain; it would doubtless depend upon the individual concerned and the representations made to him.

### Abroad

The function of the magistrate or the chief of police of the district in which an accident has occured in a foreign country is, in my experience, much the same as that of the English Coroner or the Scottish Procurator-fiscal. He is concerned primarily to determine who is dead, to establish that there are no criminal aspects to the disaster, to arrange for the registration of the deaths and the disposal of the bodies of the victims. The identity of the individual bodies may or may not be of consequence to the local legal authority in other countries; on some occasions I have found that the local 'Coroner' had required little more than a list of those presumed to be on the aircraft and to know whether the number of bodies recovered was in agreement. If so there was ready acceptance for the purposes of certification and disposal that those named on the passenger and crew list had all died.

When a British aircraft has crashed abroad and there has been close liaison between a national commission of inquiry and the local legal authority, and when the local legal authority has appointed a pathologist to conduct an examination of the victims, I have found that my participation in all aspects of the medical and pathological examination has been welcomed. On some occasions there has been little or no co-ordination between a national commission and the local legal authority; the latter has been interested in the identity of the victims and the investigation of the accident only to a very slight extent and has been prepared to accept a universal cause of death in terms such as 'multiple injuries', established from a cursory examination of a few bodies; and the Commission of Inquiry, having no medical members, has concentrated primarily upon the aircraft wreckage. It has then fallen to the lot of the British pathologists to explain tactfully to the local 'Coroner' the importance of a detailed examination of the bodies and their individual identification from the point of view of the accident investigation. In the majority of such instances, these representations have been received sympathetically and such facilities as it has been possible to offer have been provided for us to carry out the examinations ourselves; our findings have then been accepted by the local legal authority with little or no hesitation. Some of my colleagues, however, have been less fortunate when dealing with certain accidents not reviewed in this book; when co-operation is not forthcoming, there is very little that can be done about it.

## THE POLICE AND THE INITIAL RESCUE OPERATIONS

Those who arrive first on the scene of an air disaster and those who take charge of the accident site during the first few hours are the people upon whom the success of an aircraft accident investigation depends to a much greater extent than may be generally realized. Their actions may ensure the preservation of valuable evidence; they may cause it to be irretrievably lost.

When an accident occurs elsewhere than in the immediate vicinity of an airfield, members of the public are usually first on the scene. They often attempt, very properly, to rescue survivors. Occasionally they are guilty of looting or souvenir hunting; I have known an important aircraft instrument to be temporarily lost in this way and for personal possessions to be stolen from the bodies of victims. Trained personnel invariably arrive within a short time of the accident, and whether they be police, firemen, Red Cross workers or others, no consideration should or does take precedence over the rescue of survivors.

Once it is certain that no survivors remain to be helped, it is most desirable that neither bodies nor wreckage should be interfered with until competent persons arrive to organize the recovery operations in a correct manner. My experience is unfortunately, that those early on the scene, even police and firemen, are apt to rush into the business of recovering the bodies of the dead, into a search for clues to their identity and into arrangements for their speedy removal to the nearest mortuary. This stems doubtless from an understandable desire to clear up as quickly as possible the human debris that bears abhorrent witness to man's fallibility; but it is very important that haste in this matter should be avoided.

Precipitous action in removing bodies from the scene is quite likely to happen in Britain; it has happened abroad following most of the accidents that I have investigated. If it is to be avoided and the I.C.A.O. agreements and recommendations are to be put into practice, member states must ensure, not only that their local legal authorities such as Coroners or magistrates are informed of the importance of the correct procedures, but that the police are properly trained. It would be impossible to instruct all the different types of persons who may appear at the site immediately after an accident but the police are almost always at the scene within a very short time; it is they and only they who will regularly be in a position to ensure that the correct actions are taken.

All police know the importance of security and they almost always secure the accident site from interlopers at the earliest opportunity. They need to be taught, in addition, that following an aircraft accident dead bodies should be left where they are until they have been labelled, photographed, and their locations either staked or accurately mapped or both, unless there are urgent overriding indications to the contrary.

Eventual removal should be supervised at the very least by a policeman—preferably by the investigating pathologist. This is especially important if many bodies are heaped in one part of the wreckage and if there has been much burning. In my opinion the bodies should be removed without any attempt to begin a detailed examination at the site. On this point I disagree with the advice given in the I.C.A.O. Manual of Accident Investigation which states that 'the identification should begin at the scene of the accident to the extent that circumstances permit'. I have experienced too many complications and problems arising from this advice being followed; several will be discussed in Chapter 21 in connexion with the identification of the casualties. I believe that the only examination that should be undertaken at the accident site, is that necessary to ensure that a single body and that which unquestionably belongs to it, is transferred to a suitable container. Ideally the container should be a strong body-bag made of thick durable plastic sealed with zip fasteners; a large sheet of thick polythene or jackinette is adequate; least desirable is a hastily constructed coffin with defects through which important material may be lost.

## LOCAL PATHOLOGISTS AND THEIR FACILITIES

As stated, whenever pathologists are appointed by local legal authorities to examine the bodies of the casualties, whether in Britain or abroad, I have found invariably that it is very easy to reach a mutual understanding so that the examinations are carried out jointly to satisfy the requirements of all concerned. The ease with which the examinations have been conducted, however, has varied very greatly; it has depended primarily upon the buildings available for use as mortuaries.

Any building with one or more large rooms will suffice as a temporary mortuary if it can be adequately guarded. The thorough examinations of the bodies that are often necessary to establish their identities and the detailed internal and external examinations that are necessary to ensure that all medical evidence of possible importance to the accident investigation is adduced, demand an adequately equipped autopsy room. All too frequently I have had to work in surroundings that have been far from ideal; indeed they have often been totally inadequate. On some occasions this has been inevitable having regard to the remoteness of the places where the accidents have occurred. On other occasions I have felt that planned co-operation between police, Coroners or their equivalent in adjacent districts, and those in charge of mortuaries in those districts, might have led to much more suitable accommodation being made available. The facilities for pathologists to carry out their examinations and to store bodies temporarily prior to examination should be the best available; small and inadequate public mortuaries should be avoided when better equipped hospital or other mortuaries are within a reasonable distance, even though these be located in another jurisdiction. Coroners in England and Wales have the authority to move bodies into an adjacent area should it be necessary to ensure that adequately equipped premises are used (Purchase and Wollaston, 1957d) and I feel this provision should be readily invoked whenever a mass disaster—especially an aircraft accident—occurs. The one difficulty which arises from the use of mortuary facilities in a hospital is that for a period they cease to be available to those who usually use them. Pressures, therefore, bear upon the pathologists to complete their examinations with the minimum of delay.

When the numbers of casualties are large and the climate warm, refrigerated storage for bodies is invariably insufficient. Alternative means of preservation can be arranged most efficiently when there has been previous planning—again, a matter I feel for the police; at best refrigerated trucks can be hired, at worst local sources of blocks of ice need to be tapped with the minimum of delay. In tropical and subtropical climates speed in the examination and disposal of bodies is highly desirable, if not essential; it is in such geographic locations that storage and autopsy facilities are commonly least satisfactory.

## THE RELATIVES OF THE DECEASED

The initial and subsequent reactions of the relatives of the deceased vary considerably. Some cling to hopes of miraculous survival and will only accept the truth upon being convinced that the body of the person with which they are concerned has been identified beyond doubt. Some relatives make haste to the scene of the accident and demand to be allowed to help in the identification of their kinfolk. Sometimes an overwhelming desire to be finished with the whole sad affair is felt and this may lead to unreasonable and vociferous complaints to Members of Parliament or other authorities when a body is not promptly released for disposal. Religious beliefs are an important reason for relatives being impatient of delay. Pressure is thus brought to bear from these quarters upon the doctors to complete their investigations without delay.

At a slightly later stage the relatives become concerned to receive a death certificate; this is the key to the settlement of the deceased's affairs. When a person disappears and his or her dead body is not recovered and identified a death certificate cannot be issued. In most countries when there is strong evidence that death of a certain person has occurred, as in an aircraft accident, a verdict of assumed death can be obtained; in some countries, however, there is a statutory delay before such verdict can take effect. Keiser-Nielsen, Frykholm, and Strøm (1964) reported that in Sweden the delay was 3 years but in other countries such as Norway and Denmark, only 1 year. In Britain there is no statutory delay (*see* Chapter 24).

When more than one member of a family have died in the same accident, the order in which they died is a matter of concern to relatives and their legal advisors, since upon this may depend the disposition of the deceaseds' property. Section 184 of the Law of Property Act, 1925, provides that where two or more persons die in circumstances rendering it uncertain which of them survived the other or others, their deaths shall for all purposes affecting the title to property be presumed to have occurred in order of seniority; the younger shall be deemed to have survived the elder. This is known as 'the Rule of Commorientes'; it does not apply if the two persons are husband and wife and the elder of them died intestate, when the Rules of Intestacy apply, as if the younger had not survived the intestate. When both have executed a will or when the persons concerned are not husband and wife, the presumption made in the Rule of Commorientes can only be excluded if there is 'evidence leading to a defined and warranted conclusion that one person died before the other' (Marshall, 1963).

Martin and Mason (1969) have commented recently upon the inequities of the law on commorientes, but as they point out criticism of this is not new. However, the law may well not be amended for some considerable time, and in the meantime it must be accepted as it stands. It is, of course, a matter for lawyers and the courts to determine in a given case whether there is evidence to exclude the presumption of commorientes. Nevertheless, since, after many aircraft accidents, only the pathologist will be in a position to adduce relevant evidence, it is, in my opinion, essential that he should appreciate the importance and consequence of his expert opinion on the matter and the circumstances in which his opinion is likely to be significant.

Should A be found to have died from multiple injuries including a lacerated heart but B from the combined effects of multiple injuries and asphyxiation due to a post-crash fire, having oedematous lungs, carbon deposition in the lower respiratory tract and a blood carboxyhaemoglobin of 24 per cent, it is probable that all would agree this to be good evidence that A died before B. However, if B died from cerebral laceration and the only evidence of his survival for a period after the accident was found to be the presence of extensive pulmonary fat and bone-marrow embolism, the evidence that B survived A becomes very much more tenuous. The pulmonary embolism could have occurred within a matter of seconds of the lethal injury and would have depended for its production upon the maintenance for a brief period of an intact and functioning circulation but not necessarily an intact and functioning central nervous system.

What is death? The shorter the time interval there appears to have been between two persons' deaths, the more important becomes a definition of death, a subject already causing great concern in relation to the subject of organ transplantation (Simpson, 1967; Gordon, 1967, 1968; Shapiro, 1967, 1968; *British Medical Journal*, 1968). Gordon (1968) wrote 'it may be stated categorically that the forensic pathologist is not entitled to speculate about the mechanism of death on the basis of findings at necropsy (i.e., on the basis of anatomical or naked-eye changes) or on the basis of conventional microscopic or other laboratory investigations'. If this view is accepted then the forensic pathologist ought not to 'speculate' upon the relative timing of death of two persons who, from circumstantial evidence, died at approximately the same time.

It would seem wise for a pathologist to consider whether any evidence he could offer on the question of survivorship in a given case could conceivably be accepted as sufficient to lead to a 'defined and warranted conclusion that one person died before the other'; if *he* cannot feel sure that one person died before another, it is unlikely that a non-medical person will find his evidence unequivocal.

It would also seem wise for him to ascertain in a given case what opinions might affect this issue. It might be only if A were shown to have survived B that the disposition of property would differ from that if the Rule of Commorientes were applied; it might be clear to the pathologist that A did not survive B, but he might spend much time on the problem of whether B survived A, unless he determined that this was immaterial in the particular instance.

It is an advantage if a pathologist words a certificate on this matter in the appropriate way. Originally I certified that I had found no evidence to show that A and B had died other than contemporaneously; this was not what was required. Marshall (1963) reported that there was much conflict of judicial opinion as to whether, if there was evidence of simultaneous death, the Rule of Commorientes should apply. In the House of Lords it was settled thus: 'Can you say for certain which of these two persons died first? If you cannot say for certain, then you must presume the older to have died first. It is immaterial that the reason for your inability to say for certain which died first is either because you think they both died simultaneously, or because you think that they died consecutively, but you do not know in what sequence'. Although my earlier certificates were not, therefore, useless I now word them to the effect that either I believe A to have died before B, or that I can find no evidence as to which person died first; I do not now say or imply that I think they died simultaneously.

In due course a number of relatives will become especially interested in the cause of the accident; they will have considered the possibilities of litigation and the chances of recovering a greater amount of money in compensation than is normally paid out by the airline insurance companies. However, this is not a matter of direct concern to the pathologist except insofar as he will occasionally receive requests from solicitors to provide evidence as to the amount of pain and suffering an individual endured before he died.

## THE AIRLINE

Of paramount importance to the airline operators is the cause of the accident; especially is this so when the company is operating other aircraft of the same type. For commercial reasons it is very much in the interests of the airline that the investigation should be completed with as much despatch as possible. If the accident is abroad, the airline is very anxious that the bodies be repatriated and returned to relatives for disposal as quickly as possible; the disaster is still very much a news item for the national press until this has been done and this is bad publicity. There is, therefore, an understandable degree of pressure exerted by the airline upon those responsible for the medical and pathological investigation to complete their work with a minimum of delay. It is my experience, however, that the officials of the vast majority of airline companies fully appreciate the importance of a thorough medical and pathological investigation; their co-operation is very readily secured.

## ILLUSTRATIVE CASE HISTORIES

A few case histories will serve to illustrate some of the points to which reference has been made.

*Example* 1

This accident occurred in the vicinity of an airfield in open country several miles from the nearest town. The local airport fire brigade extinguished the fire and, shortly thereafter, the bodies were removed from the wreckage without being photographed, without being numbered or labelled in any way and without any record being made of their individual positions. The cadavers were then stripped of identifying personal effects under the supervision of the local medicolegal authorities but without any records being made as to the bodies from which the various items of property were removed. The bodies were then consigned unceremoniously to a hospital mortuary, later removed to a second mortuary and finally placed in a refrigerated room in a third mortuary. There they were handled by, among others, relatives searching for the body of a local passenger and a dental surgeon from a foreign military organization, commissioned to try to identify a number of his compatriots who had been on board.

Although the State in which this accident occurred was a member of I.C.A.O., it was obvious that the local authorities were not aware of the potential value of pathological examinations of the victims of an aircraft accident. According to their own legal requirements it was only necessary to establish who had been killed, not which body was which. The philosophy of the people of the country concerned was that a body after death is but an empty shell to which little or no respect is due; it did not matter therefore, in their view, whether or not bodies were mixed up in a heap in a mortuary prior to simple disposal such as burial in a communal grave.

The only fortunate thing was that the efficiency of those who had removed the personal possessions and clothing from the cadavers, left something to be desired. Several items of jewellery had been overlooked, fragments of characteristic clothing remained on some partially incinerated bodies and this together with dental evidence and the fact that a few of the casualties had not been burnt and were easily identified visually, permitted identification of all the bodies in due course. Once our wish to make full autopsies was known to the local authorities, every facility was placed at our disposal.

*Example* 2

In marked contrast to the first example, the police placed a guard around the accident site at the top of a mountain (*Figs*. 60, 61) as soon as they had established that there were no survivors. No one was allowed to interfere with the wreckage or bodies until a commission of inquiry had been appointed and the members of this commission, the British accredited representative and his advisers had all assembled at the nearby town. The local forensic pathologist appointed to the commission and I were the first to be taken to the accident site. We were transported as far up the mountain as possible by helicopter. Indeed, this was the only part of the investigation of which I did not wholly approve; the helicopter was small, and was designed for a pilot and one passenger. In the event, the pilot took off with two pathologists squeezed together inside one safety belt, feeling neither comfortable nor safe as they approached the mountain partially obscured by rain cloud!

After reaching the summit on foot, we were able to make a complete examination of the site and map the positions of all the human remains and the main pieces of aircraft wreckage. By the time this had been completed, Red Cross volunteers had climbed the mountain with stretchers, polythene sheeting, labels, and string. The pathologists supervised the labelling and photographing of the bodies, their recovery and packaging for removal to the main mortuary in the town. This was an ideal way to approach an accident investigation but as there was a delay of some 36 hours from the time of the accident to the pathologists' arrival at the accident site, it was clear that this procedure was possible only because the climate was suitable and the location of the accident sufficiently remote for satisfactory security arrangements to be made.

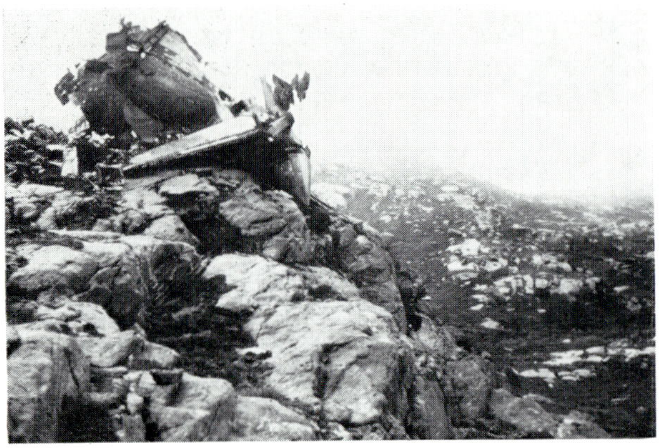

*Fig.* 60.—A view at the scene of the accident described as 'Example 2'. It occurred on top of a mountain in a temperate climate.

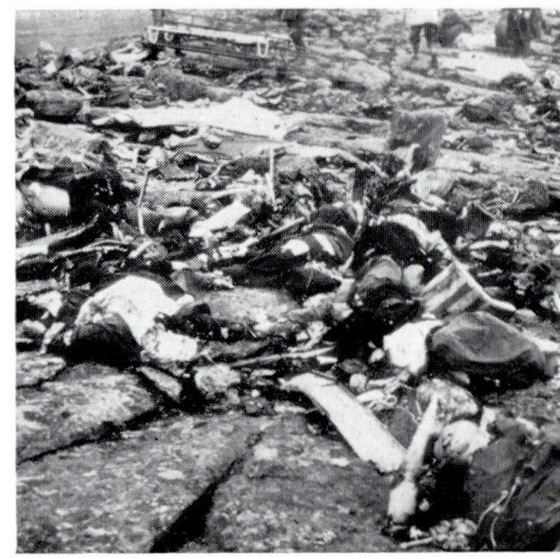

*Fig.* 61.—The first rescuers to reach the scene in 'Example 2' found no survivors; they therefore did not interfere with the human or aircraft wreckage. A police guard was mounted until the accident investigation team was assembled. The pathologists then supervised the mapping and photographing of the bodies, their recovery and packaging for removal to the mortuary.

*Example* 3

The local authorities set about the initial investigation of this accident in a most methodical way. The aircraft wreckage and the bodies had been scattered over a considerable area of countryside and several search parties were formed. Each search party was given a number and was instructed to number the bodies serially as found, prefixed by the search party number. Thus the cadavers came to be labelled 1–1, 1–2, 1–3, and 2–1, 2–2, 2–3 and so forth. Each search party was responsible for recovering the bodies found and taking them to a search headquarters set up in a field beside the most suitable access road to the area. As the bodies were delivered to the search headquarters they were put into temporary coffins which had been hastily ordered and constructed in a nearby town. The coffins were appropriately labelled with the bodies' numbers. Unfortunately, the number was sometimes put on the loose lid of a coffin and sometimes on the side of the box itself.

At a later stage, those in charge of the field headquarters deemed it desirable to check how many bodies had been recovered for comparison with the total believed to be on board the aircraft. As there were several stacks of coffins, some empty, some full, and as there was constant activity as search parties returned, the accurate counting of filled coffins was facilitated by marking them with a new system of serial numbers; again the numbers were placed indiscriminately on lids or the sides of the coffins. In due course, it was decided that the coffins should be removed to temporary storage; two nearby places of worship were chosen—two because one could not accommodate all. The priests in charge were anxious to know the number of coffins committed to their charge and, in checking them, also added their own sets of numbers.

The next step was for the police to begin an examination of the bodies in the temporary mortuaries. Space was limited and several parties were at work; there is some doubt about whether the lids removed from the coffins were always returned to the correct boxes. Clothing and personal property were removed from many of the bodies, placed into bags and returned, at least in most instances, to the appropriate coffins.

At this stage of the investigation the British team arrived. It was realized that it would be impossible to carry out a proper investigation in the temporary mortuaries in which the bodies were housed; there was insufficient space, inadequate light and no water. Fortunately diplomatic exchanges at a high level resulted in the whole of the medical investigation being put into the hands of the British pathologists; they were offered the excellent facilities of a mortuary at a base some 80 miles from the accident site. All the bodies were transferred to this mortuary and those which could not be accommodated inside immediately were stored in a number of refrigerated vans hired for the purpose and parked outside the mortuary. Despite the complications of the several numbering systems, it proved possible eventually, though not without difficulty, to identify the bodies of all the victims.

*Example* 4

The local pathologist in charge of the medical investigation of this accident was extremely experienced in forensic medicine but had not dealt previously with an aircraft accident investigation. He began by setting up facilities for an on-site examination of the bodies; this was conducted in the open. As a body was found it was brought out to the examination area, labelled, and photographed. A typist then recorded a dictated description of the location in which the body was discovered and the findings of an external examination of clothing, personal property, and the body itself. In some instances the property and clothing were removed but when this was done they were placed in a bag which was thereafter kept with the body. The body was then placed in a coffin and removed to a temporary mortuary in the city several miles away. This procedure continued for a full two days during which a number of pathologists worked in relays; but not every pathologist examined the body at the site with equal care.

Meanwhile in the temporary mortuary, a spacious building but with a somewhat inadequate water-supply, several other pathologists were conducting a second examination of the bodies. They did not have available the records made at the accident site. This resulted in several instances in duplicate records being prepared; in other cases, records were incomplete with important points overlooked at both examinations. The fact that throughout the second examination the bodies were not removed from their temporary coffins and clothing still on the bodies was left in situ, contributed to the inadequacy of the procedure.

It was difficult for the two British pathologists to contribute to the medical investigation during the first forty-eight hours. Not only was there intense activity going on in two places miles apart, but there was a very considerable language difficulty. In the event, it was decided that the best procedure was for us to try to observe all that was taking place in the temporary mortuary and, so far as it was possible, to make our own external examinations of all the bodies as they were having their second examination by the local pathologists. On the third and fourth days, the pathologist in charge was ready to sit down and discuss the findings in each body from his two sets of notes and compare these with our findings.

Where there were discrepancies or matters of doubt, the body was re-examined. Over several days the records of injuries sustained by each victim as judged by external examination only were completed; the identities of a number of bodies were established. Since it was clearly impracticable to arrange for full autopsies on all the casualties, it was agreed that this should be done only on the bodies of the operating crew (which fortunately could be fairly easily identified on this occasion) and a representative proportion of the passengers and cabin crew.

This accident was one in which mechanical trauma and the effects of a post-crash fire were very considerable and the circumstances of the accident were such that there was relatively little of interest with regard to survival and escape. In the circumstances, therefore, the enforced limitation of the pathological investigation was not particularly serious.

In my opinion, the commencement of the examinations of the bodies at the accident site should be avoided. On this occasion there were several points which were never reconciled between the report of the examination of a body at the site and the report of its later examination. For example, the first report on a certain badly incinerated body stated that a ring was found on the third finger of the left hand. The notes of the second examination of this body indicated that the left arm was completely missing but the charred right arm was present. The container with the personal property and clothing removed from this body during the first examination, contained a gold ring but nothing to indicate from which hand it had been taken. The importance of minor clues to the identification of a body will be discussed in the next chapter; unless examinations of bodies are carried out methodically and very careful records made, confusion is bound to arise.

I firmly believe that all that should be done at the accident site is a properly supervised recovery of each body together with that which definitely belongs to it. If during its recovery a piece of burnt clothing is accidentally pulled off a body but it is clear beyond any doubt that the clothing did come from that body, then a note should be made to that effect and attached to the material which should be placed in a separate small container and then attached to the body; later the contents of the pockets can be used as reliable clues to the body's identity. If, however, the body is one of a pile of burnt bodies and the piece of clothing concerned has been completely burnt off one of them but it is not certain off which, then on no account should the clothing in question be placed with any particular body. Again, it should be put into a separate container and a note made of the numbers of the several bodies with which it was associated. Nothing should be removed from the bodies at the site; no examination should be made; each body should be placed in an appropriate container and transferred to the best mortuary in the vicinity.

*Example* 5

This accident occurred when the aircraft struck a snow-covered mountain and disintegrated. Two avalanches were caused and these swept the wreckage and most of the bodies about 2000 ft. down the mountain to come to rest on a steeply inclined slope (*Fig*. 62). The wreckage was located from the air and the police were taken to the area by helicopter. Relays of police worked for the next 12 days searching an area of mountainside approximately 400 × 70 metres. They dug over snow which was in many areas up to two metres deep. They recovered well over a hundred parts of human remains, labelled each one, mapped the positions at which they had been found (*Fig*. 63), placed them in separate polythene sheets and had them transferred by helicopter to the nearest airfield and thence to the pathological institute in the adjacent city.

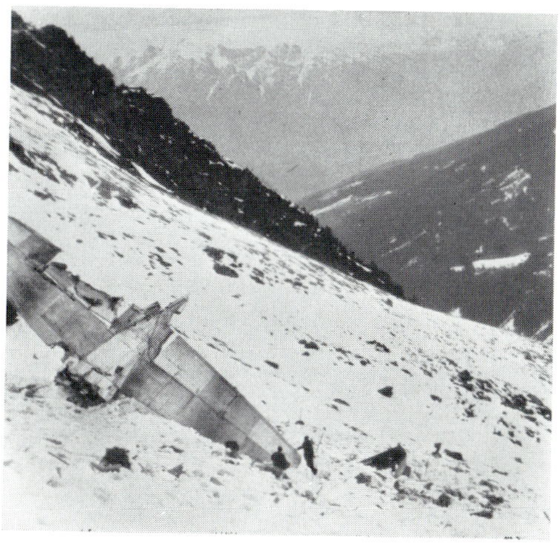

*Fig*. 62.—The site of the accident mentioned in 'Example 5'. The wreckage came to rest in deep snow on a steeply inclined mountain slope.

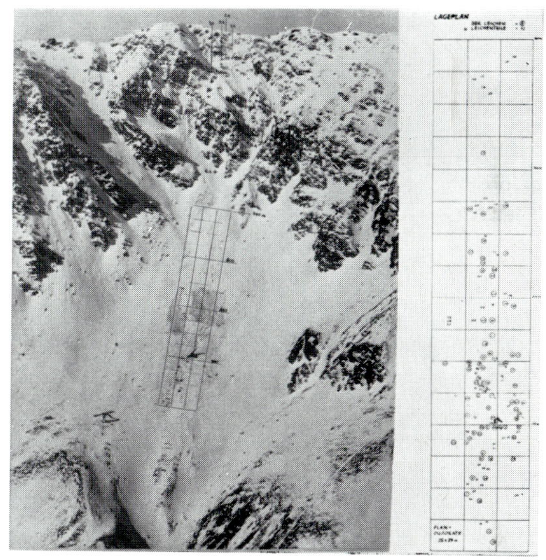

*Fig*. 63.—An aerial view of the site of the accident in 'Example 5', showing the location of certain bodies near where the aircraft first struck the mountain and the area on the lower slope where most of the bodies were found. An adjacent plan shows the exact location of each piece of human remains recovered. (*Reproduced from Stevens* (*1965a*) *by permission of the Editor 'Aerospace Medicine'*.)

The British accredited representative and his advisers arrived as the first bodies were being brought down from the mountain. Some initial difficulties arose, largely due to language difficulties, between the chief of police, the local forensic pathologist, and ourselves; these were resolved quite quickly and detailed examinations of the bodies then proceeded in a very methodical manner. The bodies were all well frozen before their arrival at the institute which had ample cold storage space in the cellars. The pathologists selected the order in which the recovered bodies should be examined; only specimens that constituted more than half a body were selected in the first instance; any separate pieces such as limbs or parts of limbs were placed in a refrigerated room for examination at a later stage.

A selected body was finger-printed and then transferred to the spacious autopsy room. It was immediately given a new cadaver number so that there should be no confusion with the original identifying numbers. The series of cadaver numbers started at 401 and printed labels were used (*Fig*. 64). The body was fully photographed.

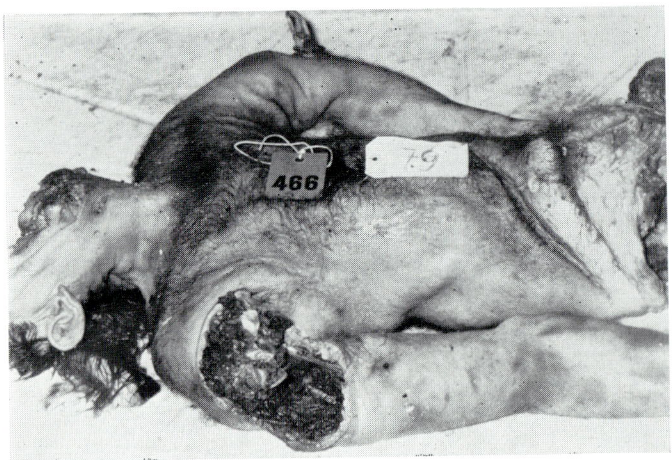


*Fig*. 64.—The second step in the examination of a body in the mortuary was the allocation to it of a cadaver number provided the 'body' constituted more than half a body. A series of numbers was needed, distinguishable from that used by the recovery teams at the accident site, for their numbers referred not only to whole bodies but to fragments of human remains. (*Reproduced from Stevens (1965a) by permission of the Editor 'Aerospace Medicine'*.)

Then police and pathologists jointly removed and examined any clothing and personal possessions; samples of each garment and any portions bearing laundry marks, manufacturers' labels or other potentially important clues to the identity of the owner were retained and affixed to a special record card labelled with the cadaver number. All personal property was listed, described and sealed in a container also labelled with the appropriate cadaver number. The body was then rephotographed and special photographs taken of any notable features such as tattoos or scars.

A full external and internal post-mortem examination followed and a detailed record was made of the dental state of the body. As two autopsy tables were available two teams worked concurrently; each consisted of a local pathologist, a British pathologist, a local policeman and a British undertaker who acted as a clerical assistant.

Comprehensive radiography of the remains was not indicated in this particular accident but some radiography of certain bodies to assist in the assessment of age was undertaken. A portable X-ray machine was used in the autopsy room for this purpose.

Specimens were taken for histology and toxicology as necessary. Thereafter the body was despatched to the cellars to be embalmed and coffined. In my opinion, each body should be thoroughly examined jointly by police and pathologists with full photographic and written records at a single operation; it should be a rare necessity for any re-examination to be required after the body has been despatched to be embalmed; the only exception to this rule is that at a late stage it may be necessary to compare a separated part with a body missing that particular part to see whether or not it matches.

Over the course of 12 days, 81 bodies and some 50 or more parts of bodies were examined in this way. The 81 bodies were all identified and it was concluded that 2 bodies only had not been recovered; they were subsequently recovered some months later having been washed to the lower slopes of the mountain in the spring thaw.

## DISCUSSION

It is hoped that sufficient emphasis has been placed throughout this chapter on the importance of planning in advance for the tasks to be undertaken in the event of a large fatal aircraft accident investigation. The preparation of such plans should be made, in my opinion, on a police regional basis; as indicated the police are the cornerstone of the whole structure of a disaster plan. Any plan conceived, if it is to be really effective, must be fully discussed with and have the approval of, Coroners, pathologists, hospital and mortuary administrators, the fire brigade, the local Red Cross or other rescue organizations and local undertakers. Many contingencies must be anticipated and provided for; these will vary from country to country and district to district. Central stores of waterproof printed labels, blank labels, indelible crayons, wooden or metal stakes, body bags or polythene sheeting, small polythene bags and similar items should be prepared. Occasional exercises need to be held so that all concerned are kept aware of the arrangements made and the part that they will be expected to play. If this is done the actions taken in the first few hours following an accident, pending the arrival of the expert investigators, will facilitate the subsequent investigations and not jeopardize them.

One of the more difficult aspects of the subsequent investigations is the individual identification of the bodies of the casualties. To a large extent this also can be facilitated by some pre-planned organization; this will be discussed further in Chapter 23.

# Chapter 21

## THE IDENTIFICATION OF THE BODIES OF THE DEAD—1

### GENERAL COMMENTS

THE sociological and legal justification for the identification of the bodies of the dead has been argued by several authors including Brown, Delaney, and Robinson (1952); Mercer, Reid, and Uttley (1954); Frykholm (1956); and Keiser-Nielsen, Frykholm, and Strøm (1964). I fully subscribe, as I have said elsewhere (Stevens and Tarlton, 1966), to the view that the identification of the victims of any disaster is a public duty. I am not sure however, that I would go so far as Keiser-Nielsen (1967) who referred to Article 6 of the United Nations' Universal Declaration of Human Rights adopted on 10 December, 1948, by the United Nations General Assembly which stated, 'Everyone

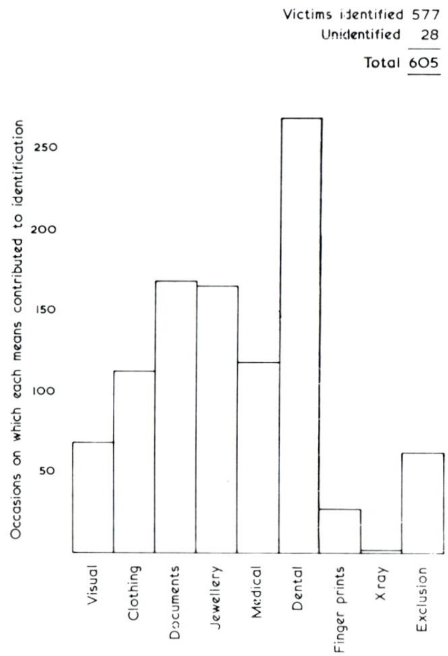


*Fig*. 65.—Histogram showing the means of identification of the bodies from 13 fatal public transport accidents and the relative values of the various types of evidence.

has the right to recognition everywhere as a person before the law'; he suggested that this may be held to imply that a citizen of a U.N. Member State has a right 'to possess his personal identity unquestioned', even after death; thus Article 6 of the Declaration, he felt, could be interpreted as an international law prescribing that identification of the dead must be carried out whenever possible.

It will be apparent from the foregoing sections of this book that the identification of the bodies of the victims of an aircraft accident is always a prerequisite for the determination of whether there is a main or contributory medical cause for the accident; it is also frequently essential if the pathological evidence is to be of maximum use in the reconstruction of the events in the aircraft before, at and immediately after the accident.

Several types of evidence may help to establish the identity of a body; some are more reliable and specific than others. Essentially personal characteristics such as fingerprints and the dental state are the most reliable evidence; circumstantial evidence such as the clothing on a body and the personal property found in the clothing is inherently less satisfactory and may, on occasions, be misleading. Considerable experience in this work has convinced me that, whenever possible, evidence of two or more kinds should be sought before the identity of a body is accepted; every case must, of course, be considered on its merits.

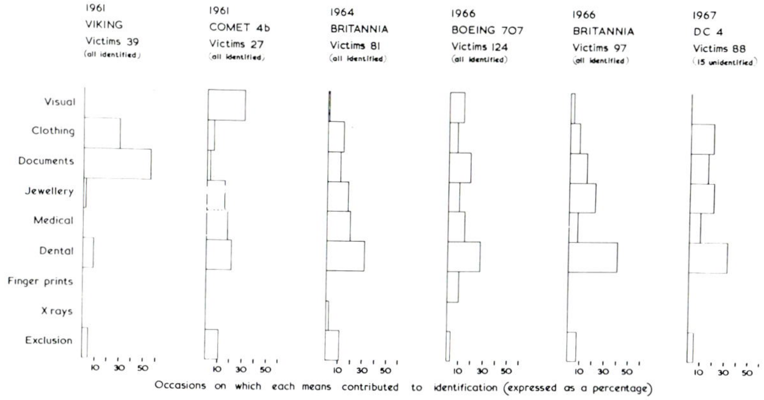


*Fig.* 66.—Histograms of the means of identification in several accidents showing how the patterns differed as a result of the circumstances peculiar to each accident. In the Viking accident mechanical trauma was very considerable but there was no fire to destroy clothing and documents; most of the travellers were young males with little medical or dental evidence to distinguish between them. In the Comet accident many died from asphyxiation from the fire without being burnt; they were visually recognizable. In the 1966 Britannia accident mechanical trauma and fire destroyed clothing and documents in many instances but it proved possible to obtain dental records of most of the travellers and dental evidence was even more useful than usual. In the Boeing 707 accident many of the victims were Americans; in many cases their finger-prints were readily available.

*Fig.* 65 shows the relative values of the various means of identification as experienced in 13 public transport aircraft accidents. It must be emphasized that the appearance of this histogram is influenced by many chance factors. For example, the usefulness of dental evidence depended as much on the availability of ante-mortem dental records as the preservation from mechanical destruction of the jaws of the victims; distinctive clothing may be of as little value as a clue to the identity of the wearer if there is no friend or relative to give an accurate description of it, as if it had been destroyed in a post-crash fire. Histograms prepared for individual accidents show that the relative values of these various means of identification are influenced by the degree of mechanical trauma to the bodies, the extent of a post-crash fire, the availability of information about passengers, and such factors as their social class, nationality, and age (*Fig.* 66).

As would be expected, sex influences the relative values of certain of the aids to the identification of bodies (*Fig.* 67); documents and personal property are frequently found intact in clothing on men's bodies but women use handbags and these are lost

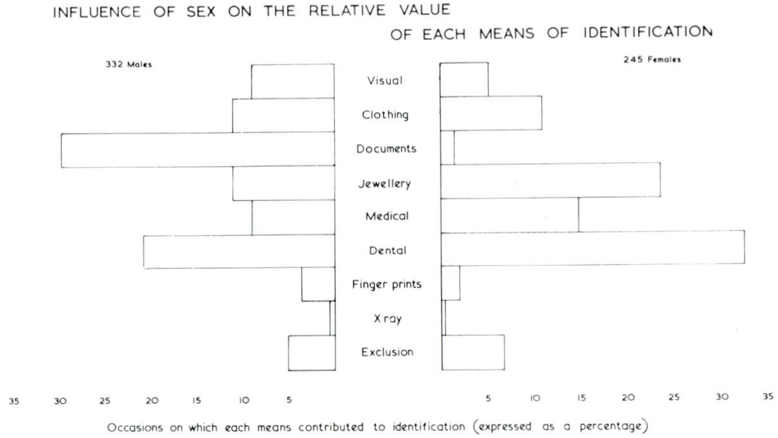


*Fig.* 67.—A histogram showing the influence of sex on the relative value of each means of identification. As might be expected jewellery is of more value in females than males, documents of much more use in males than females. Women are, in general, more conscious of dental hygiene and seek dental treatment more frequently than men; hence dental records are more frequently available in females than males.

in an accident. Women are more concerned with dental care than men; dental records are therefore much more frequently available for women than for men.

## VISUAL IDENTIFICATION

Visual identification is the standard means used by the police to prove the identity of a body subject to a coroner's inquiry. When the body has not been involved in a mutilating accident, visual identification is perfectly acceptable. I have found a strong inclination, however, for the police in this country to try to obtain visual identification of accident victims even where mutilation has been severe. The mechanical trauma and the effects of fire are often so severe in modern aircraft accidents that visual identification is frequently impossible and any attempt to use it is fraught with the danger of error. It is not always possible to rely on visual identification of the living as was well shown in the case of Adolph Beck (Morland, 1950) who was incorrectly recognized by 15 out of 17 persons as the man who had defrauded them. Incorrect identifications of the dead have been reported by several authors including Strøm (1935) and Strøm and Toverud (1940), both quoted by Gustafson (1966b); Brown, Delaney, and Robinson (1952); and Frykholm (1956).

I have experienced several cases of false positive identification and one of false negative identification during the last few years. *Fig.* 68 shows the partially incinerated body of a young girl wearing a necklace and a ring. These items of jewellery were removed and shown to a woman at the police station; she identified them without hesitation as the property of her daughter. The mother insisted upon viewing the body and on seeing it, appropriately draped so as to minimize her distress, she categorically denied that the body was that of her daughter. It was not until she had removed all the coverings and had seen the fragments of some distinctive trews which had not yet been removed from the body, that she would admit that the body was that of her daughter.

Facial features can be easily distorted after death. The only injury to the head sustained by a certain casualty was a laceration of the forehead. The body had lain

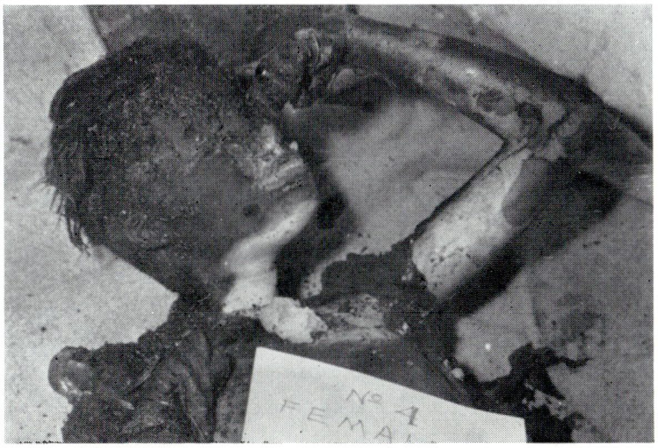

*Fig.* 68.—The incinerated body of a young girl identified on the basis of the jewellery she was wearing; on viewing the body her mother denied that it was that of her daughter and was convinced only with difficulty.

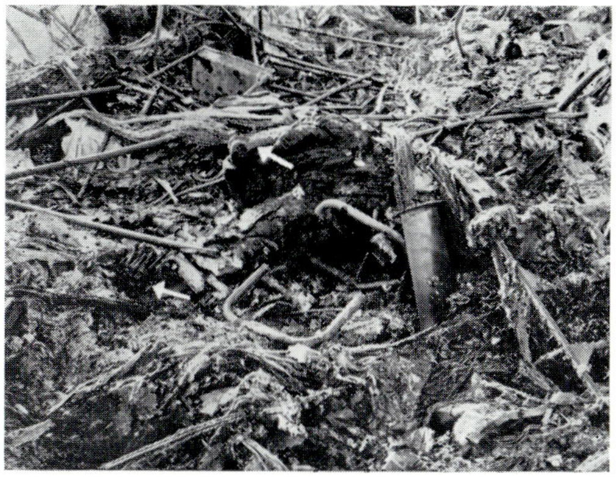

*Fig.* 69.—The burnt-out wreckage of an aircraft showing a partially incinerated body. The police initially accepted the identification of this body by an airline official whose conclusion was based on the position of the body in the wreckage.

in the snow on a mountainside at an altitude of 7000 ft. for some three days before it was recovered; it had been sunny during this period and the resultant changes were such that attempts at recognition by close relatives were, in my opinion, unjustifiably traumatic for them and likely to be unprofitable or misleading for the investigators. Comparison of a passport photograph with a body by a person not emotionally involved may sometimes provide a useful clue to identity—this was so on this occasion.

Such a comparison must be used as a clue only; having attempted such comparisons on a number of occasions I know that it is often extremely difficult and may be very misleading.

Visual identification usually implies the recognition of facial features. Occasionally, when facial features have been completely unrecognizable, we have allowed a relative to view a particularly distinctive feature such as an unusual birthmark, to obtain confirmation of a suspected identification. This too must be a carefully controlled procedure. Mason (1967) described a case in which a relative examined a number of bodies in the presence of a policeman and observed a piece of metal protruding from the arm of one of the bodies; he identified this body firmly as that of his brother because his brother had had a metal plate inserted into his arm to secure a fractured bone. The visual identification was accepted and the possibility of an error was discovered only just in time. In fact, the body was not that of the man's brother; the metal protruding from the arm was a piece of aircraft metal—in any case, it was in the wrong arm!

A variation upon the theme of incorrect visual identifications was provided by accident number 183. In this instance aircraft wreckage was largely destroyed by fire and the bodies of the occupants incinerated (*Fig*. 69). Nevertheless, the police initially accepted the identifications accorded to the bodies by an aircraft company official on the basis of their positions in the wreckage. All but one of these tentative 'visual' identifications later proved incorrect.

## PERSONAL PROPERTY

All textbooks of forensic medicine discuss the value of clothing found on a body, the contents of pockets, and the presence of rings and other jewellery in the identification of unknown bodies. The many different ways in which these articles may be helpful clues to identity have been exemplified in my experience. The view might well be taken that the examination of all this material and its use in identification should be entirely a matter for the police. I disagree; in my opinion it is a matter for a team which should jointly examine the bodies—a team consisting of at least a pathologist and a policeman, ideally also a dentist, and occasionally other experts. For this reason a number of cases will be quoted to show the snags that can occur in practice, the particular value of the 'joint examination' approach and certain of the more interesting ways in which circumstantial clues to identity found among personal property associated with a body have been followed up.

### Clothing

Clothing is retained on the bodies of casualties of aircraft accidents to a very variable degree; it may be completely destroyed by fire or garments may be badly torn or lost from blast effects either from explosive forces at ground impact, when an aircraft disintegrates at altitude or during a subsequent free fall. Fragments of clothing retained on a body are often damaged by heat, foam, rain, blood, and other body fluids; it can be quite difficult to record a correct description of garments or the material of which they are made. This may be especially difficult with men's suits. Incidentally, it might be expected that the relative lack of variety in men's clothing would make it of less value than female clothing in identification work; *Fig.* 67 does not confirm this.

Body number 405 from a certain accident was tentatively identified as that of Mrs. 'J' on some relatively weak circumstantial evidence—a ring on the finger seemed to fit a rather vague description given of the ring worn by this passenger. The dress on the body was of distinctive material and a telephoned description of the dress Mrs. 'J' had worn on the day of the accident was given by a neighbour. The description was so unlike the dress found on the body that it was considered to exclude the tentative identification.

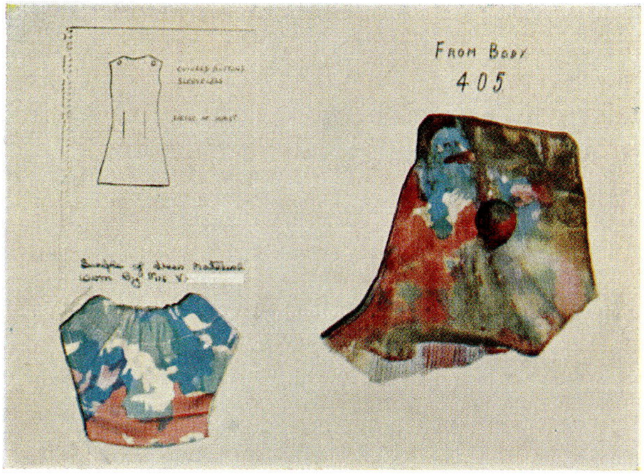


*Fig.* 70.—A fragment of dress taken from the victim of an aircraft accident, compared with a specimen of material taken from the passenger's home by a neighbour. The two pieces of material clearly match but previous descriptions of the material over the telephone by the neighbour had led to the repeated dismissal of a tentative identification that eventually proved to have been correct.

Some days later a few bodies only remained to be identified; body number 405 had to be reconsidered as possibly that of Mrs. 'J'. Twice more telephoned descriptions of the dress that this passenger had worn were taken to rule out the identification. Because of the persistent inquiries, however, the neighbour concerned went to the casualty's home, obtained a sample of the material she had been trying to describe and a pattern of the dress and sent these to us. One glance was sufficient to confirm the suspected identity of body number 405 (*Fig.* 70).

I have found that a relative's telephoned description of clothing worn by a passenger has frequently thrown doubts on the correctness of a tentative identification; if it is possible to show the relative a sample of the material recovered from the body, instant recognition may confirm the suspected identity.

In a certain accident that involved a large number of schoolboys, the difficulty in differentiating between many children of the same age and sex was simplified because the trip had been planned for many weeks and the parents had seen the children off at the airport; the clothing that each child had worn was known and described in great detail. On the other hand an accident to an aircraft carrying adult tourists, including many husbands and wives flying between cities abroad, was one in which clothing was singularly unhelpful; in spite of the fact that much of it had been retained, relatives had little idea of what clothes the casualties possessed, much less what they had worn on the day of their death.

Especially careful examination of a badly incinerated body is necessary if important evidence of identity in the form of charred fragments of clothing is not to be overlooked. Such a body must be examined by one used to handling such specimens—a pathologist; a policeman cannot be regarded as adequately trained for such tasks. On one occasion a tiny charred fragment was recovered from the nape of the neck of a grossly incinerated cadaver; a careful examination with appropriate illumination showed it to bear a name tape. The name could be deciphered but this item of evidence was a clue—not proof of identity; it transpired that the shirt worn by this body had been borrowed from an elder brother. Borrowed garments, secondhand clothing, and clues derived from such small articles as handkerchiefs which can be transferred or misplaced easily are important sources of error in the work of identifying the bodies of the dead (Simpson, 1965).

No source of information about a victim which might help in the identification of his or her body should be overlooked. Loose property at the site of an accident may be of value in this regard. A male body clad in light blue jeans was tentatively identified on dental evidence following accident number 261; the dental evidence was not sufficiently strong to be considered conclusive. The parents of the man whose body it was thought to be said that their son owned a pair of blue jeans and that he had taken them on holiday with him; they were quite certain, however, that he would not have worn the jeans to travel but would have worn his dark brown suit instead. So sure were they about this that the tentative identification was not accepted until the passenger's suit case was recovered from the wreckage; it was found intact and relatively undamaged and contained the dark brown suit but not the jeans.

### Documents

A driving licence found in the jacket pocket of a male body from accident number 187 emphasized the importance of not accepting uncritically any circumstantial evidence of identity. The driving licence in the name of Mr. 'A' was the only document in the outside jacket pocket. Its discovery caused something of a minor stir among the investigators for only a few hours previously the body of Mr. 'A' had been identified with confidence, embalmed and coffined in preparation for repatriation. Quite quickly, however, more documents were found in other pockets; these were all in the name of Mr. 'R' and, in fact, ample additional evidence was found to establish the identity of the new body as that of passenger Mr. 'R'. It remained to explain the presence of the other passenger's driving licence in Mr. 'R's' pocket.

The two men were unknown to each other and had not sat near to one another in the aircraft. Those responsible for recovering the bodies insisted that they had not found the licence loose at the accident site and had not placed it in Mr. 'R's' jacket pocket. This denial was accepted without hesitation for there had been very good evidence throughout the investigation that those responsible for the search and recovery operation had been well trained and had carried out their work meticulously. The explanation for the anomaly was a matter for conjecture; just possibly the owner had dropped it from his wallet while in the toilet, Mr. 'R' had found it and put it in his pocket with the intention of handing it to the cabin staff but had had no opportunity to do this before the aircraft crashed. On many occasions I have examined bodies that have retained only small fragments of clothing and have had but one document in the sole remaining pocket; this case shows the caution that must be exercised before uncorroborated evidence of this type is accepted.

Documents found on a body may give only an indirect clue to its identity. A male body from accident number 261 was found to have in its possession a London Underground railway ticket with a name and address written on the back. When the person named was contacted it was found that she knew but one passenger on board the aircraft that had crashed; a tentative identification could therefore be made and subsequently ample confirmatory evidence was adduced. On another occasion (accident number 255) a partially burnt address book was said to have been found lying exposed on a charred body, apparently having come from an inside jacket pocket. Inquiries from several of the people listed in the address book made it clear that the book could have belonged only to one particular passenger. A tentative indentification was made but other evidence completely excluded the body in question as that of the owner of the book. It was later shown that the body of the owner of the book had been found on top of the body with which the book had been associated by those who had recovered the human remains.

### Jewellery and Other Personal Effects

The particular value of jewellery in the work of identification is obvious; although watches and necklaces are frequently broken and lost in an accident, they are sometimes retained on the body; rings are often inscribed or of distinctive design, resist mechanical damage and fire especially well and have been found most valuable as an aid to identification.

Difficulty sometimes occurs if all the close members of a family have perished in the same accident even though distinctive items of jewellery have been discovered. On these occasions clues present have to be followed up in much the same way as indirect clues in documents. For example, a female body in accident number 255 had a bangle with a variety of charms on one wrist; one charm was designed in the form of initials. A study of the passenger list showed that the initials corresponded with those of a man who had been travelling with his wife and daughter. Numerous inquiries of neighbours and friends of this family eventually produced the confirmatory evidence that the girl had among the charms on her bracelet one with her father's initials.

Keys have been helpful in providing indirect clues to identity on several occasions. The Automobile Association has helped by giving the name of the member to whom a numbered telephone-kiosk key had been issued (accident number 139); keys found in the coat pocket of a body in accident number 261 were shown to fit the front door of the passenger whose body it was thought to be; this confirmatory evidence made a tentative identification certain beyond any reasonable doubt.

As with clothing and documents, the examination of personal property and the follow-up of clues that derive therefrom are largely a matter for routine police work. However, as in the search for minute burnt fragments of clothing on a body, so occasionally it is only a specialist's examination which will detect other objects which can prove useful clues to identity. *Fig.* 71 shows a radiograph of an extremely traumatized headless and limbless torso. The curious moon-shaped object was sought by dissection and proved to be the fastener on a partially burnt wallet containing the remains of a cheque book; it was deeply embedded in the lacerated and charred muscle of the buttocks. It is very probable that this would not have been found but for the radiographic examination.

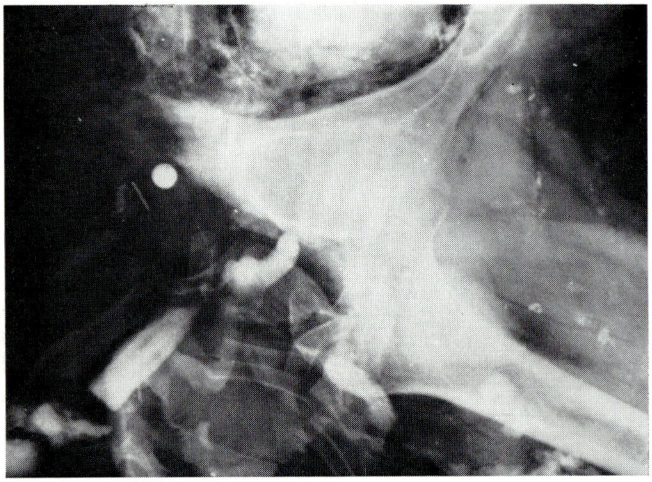

*Fig.* 71.—Radiograph of a badly mutilated and incinerated torso showing a peculiar full moon-shaped object. A search was made for this amid the charred muscle of the buttocks and a fragment of leather cheque-book case was found. The round object was the fastening stud. The recovered property led to the identification of these human remains. (*Reproduced from Stevens and Tarlton (1963) by permission of the co-author and the Editor 'Medicine, Science and the Law'.*)

Accident number 255 produced another example of the value of loose property found at an accident site. Body number 94 was found to be wearing a silver locket on a chain around the neck; the picture inside was of a bearded man. In a purse found among the wreckage was a photograph of the same man; other documents in the purse indicated the name of its owner and hence the probable identity of body number 94. Since this passenger's husband was also on the aircraft, the beard provided a useful clue to his body.

## MEDICAL EVIDENCE

Medical evidence of identity includes the sex of a body, an estimation of its age, stature, the colour of its skin, eyes, and hair and the demonstration of external identifying marks such as naevi, tattoos and traumatic or surgical scars. An internal examination may reveal a disease diagnosed in life; a body from accident number 187 was found to have Hodgkin's disease; this was the first clue to its identity and confirmatory evidence was not difficult to obtain. A detailed post-mortem examination on a partially incinerated body may reveal the presence of a post-surgical state although the scar of the operation may have been destroyed. The importance of all or most of these clues to the identity of a body is discussed in standard textbooks of forensic medicine; its further discussion and exemplification here is unnecessary although many examples are available in our material. One unusual problem was encountered, however, and deserves a brief comment, if only because it emphasizes once more that no evidence on any aspect of an aircraft accident can be accepted at what might be described as its face value.

*Fig.* 72 shows a body with male external genitalia but a prominently female configuration of the breasts, painted finger nails and shoulder-length dyed blonde hair. There were surgical scars on the lateral aspects of the breasts and palpation revealed

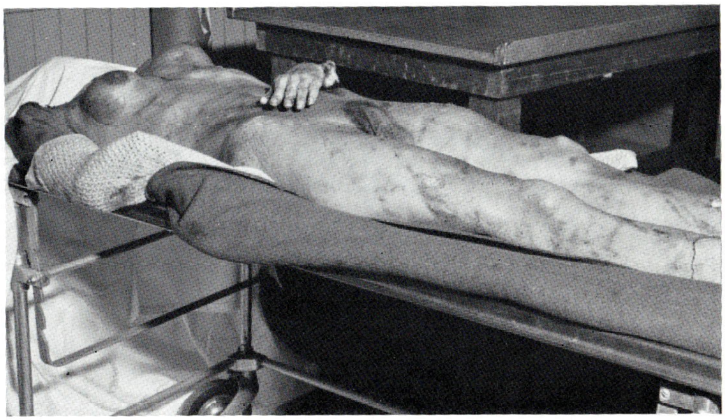

*Fig.* 72.—A body with male external genitalia. This body had been clothed in female garments, had long painted finger-nails and had had bilateral mammoplasty with prosthetic implants.

that their contour was maintained by pliable prostheses of some type (a dissection to discover the nature of these prostheses was not carried out). The body had been wearing female clothing. There were four other transvestites on board this aircraft; some had worn only female clothing and some female underclothes beneath male external garments. Had these and other bodies from this accident been traumatically bisected—and mechanical trauma of this extent is by no means uncommon in aircraft accidents—the problem of matching the separated halves, making a correct total count of the male and female bodies recovered and a satisfactory comparison with the passenger list could have been considerable.

## RADIOGRAPHY

The value of radiography (other than dental radiography) in the identification of the dead has been reported on numerous occasions both for a single body or small groups of bodies arising from crime (Beddoe, 1956; Greulich, 1960) and large numbers of bodies that have resulted from a mass disaster (Singleton, 1951; Brown, Delaney, and Robinson, 1952; Demy, 1963). The cranial air-sinuses may have very characteristic outlines in a particular individual (Culbert and Law, 1927; Schuller, 1943) but this is of limited value in the context of air crashes where gross damage to the skull is common.

I have not found it necessary to use radiographic evidence to any great extent to identify victims of aircraft accidents; on a few occasions radiographs have been used to assess age; in children especially, films of the carpus, the knee, the hip, and elbow can be helpful in this respect. It is important, nevertheless, to keep in mind the potential value of radiography to produce specific evidence of identity; if facilities permit, there is much to be said in favour of the systematic radiographic examination of every cadaver as suggested by Fully, Coblentz, Dessertine, and Dérobert (1965). I would be inclined, however, to restrict the procedure to those bodies that appear likely to prove difficult to identify because of the extent of damage by mechanical trauma and fire, both to the body itself and its associated possessions, and to those occasions when full radiographic examination of all casualties is required as part of a search for evidence of sabotage (Chapter 5).

The case of light aircraft accident number 207 demonstrates that radiographic evidence can occasionally prove to be a useful and reliable sole means of identification. An unclothed, headless and limbless body was washed up on the seashore some twelve weeks after the accident. Post-mortem radiographs of this body were compared with ante-mortem films of the missing pilot. The radiologist (Stevens, 1966b) reported that there were so many points of similarity that a positive identification was beyond any reasonable doubt, an opinion that was accepted by the coroner and his jury at the subsequent inquest.

## FINGER-PRINTS

Finger-prints have been of limited value in my experience of identification procedures following aircraft accidents. It is not always possible or easy to obtain prints from the victim of an aircrash; hands may be amputated and missing completely; the soft tissues of the fingers may be destroyed by fire. If there is less than complete destruction, however, it may be possible to obtain satisfactory prints, either from partially desquamated epidermis or by the use of special techniques (Brown, Delaney, and Robinson, 1952; Cunha, 1952).

Often no records are available for comparison with the finger-prints of a cadaver; in the United Kingdom only criminals and merchant seamen have their finger-prints recorded routinely. In the United States of America a high proportion of the population have their finger-prints filed either by the Federal Bureau of Investigation or by one of the departments of an individual state; when an aircraft accident has involved American citizens, we have found finger-prints useful and the column in *Fig*. 65, p. 140 results almost entirely from the American subjects killed in the 13 accidents.

On two occasions I have asked the police to search the homes of an unidentified British passenger or member of aircrew for finger-prints to compare with those taken from an unidentified cadaver whose identity we have had some cause to suspect. On one occasion this proved helpful, on the other matching prints could not be found.

## SEROLOGY

The usefulness of blood grouping in the differential identification of passengers killed in an aircraft accident has been described by Frache, Carella, Murino, and Fucci (1954). I have had little experience of this means of identification and have not required to test its value in the majority of large aircraft accidents. On the one occasion that it appeared possible that the knowledge of a particular body's blood group might help, it was not possible to group the tissues because of interfering substances produced by bacterial growth during post-mortem putrefaction (Dodd, 1966). The body that was identified by radiographic means several weeks after a light aircraft accident proved to be of blood group B. The wife of the pilot whose body it was thought to be could not help very much; she thought that her husband had been of blood group B but was not certain; all attempts to find documentary evidence of his blood group failed.

# *Chapter 22*

# THE IDENTIFICATION OF THE DEAD—II

## DENTAL EVIDENCE

### INTRODUCTION

FORENSIC odontology has been a recognized specialty in Scandinavia for many years. In Norway since 1948 an identification commission comprising at least a policeman, a doctor (usually a pathologist) and a dentist has been appointed by a prefect of police whenever the necessity has arisen by reason of a mass disaster or crime (Keiser-Nielsen, Frykholm, and Strøm, 1964). Although the value of dental evidence in the identification of the dead has been recognized for many years (Reid, 1884; Thompson, 1897; Amoëdo, 1899; Humble, 1933; Schirnding, 1934) and in more recent years has been the subject of many reports including those of Van Leeuwen (1948); Simpson (1951); Grant, Prendergast, and White (1952); Strøm (1954); Wyckoff (1957); Pedersen and Keiser-Nielsen (1961); and Keiser-Nielsen, Frykholm, and Strøm (1964), it is only in very recent times that forensic odontology has excited more than sporadic interest among dentists in Britain, but a number of local forensic odontological study groups have now been formed such as that based on the Dental Hospital, Liverpool. It was not until 1966 that a book on forensic odontology appeared in English—and even then the author was a Scandinavian, Gustafson (1966a).

In British aircraft accident investigation during the years covered by this report, it has fallen to the aviation pathologist to make a study of dental evidence as an aid to identification; in the earlier years the invitation for a Royal Air Force pathologist to participate in civilian aircraft accident investigation was something of an experiment; any suggestion that a dentist should be included in the team would certainly have been received with little enthusiasm.

It is difficult to refute the assertion by Sims (1968a) that the subject of forensic odontology is extremely complex and that 'there is no place for the amateur, no matter how enthusiastic'; however, the histogram (*Fig.* 65, p. 140) shows that despite the absence of a qualified dentist, dental evidence has been the most useful single means of effecting identification in my series of victims from aircraft accidents. Furthermore there is no doubt that the enthusiastic amateur is to be preferred to the disinterested expert such as the dentists in two cases described by Gustafson (1966c). It was my misfortune to go to an accident abroad and find on my arrival that eight dentists were already engaged upon the examination of the dental evidence in the cadavers. Working concurrently with the local pathologists, they completed their examinations and records within 48 hours. During the succeeding days both local and British pathologists agreed upon the identities of certain bodies from the sum of various items of non-dental evidence; these bodies, their examination completed, were embalmed and sealed in lead-lined coffins for repatriation.

Before these coffins had been despatched, dental documents of many of the passengers and crew were received by the investigating team and it so happened that some of the records received in the first batch related to bodies already identified. As a precaution these ante-mortem records were compared with the dental evidence found by the dentists in the already identified bodies; in two or three instances there was complete disagreement. For example, one passenger's dental records stated that she had had several teeth extracted and that several other teeth had amalgam restorations. The dental findings recorded in the body identified as hers were 'all teeth present except for four third molars; no restorations present'. The coffin had to be opened and the teeth re-examined. The dental state was found to be as recorded in the passenger's ante-mortem records and not as recorded by the dentists examining the cadaver. After the discovery of several more incorrect recordings of the dental state of the cadavers, it became clear that it was necessary to check all the work done by the eight dentists.

It transpired that there was an explanation though not an excuse for their inefficiency. Apparently the general standard of dental records in the country in question was poor and the dentists could not believe that the unpleasant task that they had been given was going to be of any value whatsoever in the identification of the casualties. It was a very considerable surprise to them when they found the relatively high standard of the dental records that were received from Britain.

I believe that it is important to distinguish between two different problems. The first is the identification of one or more bodies the likely origin of which is completely obscure. It is probable in these circumstances that they will be associated with crime or suspected crime; the potential importance of the finer and more subtle points of evidence to be adduced from an examination of the teeth and jaws are such that the skill required will be beyond the capabilities of a non-dentally trained person; the expertise of a forensic odontologist will be highly desirable if not essential. The second problem is the differential identification of bodies from a limited group, the composition of which is known with complete or almost complete certainty; the competence required in the examination of the teeth in this context is likely to be, in my opinion, well within the capabilities of any interested forensic pathologist.

## Dental Nomenclature

Frykholm and Lysell (1962) reviewed the many systems used by dentists to record teeth and tooth surfaces. They discussed more than a dozen different notations for permanent teeth, an even larger number for deciduous teeth and five systems for indicating tooth surface. In some countries, such as America, several of these systems are in current use; in Britain only one system is found. It can be confusing when dealing with a mass disaster in which people of many nationalities are involved, to receive telegraphed dental information based on a variety of nomenclatures.

Zsigmondy's system is used in Britain; in this the teeth are numbered in each quadrant from 1 to 8 from the central incisor to the third molar. When a particular tooth is referred to in manuscript the number is placed in an angular symbol to indicate the quadrant in question. This has the great disadvantage that the angle cannot be spoken simply and cannot be transmitted by ordinary telegraph or typed without a special typewriter. Early in this work I adopted the Haderup nomenclature as recommended by the International Dental Federation. In the Haderup system, the teeth are numbered from 1 to 8 in each segment from the central incisor to the third molar as in Zsigmondy's system; the upper jaw is indicated by the '+' sign and the lower jaw by the '—' sign. The right upper segment is indicated by the '+' sign appearing after the tooth number and the left upper segment by the '+' sign appearing in front of the tooth number. Similarly the '—' after a number indicates the right mandibular segment, the '—' in front of a number indicates the lower left segment. I have used this system to record the dental findings in cadavers; it is particularly useful when dictating to an assistant. When necessary, dental information received in any other nomenclature has been 'translated' into the Haderup system for purposes of comparison.

### Comparison of Dental Records with Dental Evidence in Cadavers

Dental identifications are most frequently made simply by finding similarities between the teeth present and restorations recorded in a known person's chart and those present in an unidentified cadaver. *Fig*. 73 shows a case in which no less than

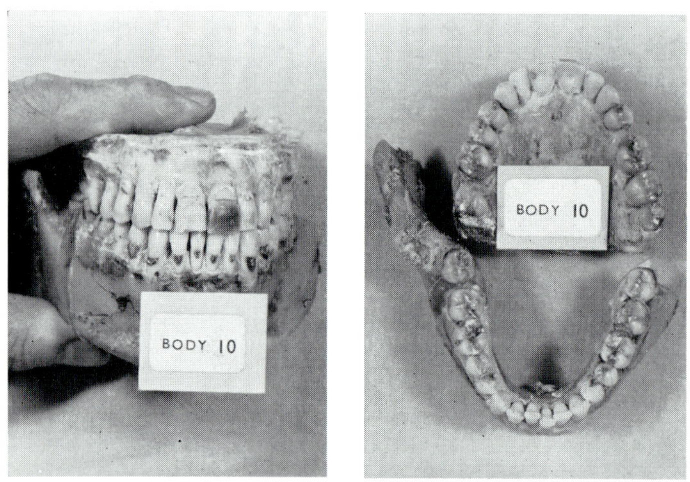


*Fig*. 73.—Views of the jaws of a cadaver in which 52 amalgam restorations in the teeth matched the ante-mortem records available of a certain passenger believed to have been on board the aircraft.

52 amalgam restorations were found in a body and these could all be matched in the dental records of a certain passenger; there were no discrepancies and a positive identification was absolutely certain. Such strong evidence is rarely obtained; far fewer similarities are usually present between records of the known person and the findings in the unknown body.

It is impossible to state precisely what number or combination of similarities constitute acceptable evidence of identification—each case must be judged on its merits. Wyckoff (1957) said that should there be several similarities in restorations by teeth and surfaces between the findings in the unknown and the known person's records, then, even though those restorations be in commonly filled teeth, their combination may be accepted as strong evidence in making an identification. It is important that dental evidence should not be considered in isolation but rather in combination with other evidence of the various types that have been discussed; the fewer the number of points of similarity in the dental evidence, the greater the need for other confirmatory evidence.

In 202 (86 per cent) of 235 occasions when simple comparison of dental evidence in a cadaver with passengers' or crews' records suggested the possibility of a correct match, the number of points of similarity exceeded 7; on only 8 of the 33 occasions when there were 7 or less points of similarity, was the dental evidence the only available evidence for consideration. On these 8 occasions the relatively few points of similarity were either sufficiently distinctive or their combination sufficiently unusual for the evidence to be considered strong enough for a confident identification.

For example, only three small fragments of jaw were found in body number 38 from accident number 261. As is seen in the chart (*Fig.* 74) the upper third molars had

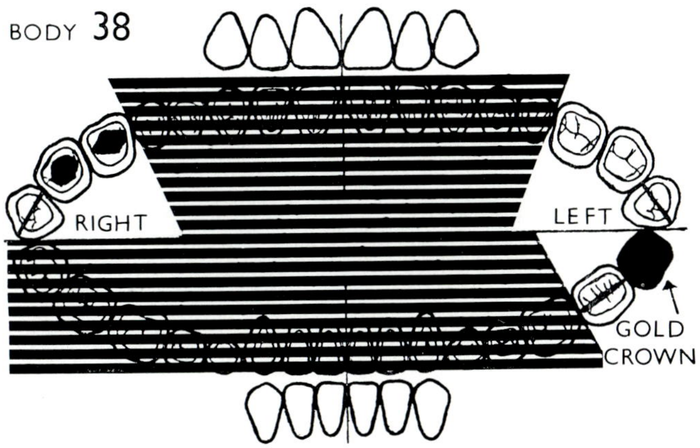


*Fig.* 74.—The findings in the fragmented jaws of an aircraft accident victim. There were four points of similarity between these findings and the dental information supplied about a particular passenger. It was considered that the three particular missing teeth and the gold crown on the third molar was a sufficiently distinctive combination to be acceptable evidence of identity in this case.

been extracted; the upper first and second molars were all present, those on the right having occlusal fillings; the left lower third molar had a gold crown and the left lower second molar had been extracted. It was unfortunate that one of the passenger's dentist had read of her death in the newspaper, had extracted her record card from his file in case it should be needed but it was inadvertently destroyed by an assistant. However, the dentist was able to say with certainty from memory that the passenger had had the two upper third molars and the lower left second molar extracted, that he had prepared a gold crown for the left lower third molar and that the other upper molars were present—but he could not say whether they had any fillings. Confirmation of most of this was obtained from the records of the Dental Estimates Board. There were, therefore, four points of similarity between the information about this passenger's mouth and the findings in body number 38. It was considered that the combination of three named missing teeth and a gold crown on a third molar was sufficiently strong evidence of identity in the circumstances. There was some additional support for this conclusion in that no other gold restoration was found in any other victim's mouth and this was the only female passenger whose records showed a gold crown on a molar.

The use of dental evidence in my experience of aircraft accident investigations has been almost entirely comparative and not reconstructive since the former is the process particularly applicable to the differential identification of known groups, the latter of

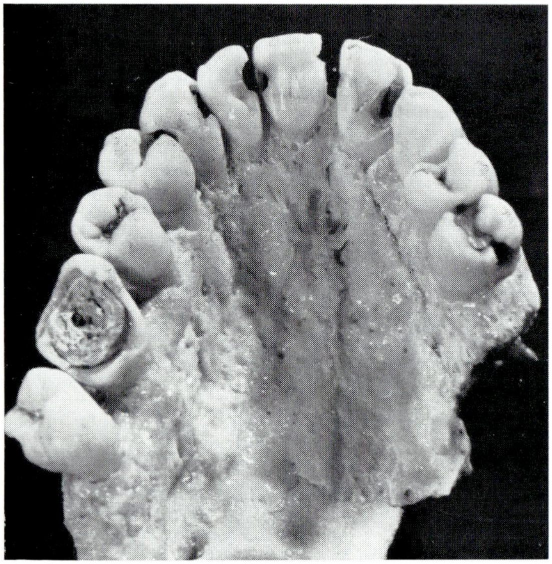

*Fig*. 75.—Appearances in a mouth that suggest that ante-mortem records will not be available. Useful dental evidence may nevertheless be forthcoming in such a case and efforts to obtain it should not be abandoned too quickly.

greatest value in relation to completely unknown bodies. However, some people just do not attend dentists, or if they do, only in emergency. When one finds a jaw such as is shown in *Fig*. 75, there is little hope that matching dental records of a known person will be discovered. Nevertheless, this should not deter one from seeking dental information about a person who rarely attends a dentist.

In accident number 231, body number 107 was thought possibly to be that of passenger 'H'. The jaws showed very gross caries in most of the remaining teeth. A dentist sent information to the effect that he had no dental records of 'H'; it was true that 'H' was nominally one of his patients as were all 'H's' family, but 'H' had not attended the surgery for several years. On being telephoned and asked for further help, the dentist could say that when last seen, 'H' had had all his front teeth present, all badly nicotine-stained, but that most of the molars and premolars had been grossly carious and in several instances only roots had remained. The account was so close a description of the state in the mouth of body number 107, that it was taken as confirmatory evidence of its identity.

Although the dentist is the prime source of information about a person's dental state, relatives or friends may be able to contribute valuable evidence about characteristics in the front teeth; even a photograph of the person smiling may be of help (Knott, 1967).

### Inconsistencies between the Chart of a Known Person and the Findings in a Cadaver

There may be several points of similarity between the records of a known person and the findings in an unknown body but there may also be, indeed there often are, inconsistencies. Inconsistencies may be of two types; those compatible with a positive identification and those incompatible with a positive identification.

Fillings present in the mouth of a cadaver but not shown in a known person's record are not *a priori* evidence to bar a positive identification. It is quite common practice for a dentist examining a new patient to record only the teeth missing in that patient's mouth and to ignore any fillings already present; any fillings the dentist himself subsequently inserts are recorded. Even a tooth missing in the unknown but not recorded as extracted in the known person's chart is a compatible inconsistency, particularly if the last recorded visit to the dentist on the known person's chart is some considerable time before the accident; another dentist may well have extracted the tooth as an emergency.

Wyckoff (1957) commented about incompatible inconsistencies as follows: 'it is mandatory that there be no incompatibilities such as restorations in the dental records of the known which do not exist in the unknown casualty if a positive identification is to be acceptable, nor any teeth present in the cadaver which are reported as extracted in the dental records of the known'. This is a sound basic principle but from time to time the total evidence in favour of a positive dental identification is so overwhelming that an incompatible inconsistency as defined by Wyckoff (1957) has to be disregarded; but this should not be done lightly. An example of the problem occurred in accident number 151.

Body number 6 was thought possibly to be that of a coloured passenger on the basis of three small areas of scorched but apparently pigmented skin found on the trunk and the soles of the feet of an otherwise charred corpse. A tentative identification was made by exclusion since only one man of a dark-skinned race was on board the aircraft. There were eight points of similarity between the restorations present in the cadaver and restorations or cavities charted in the records of the coloured passenger ('S.B.') (*Fig.* 76). There were, however, certain inconsistencies; a filling recorded on the mesial aspect of the lower right first molar and one on the distal aspect of the lower right second premolar in 'S.B.'s' chart was not found in the body of the unknown and neither was a cavity recorded on the mesial aspect of the lower left second premolar. The absence of a cavity or a restoration at the site of the recorded cavity in the lower left second premolar was easily discounted; it is reasonably common for a dentist to think that his probe has caught in a very early cavity, to mark it on the record as such so that it may be checked at the next visit and dealt with if necessary. However, the inconsistencies in the right mandible were more important and additional evidence had to be sought to try to confirm or negate the identification.

The unknown body had all 32 teeth present (*Fig.* 77). 'S.B.'s' records showed that he had had all 32 present one year before his death. The arch in the unknown was very good with good spacing of teeth and no tendency to crowding. A faint line of discoloration was noted along the gingival margins resembling the melanin deposition found at that site in many coloured races (Jakobsen, 1967). The dental findings in all the other male bodies recovered from this accident excluded any of them as being that of passenger 'S.B.' with one exception; there was good alternative evidence, however, that this one exception could not possibly be that of 'S.B.'

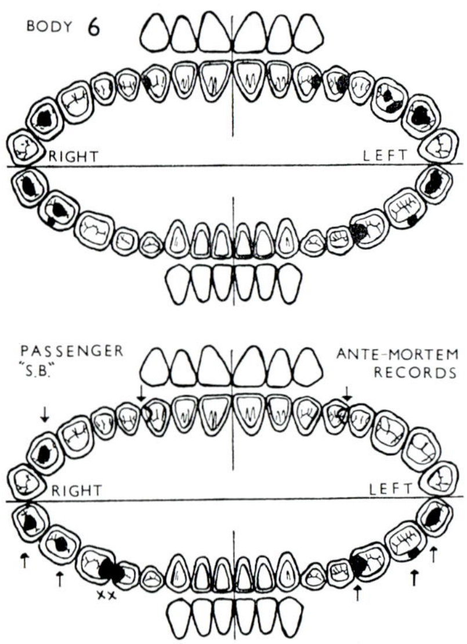


*Fig.* 76.—Post-mortem findings in body number 6 from accident number 151 compared with the chart of passenger 'S.B.'. There were eight points of similarity (arrowed) but there were two apparently incompatible inconsistencies (marked xx) in the lower right premolar and first molar.

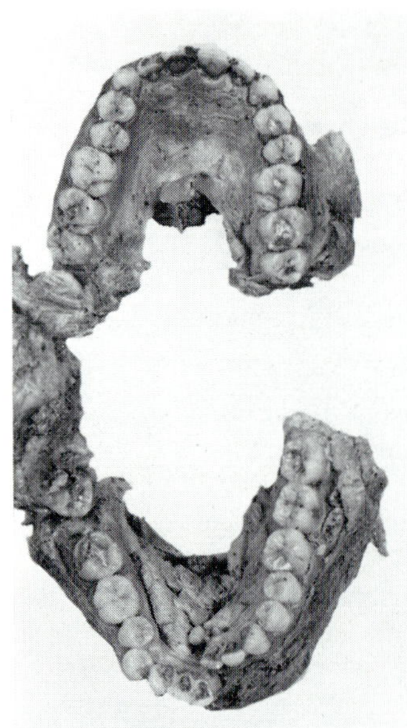

*Fig.* 77.—The jaws of body number 6 showing all 32 teeth present. There is a good arch and little tendency to crowding of teeth.

On the basis therefore of several points of similarity, the appearances suggestive of pigmented skin, the proof of quite marked melanin deposition in the gingiva (*Fig.* 78), the racial characteristics of a good dental arch and no extractions having been necessary by the age of about 25 and exclusion by dental and other means of other bodies as that of 'S.B.', it was concluded that the incompatible inconsistencies in the lower mandible should be discounted as clerical errors or errors having resulted in some other way.

It is necessary, therefore, to accept on occasion that dental records are erroneous; sometimes they are truly incorrect and sometimes they are merely misinterpretations as the following example shows. After accident number 261 the family was asked for the dental record of a certain passenger in her late twenties. The passenger's dentist was deceased but records were somehow obtained by the family and another dentist, a friend of the family, was asked to telephone the information in the records to the investigating team. Evidence from the clothing on a certain body quite strongly suggested that it belonged to the passenger in question; comparison of the telephoned dental records with the findings in the cadaver matched in respect of four fillings in commonly filled teeth but there was an important discrepancy. The upper left second premolar was reported as extracted in the passenger's chart but it was present in the cadaver; indeed all eight premolars were present in the cadaver and so a mirror-image charting error was not a possible explanation.

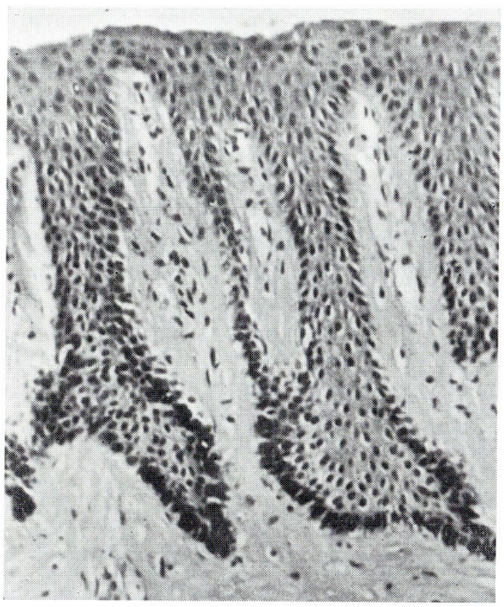

*Fig.* 78.—A section of the gingiva from body number 6. There is a lot of melanin in the basal layer. H. & E. (× 100.)

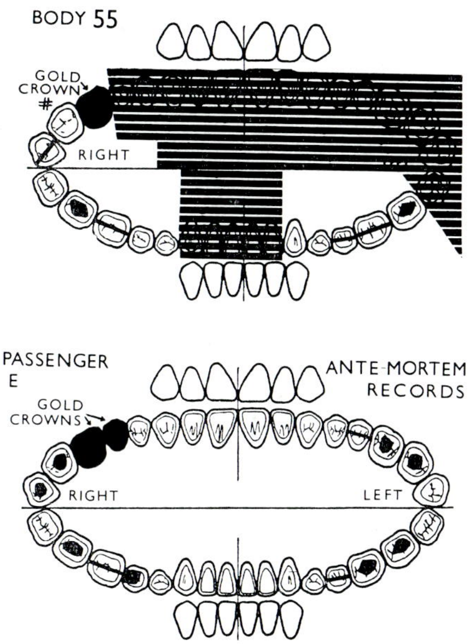


*Fig.* 79.—The dental findings in body 55 from accident 222 compared with the dental records of passenger 'E'. There was an incompatible inconsistency in the lower right second premolar.

The dentist who transmitted the information was contacted again and questioned more closely; he insisted that the records were precisely as he had stated and that there could be no confusion. He was asked to search the documents for a written note as to the date of the extraction; he then discovered that it had been when the passenger had been in her late teens and the written note indicated that the tooth that had been extracted was a retained deciduous second molar and not, as appeared to be from the pictorial chart, a permanent second premolar.

Retained deciduous molars are not very uncommon but they are sufficiently unusual to be an important clue to identity when present. An example of this occurred in accident number 222 when a much-filled deciduous molar in body number 65 was not immediately identifiable on ordinary inspection but was detectable on a radiograph; on extraction it was found to consist largely of the crown, the roots having been resorbed. Although it was not so in this case, a deciduous molar is often retained when a permanent premolar is congenitally absent; this characteristic may be familial and could, therefore, in certain circumstances, be an indirect clue to the identity of a body even though dental records of the person concerned could not be obtained.

An incompatible inconsistency occurred in a case from accident number 222. Passenger 'E's' brother claimed that he recognized a ring taken from body number 55 but as it was a plain ring he could have been mistaken. Only small fragments of jaw were found in body number 55 but there were similarities in these and 'E's' dental records (*Fig.* 79) in respect of two extracted teeth, two amalgam fillings and a gold

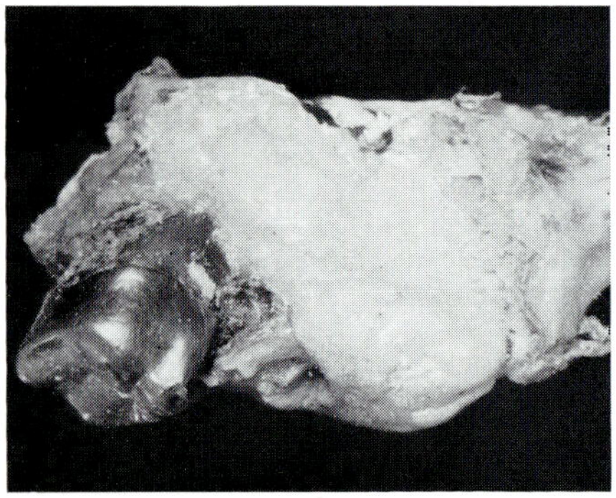

*Fig.* 80.—Fragment of the right maxillary molar region of body 55 showing a gold crown on a molar and a fractured molar which was apparently angled forwards.

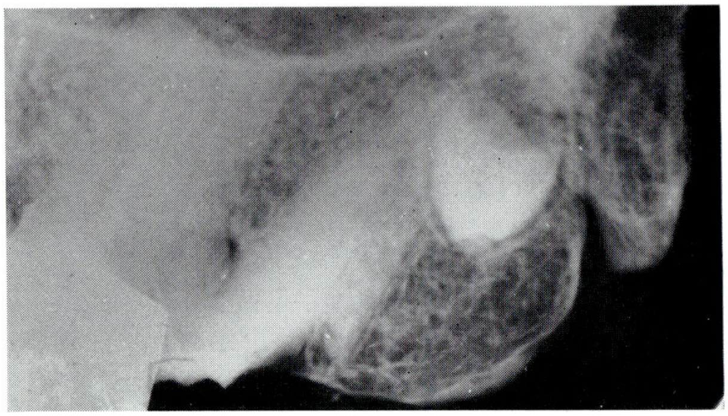

*Fig.* 81.—A radiograph of the fragment shown in *Fig.* 80. An apparently unerupted third molar can be seen. It could be that the crowned tooth was the first molar, the fractured tooth the second and that the third molar was unerupted. An alternative interpretation was that the crowned tooth was the first molar, the second molar had been extracted a long time previously, the third molar had erupted, had angled and drifted forwards and had been fractured in the accident and the unerupted tooth was a rudimentary supernumerary molar.

crown, on the upper right first molar (*Fig.* 80). The upper right second molar was shown in 'E's' chart to have an occlusal filling but this tooth appeared to have been broken in the accident.

The upper right third molar was shown in 'E's' records to have an occlusal filling and the lower right second premolar a disto-occlusal filling. A radiograph showed an unerupted upper right third molar (*Fig.* 81) and the lower left second premolar was perfectly healthy; there were, therefore, two important incompatible inconsistencies.

It could be argued that the unerupted tooth seen in *Fig.* 81 was a rudimentary supernumerary molar, that the original third molar could have erupted and had an occlusal filling and that it was the fractured tooth seen in *Fig.* 80, and that the second molar had been extracted some considerable time previously (the fractured tooth does look as though it may have been angled forwards in both *Figs.* 80 and 81). However, if it were concluded that the second molar had been extracted a long time before, this merely replaced one incompatibility by another though a less serious one. In any case, whatever the conclusion about the right maxillary molars, there was still the problem of the filling not found in the mandibular premolar. In due course, further non-dental evidence was discovered to prove that body number 55 was that of passenger 'E'. The dental inconsistencies were best explained by the dentist who, when questioned on the subject, explained that 'E' and three of his brothers were all his patients; it was quite probable, he thought, that their records had been mixed up!

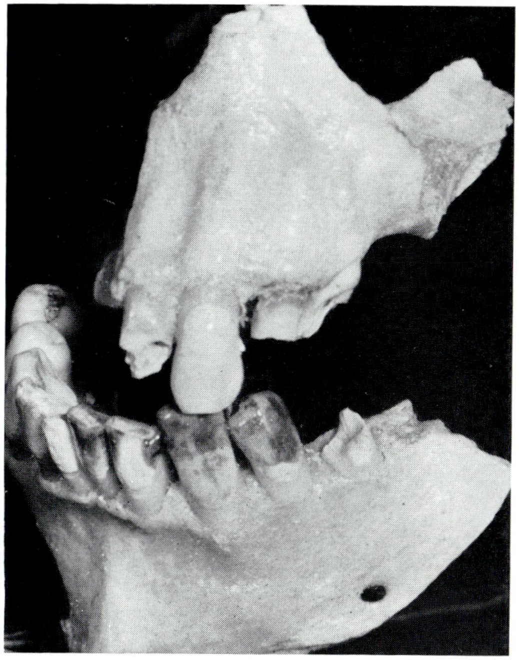

*Fig*. 82.—Fragments of jaw of body 18 from accident 231. Although the left mandible was fractured behind the second premolar, it was possible to see that the first molar had been missing.

### Difficulties encountered with Molars

The charting of molars is a frequent source of error, both for the practising dentist and, to some extent, for those engaged in the charting of teeth in cadavers for identification purposes. The first, second, and third molars have typical morphological characteristics and differ in maxilla and mandible. Variations occur and, particularly if the teeth have been subjected to extensive restorative work, it may be difficult to identify them accurately when less than three are present in one quadrant. If a second molar is removed the gap tends to close due to the drifting forwards of the third molar; after a time it may be difficult to decide whether it is the first and second or the first and third molars that are present. Some dentists are particularly careful to try to chart these teeth accurately; even the most meticulous may be misled as is shown by the following example.

Body number 18 from accident number 231 was thought to be possibly that of one of the pilots; there were similarities between the findings in fragments of the jaws and the records of that pilot. In particular, there were two amalgam fillings in the lower right first premolar and a silicate restoration in the right upper canine all on the appropriate teeth surfaces. There was one important inconsistency; although the left mandible was fractured behind the second premolar it was possible to see that the first molar had been missing and presumably extracted for some time (*Fig*. 82). The pilot's dental record showed the first molar to be present; furthermore, quite extensive restorative work had been performed on it only a few weeks previously. Discussion of this inconsistency with the dentist concerned over the telephone produced a firm statement to the effect that, if the lower left second molar was missing in the jaw, it was most definitely not the jaw of his pilot patient. Nevertheless, the dentist agreed to examine the specimen himself. On doing so he immediately recognized the shape of the arch of the upper jaw; on comparing the shading of the silicate in the canine with his records of that used on his patient he found that they matched; he recognized the amalgam fillings in the lower right first premolar as his own work. He somewhat reluctantly admitted that he must have been mistaken about the left lower first molar; it must have been extracted many years before he was first consulted by the patient; the second and third molars must have drifted forwards and angled forwards to such an extent that, with the crown of the second molar touching the crown of the second premolar, they had appeared to him to be the first and second molars.

### Recent Extractions

Complete healing of the socket of an extracted tooth takes many weeks; a radiographic assessment of the age of a recent extraction is possible (Mangos, 1941). Whenever, therefore, there is a history of a passenger or a member of air crew having had an extraction in recent weeks, the finding of a tooth socket of appropriate age is very important evidence in establishing the body's identity. Only one such instance has occurred in the accidents I have investigated.

### Anatomical Abnormalities

Rarely have I found that dentists' records detail any intra-oral features other than the presence or absence of teeth and the presence and location of restorations and prostheses. In many mouths there are distinctive features; crowding of teeth may have resulted in prominent displacement of one or more; a patient may have an epulis, a fractured tooth, markedly hypoplastic third molars, or some other anatomical feature which, if note had been made in ante-mortem records, would be very important clues to the identity of the persons concerned.

It is appreciated that the making of detailed records is time consuming and that there are limits beyond which it is uneconomical and too inconvenient for the busy practising dentist to go; nor can one advocate that dentists consciously regard each patient as a potential candidate for a dental identification following his or her death in a disaster. Nevertheless, it is probably fair to say that a record of any especially prominent or distinctive abnormality would take but little of a dentist's time and should not be in any way regarded as wasted effort. *Fig*. 83 shows three fragments of jaw from aircraft casualties with anatomical or pathological perculiarities, a record of the existence of which would have greatly assisted in the identification of the bodies of the individuals concerned.

Not all dental records I have received have been deficient; several have been as detailed as anyone could wish. For example, on one occasion not only was the position and shape of each restoration clearly marked on the chart but the dentist supplied a summary of the dates each filling had been inserted, whether they had been polished

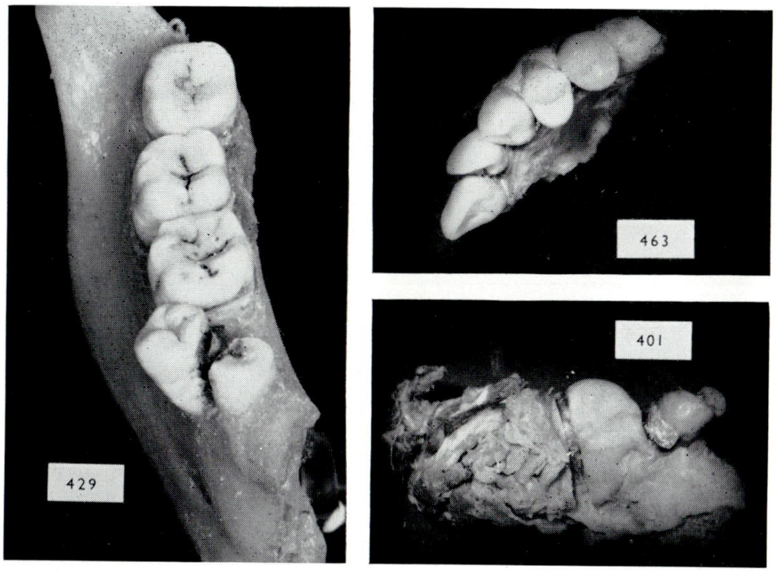


*Fig.* 83.—Three fragments of jaw from different bodies. In each there is an anatomical or pathological abnormality. Had these abnormalities been noticed in passengers' dental records they would have provided valuable evidence in the identification of their bodies. (*Reproduced in part from Stevens and Tarlton (1966) by permission of the co-author and the Editor 'British Dental Journal'.*)

and the dates upon which this had been done, a description of the mottling of the patient's teeth and the shades of the synthetic fillings he had inserted. There was a comment about the shape of the arch and the general regularity of the teeth; indeed there was little if anything about this mouth that could possibly have been helpful in identification about which we were not told.

## Distinctive Prostheses and Restorations

From time to time there are found in bodies dental restorations or prostheses which are very highly characteristic and in themselves provide very strong proof of identity whether the information about their presence in a particular person comes from professional records (*Figs.* 84 and 85) or even a relative or friend's description (*Fig.* 86). *Fig.* 87 shows an upper jaw from a middle aged female body; a son reported that he did not know which dentist his mother had attended but that she had had a prominent gap between her upper central front teeth and that she had worn an upper denture with only one artificial tooth—replacing one of the upper right front teeth. Such a description would be most unlikely to fit two people on the same aircraft; in the event (accident number 255) this evidence was used to identify one of only five female bodies remaining unidentified; the other four were easily excluded on this dental information and only one fitted the description.

When a person had become edentulous it is clearly more difficult to use the oral cavity as a means of identification unless dentures have been fitted and have been

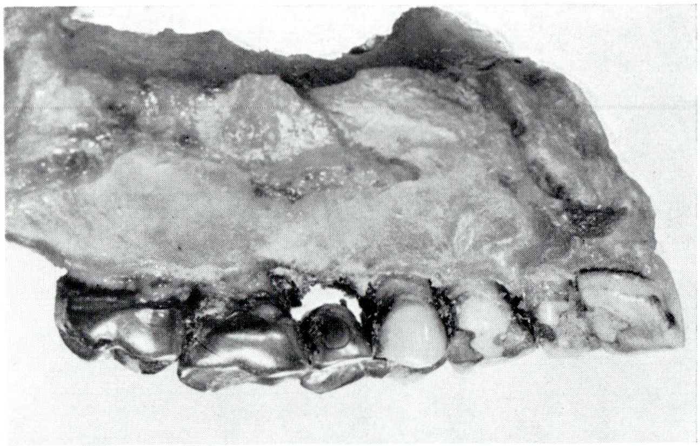

*Fig.* 84.—Distinctive gold crown and bridge work in a fragment of jaw which provided very strong proof of identity as a professional record of its presence in a known person was available.

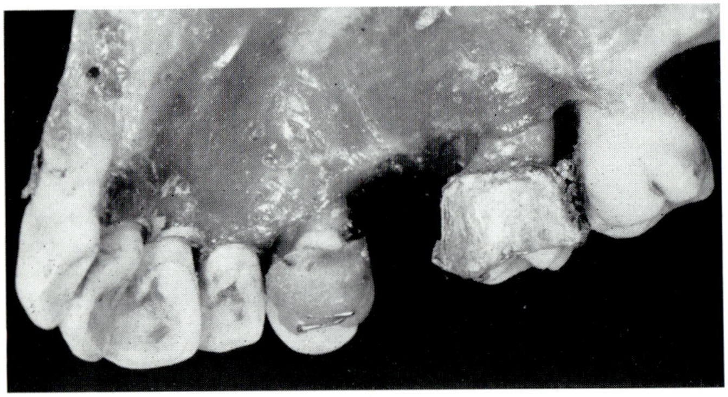

*Fig.* 85.—Another fragment of jaw with a highly distinctive combination of features. The first molar had been prepared for a crown and had a temporary aluminium ring around it; both premolars had been extracted and the gap had closed a little; the canine had a porcelain inlay. Professional records were available to compare with the findings in this body.

retained in the dead body and can themselves be used for identification purposes. Jerman and Miller (1968) stated that a survey in the U.S.A. in 1957 showed that almost one-third of people aged 35 years or more were without natural teeth; certainly a very large number of the victims of the air crashes we have investigated have been edentulous and there is no doubt that it would be of very considerable assistance to those engaged in the work of identification of the dead if a universal scheme of marking of dentures were adopted. A good deal of attention has been paid to this subject in recent years and to the need for such markings to resist destruction by the ravages of a disaster situation—in particular fire (Harvey, 1966; Jerman and Miller, 1968). Perhaps about a fifth of the bodies we were unable to identify (*Fig*. 65, p. 140) would have been identified if the dentures they wore had had identification marks.

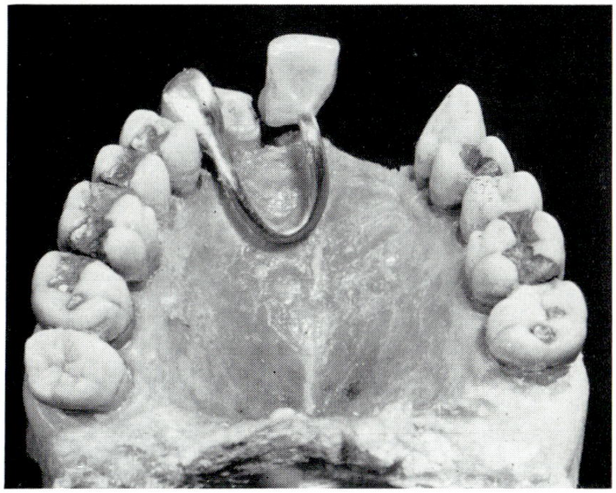

*Fig*. 86.—Another very distinctive prosthesis—a gold cantilever bridge involving a canine and an acrylic crown replacing a central incisor. Relatives were able to give a sufficiently accurate description of this distinctive prosthesis that professional records were not essential for identification purposes in this instance.

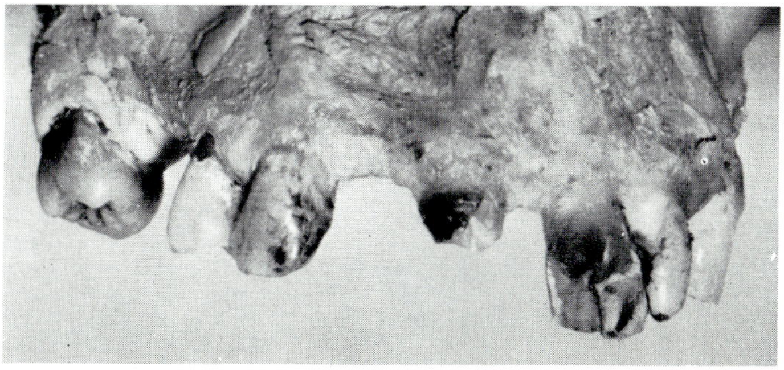

*Fig*. 87.—Body number 58 from accident number 255 was finally identified with the help of a passenger's son. He described a prominent central diastema in his mother's upper jaw and said that a lateral incisor was missing; she had worn a denture bearing a tooth in that position.

Most dentures are made of acrylic. Information, therefore, that a certain passenger on board an aircraft had had an upper denture the plate of which was made of metal, would be an important clue to the identity of any body found wearing such an appliance. Metal denture plates were found in two bodies in accident number 231. In the event one plate was gold and one white metal; full descriptions of each were obtained from the dentists who had supplied them. Questioning of relatives, had it been necessary, would probably have produced sufficiently reliable information about these dentures to distinguish between the two, not only on the basis of the type of metal used but from the teeth that they bore.

A knowledge of dental practices and materials used in different countries can often help to deduce the likely country of origin of an unknown body. While this is generally true, with the increasing migration of professional people, the type of restorative work in a cadaver's mouth may be more a clue to the origin of the dentist than his patient. There is no question but that the assessment of evidence of this type requires a true expert—a forensic odontologist.

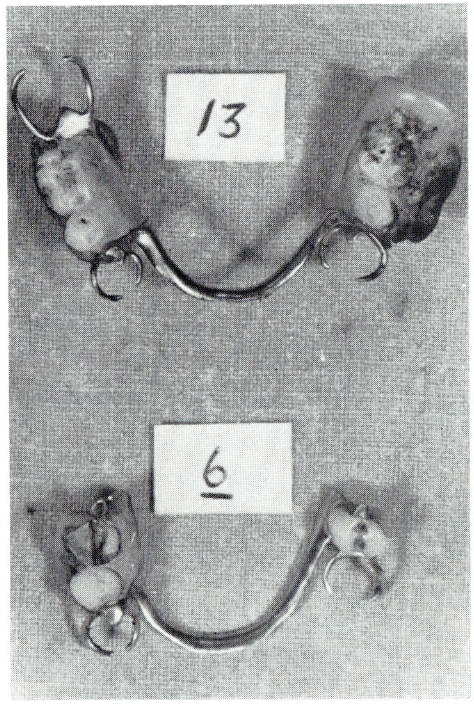


*Fig.* 88.—Comparison of dentures found in two bodies from the same accident. One proved to be British and the other American. An incorrect tentative identification was made at first because the appliance in what proved to be the British body was thought to be of American origin.

After one accident an American dentist was asked to examine the bodies and to identify the few Americans that were among the victims. He had information about some but not all of the passengers for whose bodies he searched. He was quickly successful in finding all but one; he had been given no information about the last body save that she wore a mandibular denture. He found that body number 6 had a denture which he judged was like many made in America and unlike those found in Europe; on this evidence alone he was allowed possession of the body. A few days later, having encountered some difficulty in identifying the remaining female body (number 13) as that of the only female passenger (a British lady) whose body had not been found, we found that body number 13 also had a denture (*Fig.* 88). Consultations between the American dentist and ourselves led to the identification of body number 13 and not body number 6 as that of the American; body number 6 was that of the British passenger.

Acrylic crowns are not uncommon; I have found several bodies from a single accident to have had one or more. They are nevertheless important clues in identification. It might be expected that they would be recognized quite easily—even by a pathologist. Not only have I missed one on initial examination of a mouth on a number of occasions but some of my dental colleagues have later made the same mistake when shown the same specimens; I like to consider that this speaks as much for the skill of the manufacturers of dental prostheses as for the lack of skill of the observers!

On one occasion it was necessary to retain certain specimens for further examination and, having no formol-saline available, I used some embalming fluid. When I examined the specimen some hours later I found an acrylic crown I had not originally noticed, stained bright blue. This had resulted from phenol and a dye that were present in the embalming fluid. I have tried to modify this serendipitous test for acrylic so that it could be used during an inspection of the teeth and jaws in situ in a cadaver. Unfortunately no paste or fluid I was able to prepare would react with sufficient speed to be of value; Midda (1969) has followed this up with more success and has described a disclosing spray which will demonstrate synthetic fillings or crowns speedily and reliably.

## Dental Radiographs

Dental radiographs are of immense value in the identification of the dead. To make an identification by simple comparison of the findings in the cadaver and ante-mortem records, it is usually necessary to have the whole jaws or large fragments available for examination unless, as discussed above, the fragments discovered have particularly distinctive features. If ante-mortem radiographs are available and post-mortem films are prepared from even a small fragment of jaw it may be possible to effect an identification which would be impossible with only naked-eye inspection of the teeth.

*Fig.* 89 shows what at first sight appeared to be two normal teeth in a badly broken and burnt mandible from a certain accident; closer examination after the removal of charred debris revealed specks of yellow metal at the base of the crown (*Fig.* 90). A radiograph showed that these normal-looking teeth consisted of a synthetic crown set on a metal post inserted into the root. Ante-mortem films were available from one of the pilots; on comparison of one of these films with the post-mortem radiograph a positive indentification was made with confidence (*Fig.* 91).

Films of a fragment of jaw from a body in accident number 187 compared with an ante-mortem radiograph of one of the passengers did not permit a confident identification although the appearances of the restoration were strongly suggestive of a true match. The outlines of the fillings did not quite coincide and although a difference in the angle of projection from which the films had been taken was a possible explanation, there remained an element of doubt. A careful perusal of the copious clinical notes supplied with the ante-mortem radiographs revealed a more satisfactory explanation; subsequent to the ante-mortem film, the fillings had been removed for recurrent caries and new fillings inserted. The outline of the new ones was naturally not quite the same as the original.

When there is very extensive damage to a skull from fire as well as mechanical trauma it may be necessary to search especially diligently for any fragments of jaw and teeth that remain. It may be necessary to reconstruct the jaw as far as possible and radiography of the reconstructed fragments may be helpful as in the following instance.

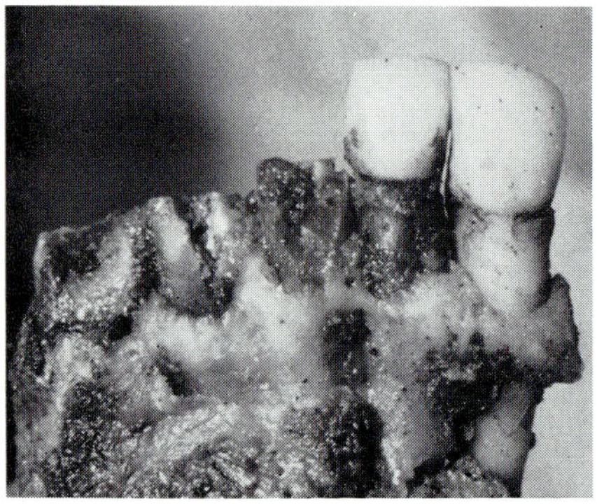

*Fig*. 89.—Two apparently normal teeth remaining in a fragmented and charred mandible. (*Reproduced from Stevens and Tarlton (1966) by permission of the co-author and the Editor 'British Dental Journal'*.)

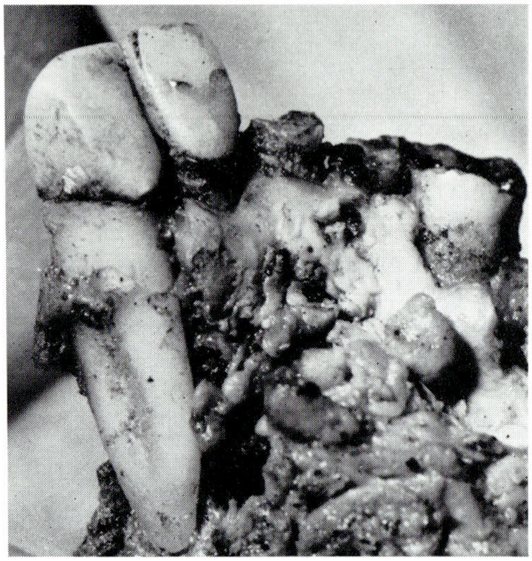

*Fig*. 90.—Another view of the specimen shown in *Fig*. 89. It can be seen that these were artificial crowns. (*Reproduced from Stevens and Tarlton (1966) by permission of the co-author and the Editor 'British Dental Journal'*.)

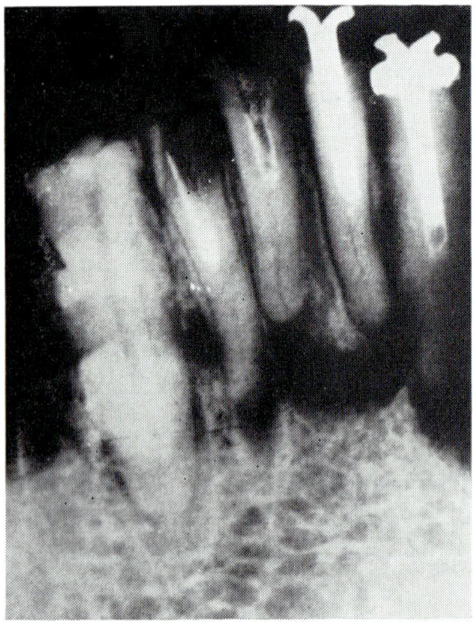

A

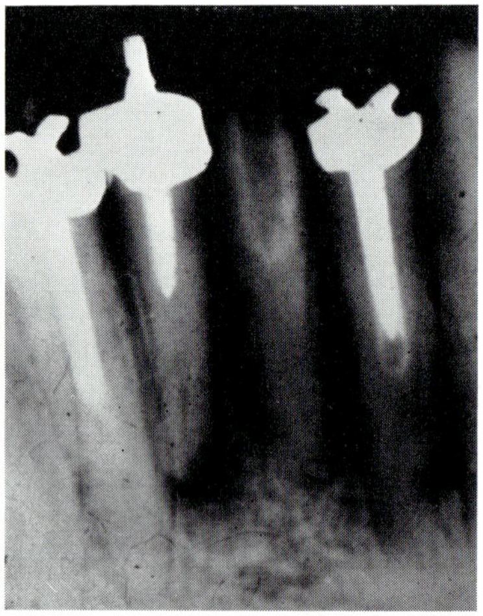

B

*Fig*. 91.—Comparison of: A, a radiograph of the specimen shown in *Fig*. 89, with B, an ante-mortem radiograph of a pilot taken a year before death. The appearances in the left lower lateral incisor provided unequivocal evidence of identity. (*Reproduced from Stevens and Tarlton (1966) by permission of the co-author and the Editor 'British Dental Journal'*.)

Body number 54 from accident number 255 was extensively destroyed; *Fig*. 92 shows all that remained of the skull. *Fig*. 93 shows the fragments of jaw that were recovered. Comparison of a radiograph of the upper left maxilla with the ante-mortem film of a certain passenger showed little resemblance. A possible explanation was that fire and

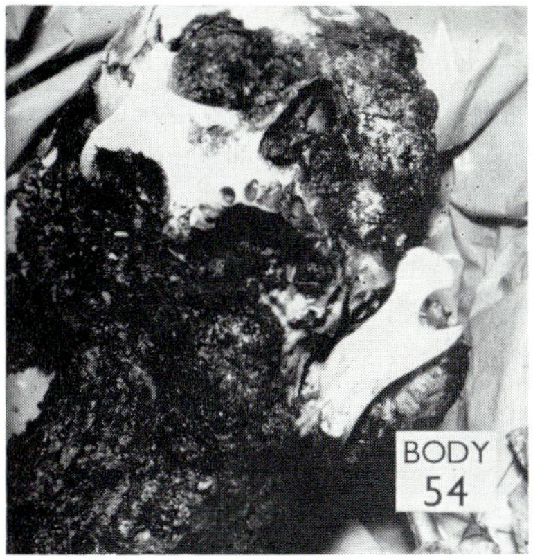


*Fig*. 92.—The charred remains of the skull of body 54 from accident number 255. (*Reproduced by permission of Professor Dr. J. Milčinski, Inštitut Za Sodno medicino, Ljubljana, Jugoslavia.*)

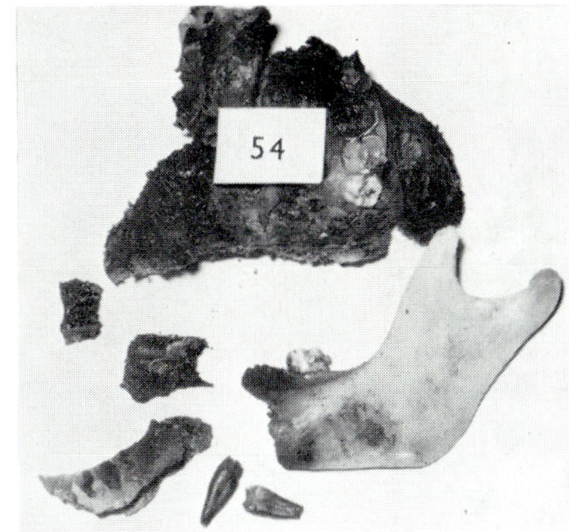


*Fig*. 93.—The fragments of jaws and teeth recovered from the head shown in *Fig*. 92.

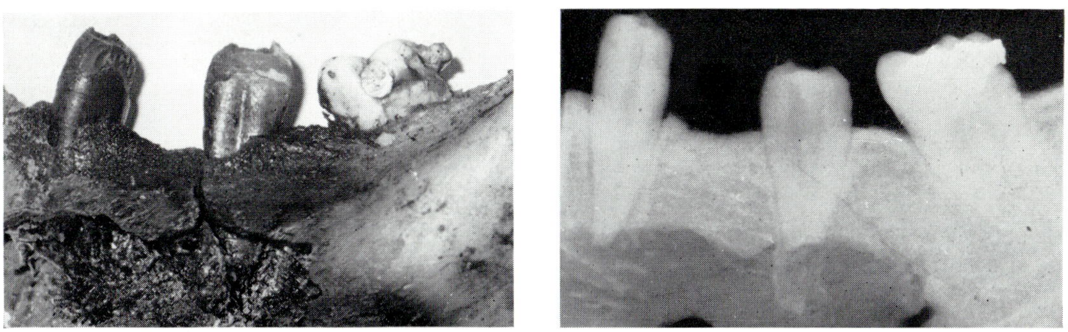

A B

*Fig*. 94.—A, Reconstruction of the mandibular fragments shown in *Fig*. 93, and B, a radiograph of the reconstructed specimen. A distinctive spacial disposition of the two premolars and the third molar is present.

trauma had resulted in the loss of fillings in the upper left premolar and molar area but this only provided an explanation for a failure in the match, not evidence to support a positive identification.

On reconstruction of the fragments of the lower jaw, a relatively unusual spacial disposition of the premolars and the third molar was discovered (*Fig*. 94); it had clearly resulted from the extraction many years before of the first and second molars. This spacial disposition matched the appearances in the ante-mortem film so closely that the fact that the restorations were not present in the premolars did not materially reduce the certainty of this identification; they had undoubtedly been lost as a result of the fire as had the fillings from the maxilla. Had it been considered necessary, detailed examination of the premolars in the laboratory would doubtless have proven that there had been fillings in these teeth.

Occasionally a radiograph of a fragment of jaw bearing a single tooth will be sufficient for a confident identification if an ante-mortem film is available for comparison (*Fig*. 95). So valuable are dental radiographs that dentists should be asked to supply

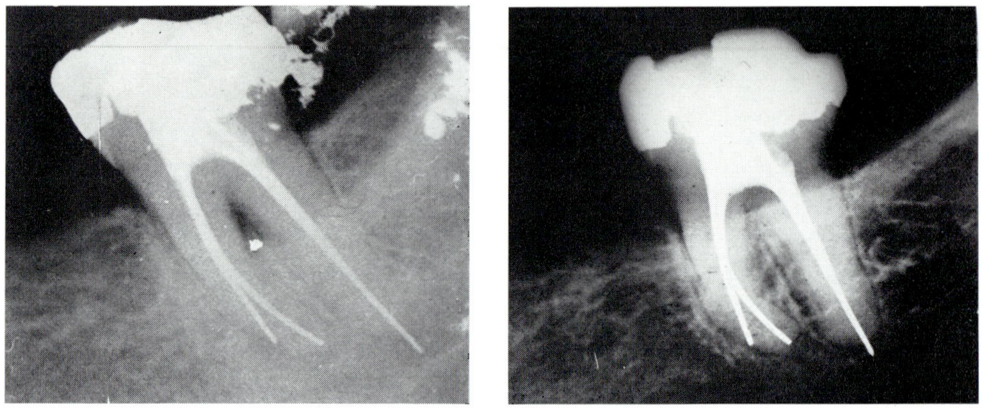

A B

*Fig*. 95.—Comparison of: A, a post-mortem radiograph of a fragment of jaw bearing a single tooth with B an ante-mortem film. It is difficult to conceive of stronger evidence of identification.

them whenever they are available in addition to other records. Frequently I have received only films and no written records or charts; they have invariably been quite sufficient.

In the uncomplicated situation where jaws and teeth have been preserved and only bite-wing radiographs supplied by the dentist, sufficient points of similarity can often be detected on comparison of the naked-eye appearances in the teeth and the ante-mortem films, but post-mortem films should be prepared for confirmation nevertheless.

### Dental Evidence of Age

The age of a body can be estimated in a number of ways. Dental evidence is of greatest value in the young; the eruption of deciduous and permanent teeth is a valuable guide as is discussed in greater or lesser detail in all the standard textbooks of forensic medicine. Radiographs help further by showing the state of calcification of crowns and roots of individual teeth. In older bodies the angle between the body and the ramus of the mandible is a rough guide to age, although as Gustafson (1966d) points out, the angle is more related to loss of teeth than specifically to age.

An assessment of age from an examination of individual teeth is a very specialized procedure (Gustafson, 1947, 1950, 1966e) and not all workers agree upon the criteria to be used (Dalitz, 1962; Miles, 1963, quoted by Sims, 1968b). This is a task only for the expert with considerable experience in the procedure involved; it has not been necessary to go to such lengths in the differential identification work in which I have been involved.

Several times it has been necessary to use dental radiographic evidence of age to distinguish between a number of children but there has always been additional evidence to take into account. Only once have I found that, all other bodies having been identified, I have been left with two female bodies, grossly incinerated and with only dental evidence to distinguish between them. On this occasion, although the jaws were substantially intact, it proved impossible to obtain ante-mortem dental records of either of the two women passengers whose bodies by exclusion they had to be. The only way to distinguish between them was on age; one passenger had been approximately 50 years old, the other in her early twenties. The task was not quite as simple as might be supposed—but it was not too difficult. Both mandibles had most of their teeth present. Body number 64 showed a greater attention to dental hygiene than body number 75 which had a good deal of calculus behind the front teeth. Body number 64 had had a good deal of periodontal disease as was shown by the pathological alveolar resorption, but this, it could be argued, could point either to the older or the younger. The staining of the third molar in body number 75 suggested that it had been in the mouth a lot longer than the third molar in body number 64 but, in fact, conclusive differentiation was made on comparison of radiographs. The roots of the second and third molars were not completely closed in body number 64 unlike those in body number 75; body number 64 was the younger and consistent with an age in the early twenties.

## Coincidence of Unusual Findings in Two Bodies

The assessment of the significance of any particular feature or combination of features found in a body is an assessment of the chance that such feature or combination might appear in two individuals within the group being examined. The

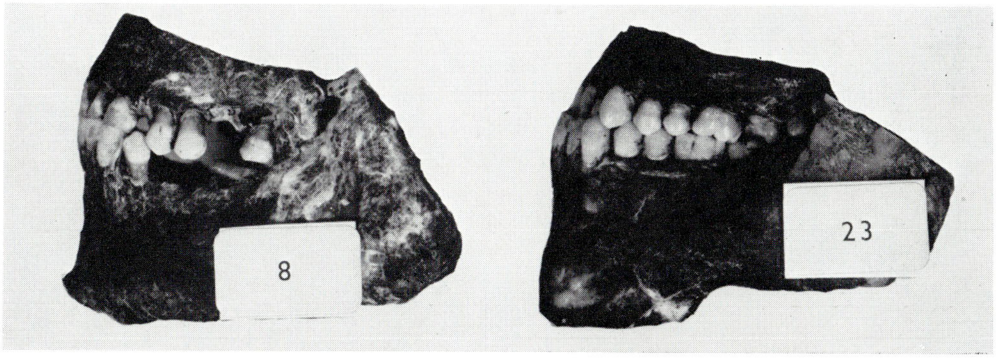


*Fig.* 96.—Jaws from two of the last five bodies to be examined in accident number 152. By coincidence two of these had protruding lower jaws. In body 8 this was of minor degree producing only an edge-to-edge bite; in body 23 the feature was much more pronounced. (*Reproduced from Stevens and Tarlton (1963) by permission of the co-author and the Editor 'Medicine, Science, and the Law'.*)

combination of features usually found is such that the chance that two bodies in a given group would show them is negligible. When commoner features are being considered and particularly when they are only few in number, the chance of coincidence is greater. An example of this occurred in accident number 152.

After two days work, five bodies remained to be examined; all were badly incinerated. Little was known about them but one was known to be rather taller than the others. This information was of doubtful value because incineration had caused gross contractures and destruction of the joints of the limbs such that it was impossible to measure the bodies' heights accurately. Nevertheless, the apparently tallest body (number 8) was selected for examination first, primarily because one additional piece of information concerned the tallest of the 5 passengers; his relatives had stated that he had a protruding lower jaw. Examination of the jaws of body number 8 did in fact show a slightly protruding jaw to the extent that there was an edge-to-edge bite. It was considered that this was unlikely to be coincidence and the body was therefore accorded a tentative identity.

The next body to be examined was number 23—selected at random from the remaining four; it was found to have an unusually prognathic lower jaw (*Fig*. 96), and it was later shown on the balance of all the evidence to be that of the passenger to whom body number 8 had originally been tentatively ascribed.

## Conclusions

As indicated at the beginning of this chapter, from my experience of differential identification of those involved in an aircraft accident, I am sure that dental identification in this context is well within the capability of a forensic pathologist providing he has sufficient interest in the subject. Occasionally he will encounter a problem with which he will need help; but everyone needs a second opinion from time to time, even in his own field of special competence.

However, with the ever increasing numbers of casualties in a single air disaster, the task of the investigating pathologist is becoming so great that one person cannot cope with it alone. I believe it is logical that a dentist should be appointed to assist whenever large numbers of casualties occur. I would say that a large number in this context is over fifty; those promoting forensic odontology as a specialty and pathologists disinterested in the subject would doubtless regard ten as a large number.

With the prospect of aircraft carrying 350–500 people within the next few years, it would appear that the example of the Scandinavian countries should be emulated in future practice in Britain; teams, each including at least one pathologist and one dentist should be formed for the investigation of every mass air disaster when the casualties exceed a given number—that number being selected on the basis of the experience and competence of the personnel currently involved in aircraft accident investigation. In fact, early in 1968, the Royal Air Force Dental Branch agreed to provide assistance with the identification of air crash victims whenever required by a Royal Air Force Pathologist.

## *Chapter 23*

# THE IDENTIFICATION OF THE DEAD—III

## PROCESS OF IDENTIFICATION BY EXCLUSION

BROWN, Delaney, and Robinson (1952) emphasized the value of using a graph in the form of a crossword puzzle during their examination of the bodies after the fire that gutted the 'Noronic' in Toronto Harbour in 1949. By relating information about a given male passenger with the findings in many male bodies, for example, it was possible to exclude many of them as being that of the particular passenger; thus the remaining bodies could be concentrated upon in an attempt to find that of the passenger in question. Although showing the value of the narrowing down of possibilities by exclusion in this way and although they had what they believed to be a reliable passenger list, these authors stressed that they were not prepared under any circumstances to use evidence of exclusion as acceptable evidence of a given identity.

Helpern (1957) considered it justifiable to use exclusion as a means of identification in certain circumstances and this is my view also. In accident number 151 only one female was believed to be on board the aircraft; only one female body was found; the total number of bodies found agreed with the total number known to be on board the aircraft; it would seem totally unreasonable not to accept the identity of the female body in these circumstances as that of the female known to be on the aircraft. Similarly in accident number 261 there was only one infant among the 88 persons on board the aircraft; although parts of only 86 different persons could be identified in the wreckage, they included the body of an infant of the appropriate age. There was no other evidence of this infant's identity but it would have been quite unreasonable not to accept its identity on the basis of exclusion.

It is my personal view that if the appropriate number of bodies has been recovered from an accident site and they match the list of persons believed to have been on board, not only in total number but by sex and on numbers of adults and children; if the crew have been identified and only two or three bodies remain unidentified; then it is permissible to identify the remainder by a combination of exclusive deduction and relatively weak items of evidence which by themselves would not justify confident positive identifications. I have used deductive reasoning of this type on a number of occasions and the following illustrates the process:—

Three female bodies remained to be identified, numbers 404, 451, and 482; the bodies of only three female passengers, 'A', 'B', and 'C' had not been identified. From the information in *Fig.* 97 it can be seen that the dental records of 'A' had been received from her dentist; on comparing the information therein with the bodies it was found that the teeth in bodies numbers 451 and 482 did not match the information in 'A's' dental records; indeed it proved conclusively that neither of these bodies could be that of 'A'. Body number 404 had been decapitated and the jaws were not present;

comparison of the dental evidence with 'A's' records was not therefore possible but by exclusion body number 404 had to be that of 'A'.

On comparison of the information received about the colour of 'B's' and 'C's' hair with the findings in the bodies, it was possible to complete the puzzle; body number

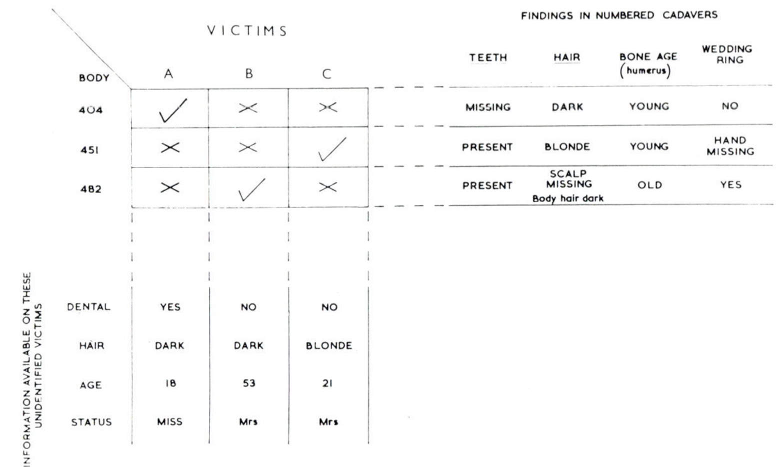


*Fig.* 97.—Diagram to illustrate identification by processes of deduction and exclusion. (*Reproduced from Stevens* (*1965b*) *by permission of the Editor 'Military Medicine'*.)

451 had to be that of 'C' because of the blonde hair, and body number 482 had to be that of 'B' by final exclusion. Reasoning of this sort appears to me to be acceptable so long as a number of additional pieces of supporting evidence are available and so long as no contradictory evidence is found. If there is any conflicting evidence, then there is no alternative but to report that the remaining bodies cannot be identified.

In the example given, the married status of the three passengers was known. 'A' was unmarried; on the left hand of body number 404 there was no wedding ring. 'B' and 'C' were both married; the left hand was missing from body number 451 but body number 482 had a wedding ring. At least there was no contradictory evidence here.

An assessment of the approximate age of each of the three bodies fitted the known age of the three passengers. The age of a body can be assessed in a variety of ways; the evidence available is often severely limited by the degree of mutilation and mechanical trauma sustained. In the example quoted, the most convenient way of comparing the ages of the bodies was by an examination of a section of humerus from each (*Fig.* 98). That in body number 404 showed a well marked epiphysial plate; 'A' was 18 years old. The humerus from body number 451 did not have an epiphysial plate but there was a very clear demarcation between the bone of the head and the cortex; this was clearly the bone of a person in the early twenties and was compatible with passenger 'C's' age—21 years. Finally the humerus from body number 482 was clearly very much older; an accurate assessment of its age was impossible but since no clear demarcation between the bone of the head and the shaft was present, it was certainly the oldest of the three bones and could well have belonged to the 53-year-old passenger 'B'.

I have found both Coroners and their juries in Britain, and the legal authorities overseas, always ready to accept evidence of identification of this type in the circumstances.

## THE COUNT OF THE BODIES RECOVERED

One of the earliest problems that arises after a mass disaster is that of how many people have been involved, how many bodies have been recovered and how many remain to be recovered. In the case of an aircraft accident there is rarely difficulty in

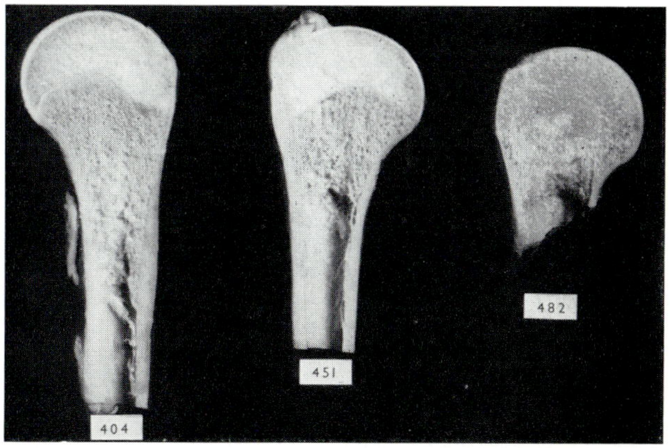


*Fig.* 98.—Sections of humerus from three bodies from the same accident (*see Fig.* 97). (*Reproduced from Stevens* (*1965b*) *by permission of the Editor 'Military Medicine'*.)

obtaining the information about the number of people involved, although it is always possible that there may have been a stowaway on board. In certain instances there may be, at least initially, some doubt about the number of occupants of the aircraft; this was the case in accident number 151—the information from Leopoldville was that only 15 persons had been on board Mr. Hammarskjöld's aircraft—but 16 bodies were found. It transpired that 16 persons were known to have been on board.

Mason and Tarlton (1965) described an accident in which the investigation consisted solely of a determination of the number of bodies recovered. The local pathologist on the third day following the accident stated that from his examinations the bodies of all 111 persons known to be on board the aircraft had been recovered. Later that day two more bodies were recovered and two days later yet another. Thus it seemed that there had been three extra persons on board the aircraft since, as it had crashed in swamp, there was little or no possibility that the accident had involved three people on the ground.

The local pathologist was firm that there could be no mistake and the airline was faced with charges that it had infringed a number of regulations including the carriage of undisclosed passengers.

Examination of all the coffins to see which contained half of a body or less, showed that coffins 93 and 94, 66 and 76, 92 and 77 could have been pairs, each pair containing portions of the same body. Those coffins were re-opened for further examination and the pairing was proved to everyone's satisfaction, thus reducing the total number of bodies recovered to the correct 111.

I have experienced another occasion when the possible bisection of a body had not been considered by those recovering and examining the remains and it was announced that all bodies had been recovered. It was not until it was pointed out that two of the 'bodies' were probably the upper and lower half of the same body bisected between L2 and L3 that a further search of the accident site was carried out and the last body discovered.

## THE ORGANIZATION OF AN INFORMATION SERVICE

Identification of the bodies of the victims of any mass disaster hinges upon the availability of information about the casualties. When an aircraft crashes on an internal flight the ordinary police lines of communication are probably the most efficient for securing the information required. It is generally accepted that this work is the duty of the police but on occasions the task has been carried out by airline personnel (Fisher, Spitz, Breitenecker, and Adams, 1965), or an *ad hoc* Red Cross committee (Brown, Delaney, and Robinson, 1952).

When a crash occurs in a foreign country and the majority of passengers are not citizens of that country, the speedy acquisition of the necessary information is one of the biggest problems encountered. It is particularly in this connexion that the benefit of a well organized disaster team is felt. An *ad hoc* organization to secure the information required wherever one may be working abroad, will invariably take some time before it produces results; it will certainly be a lengthy process if, as is suggested in the I.C.A.O. manual, families are asked to fill in a questionnaire provided by the national authorities or the airline concerned after it has been established that there are bodies which cannot be identified by simpler means.

Shortly after the Second World War, British airlines adopted the practice of employing a particular firm of funeral directors to travel to the scene of a fatal aircraft accident abroad and to conduct the administrative arrangements for the repatriation or disposal of the bodies of the casualties. When the local authorities took the usual steps to identify the bodies the firm merely had to supply the information necessary to permit registration of the deaths; permission was then given by the local authorities for repatriation of the bodies.

From time to time the firm found that the country in which the accident had occurred had little or no interest in the individual identification of the victims nor in any legal formalities; on these occasions the funeral directors were given permission to repatriate a collection of unidentified bodies.

With no local medical assistance and none of their own, the funeral directors themselves had to attempt to identify the bodies; I believe they were extremely conscientious in their efforts in this regard. They found it necessary to develop an information system within their own resources, and arrange that when their team went abroad to deal with a group of aircraft accident casualties, one member of the firm set up headquarters in London and from there, with the help of undertakers, police, and other contacts up and down the country, compiled dossiers on each casualty. They transmitted the information obtained by telephone or telegraph to the team in the accident area.

When, for the prime purpose of performing a medical investigation of the aircraft accident, we have found ourselves in a foreign country and involved in the identification of the bodies of the casualties, on most occasions we have had this firm's ready-made information service at our disposal. The coincidence of the firm of funeral directors being commissioned by the airline involved and ourselves attending on behalf of the Ministry of Aviation resulted in an increasing amount of co-operation over the years. We advised them on what additional information they should routinely seek to facilitate our work of identification. As a result, dental records and radiographs are now obtained at the outset; whenever practicable the original documents and films supplied by dentists are sent out to the accident area with the minimum of delay. It has not been unusual for us to have received dental information—in most cases actual documents and films—of some 60 per cent of the casualties within four or five days of the accident. If for any reason there is insuperable delay in the transmission of these documents, as much provisional information as possible is relayed by telephone or telegraph or more recently by the telex system.

The staff in the London office use a check-list (*Fig.* 99) for the information to be secured for both identification and death registration purposes. Duplicate forms are raised by one of the team of funeral directors at the accident site; these forms are kept in individual transparent plastic files which can be handled if necessary by a prosector's gloved hands. In these files are kept also dental charts, radiographs, photographs, copies of finger-prints or any other material collected to help to identify the body of a particular person known to have been on board the aircraft. The various sections on the check-list are numbered; this simplifies the telegraphic communication of the items of information for each item is merely prefixed by the code number.

The members of the funeral directors' field teams have acquired considerable expertise in this work having worked with police and pathologists in many countries; their clerical assistance in recording detailed post-mortem notes and dental evidence and in the handling of documents is invaluable; it contributes as much as any other single factor to the smooth and methodical progress of an investigation. On the two occasions when I have investigated accidents to other than a British aircraft and the British undertakers' information service has not been available to me, the alternative arrangements that have been made have been very much less efficient.

Whether or not there is a place for this particular firm's information service when a British aircraft crashes in Great Britain is debatable. On one occasion the coroner and the police were very glad to avail themselves of the service (accident number 231). Many of the police officers with whom I have discussed the matter have expressed the opinion that the firm's services would be valuable if only to release the police for the many other duties which arise in connexion with a large disaster. I have found it generally agreed, however, that close co-operation between the police and the firm would be better in most cases than that the funeral directors should take over the work completely.

**ACCIDENT**

Surname.............................................Mr./Mrs./Miss

**REGISTRATION PARTICULARS**

1. Christian Names.............................. 5. Religion ................................
2. Date of Birth................................ 6. Profession .............................
3. Place of Birth .............................. 7. Nationality ............................
4. Usual Residence ............................ 8. Married/Single ..........................
9. Father's Name ..................Profession.....................Nationality .................
10. Mother's Name................. Nationality .................
11. Husband's Name ...............Profession.....................Nationality .................
    Place of Birth .................

12. **Next of Kin**

    Name in full ............................ Relationship.............................

    Address.................................. Telephone................................

13. **Other Contacts**

    (*a*) Solicitors ..........................................

    (*b*) Dentist ............................................

    (*c*) Doctor ............................................

    Dental Chart { requested / obtained / sent to Field Team

**IDENTIFICATION PARTICULARS**

14. Build............................Height...................Weight.....................
15. Race ...........................................
16. Colour of hair...................................
17. Colour of eyes.............................................
18. Scars (surgical or other) and identifying marks
19. Medical History (i.e., broken bones, non-surgical illnesses, etc.)
20. Clothing, jewellery, etc.

*Fig.* 99.—A check-list used for the collection of information about those believed killed in an accident. (*Reproduced from Stevens* (1965*a*) *by permission of the Editor 'Aerospace Medicine'*.)

# MISCELLANEOUS TECHNIQUES IN THE WORK OF IDENTIFICATION

## The Recording of Data about the Cadavers

The importance of joint examination of a body by police and pathologists has been stressed in the preceding chapter. It has been my practice to raise for each body, in addition to any records made by the police, an identification protocol. The format of this protocol has been changed from time to time on the basis of our experience; the most recent variation is shown in *Figs*. 100 and 101—but different colours are used for male and female bodies.

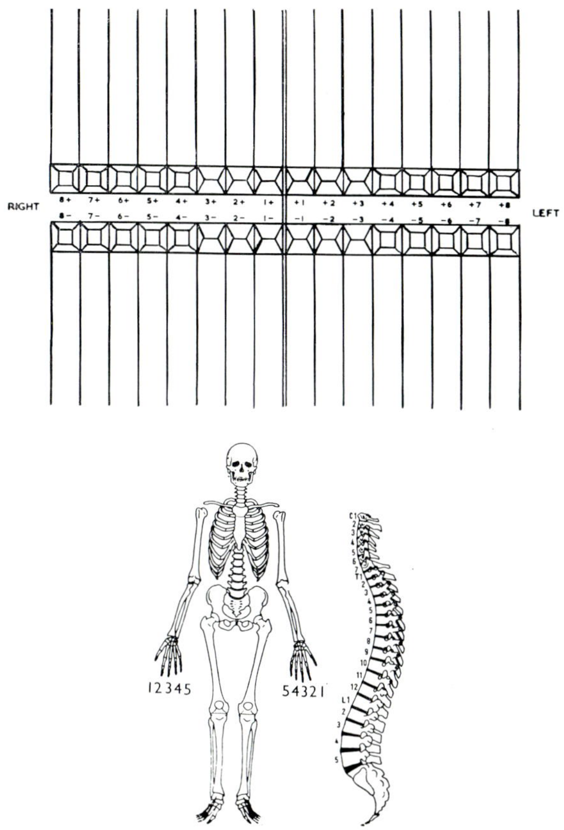


*Fig*. 100.—Reverse of the protocol shown in *Fig*. 101. The space beside the skeletal diagram is used for a description of any additional physical features noted on external or internal examination which might help with identification. This protocol is not intended for the notes of a full autopsy. (*Reproduced from Stevens (1965b) by permission of the Editor 'Military Medicine'*.)

I have seen examples of many other forms compiled for this purpose; many have been, in my view, unnecessarily complicated. It may be argued that a form for this work should provide a comprehensive check-list of every possible piece of information that should be looked for and could conceivably help in identification. Such a comprehensive form has the disadvantage that large parts will not be applicable to the

*Date of Examination:* BODY No. ..................

IDENTIFIED AS ......................

*ACCIDENT:* IDENTIFIED FROM: Documents
Clothing
Jewellery
Dental
Physical
Exclusion

---

*MALE/FEMALE* *ESTIMATED AGE*

*BUILD*

*ESTIMATED HEIGHT*

*ESTIMATED WEIGHT*

*COLOUR OF SKIN* *COLOUR OF EYES* *COLOUR OF HAIR*

*CLOTHING*

*PROPERTY and JEWELLERY*

---

*Fig*. 101.—Front of a simple identification protocol used in aircraft accident investigation. (*Reproduced from Stevens (1965b) by permission of the Editor 'Military Medicine'*.)

individual case and often there will be insufficient space for detailed descriptions where they are appropriate. I prefer to accept that the person making the examination is sufficiently experienced not to require a comprehensive *aide-mémoire*; I advocate the use of a form with a small number of broad headings and adequate space for detailed descriptions under those headings. I think it is advantageous to use a form which is one sheet of paper only; if kept in a transparent plastic file it can be handled in the autopsy room if necessary and either side examined at a glance.

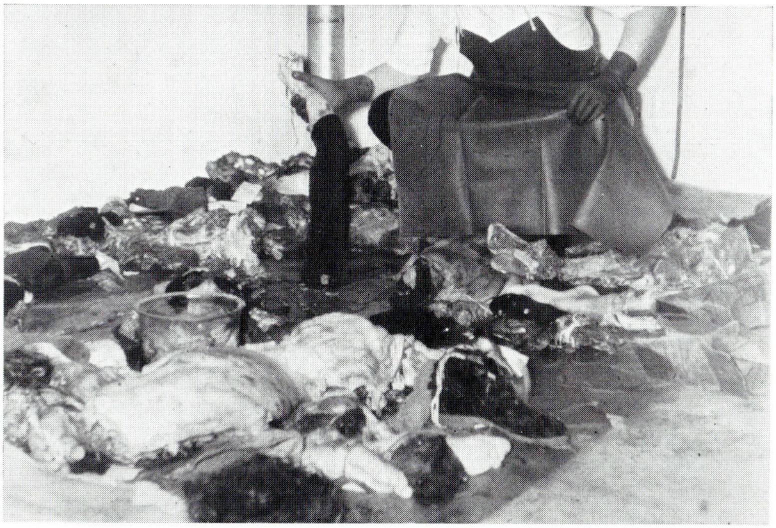

*Fig*. 102.—A collection of fragmented human remains from an aircraft accident. It is necessary to examine such material carefully, preferably after the examination of the complete and substantially complete bodies. (*Reproduced from Stevens (1965a) by permission of the Editor 'Aerospace Medicine'*.)

On one side of our protocol there are two important features—a dental chart and a skeletal diagram. The latter permits a rapid pictorial representation of the parts of a body found to be missing; if a body is bisected the level of bisection can be shown easily. Specimens consisting of more than half a body should always be examined first; it is much the most convenient procedure to leave the examination of the separated parts to the end for then it is a relatively simple task to check through the plastic files containing the records of the bodies and ascertain which ones are missing, for example a forearm amputated just below the elbow. It is usually easy to distinguish between a male and a female forearm and a particular specimen can be matched with the appropriate bodies until the correct one is found. If that body has been identified already there is no more to be done but to dispose of the arm into the appropriate coffin. If the body has not been identified there may well be useful clues in the separated forearm which will serve to identify the body. Remnants of clothing may be on the arm whereas all the clothes may have been lost from the torso; the forearm may have a distinctive tattoo or there may be rings on the fingers. The examination of 'spare parts' is a particularly gruesome task (*Fig*. 102) but one that must be done if the investigation is to be carried out thoroughly.

On one occasion it was necessary to reconstitute the face of a cadaver found at one end of an accident trail with jaws and facial tissues discovered at the other end. There was no doubt that these separated tissues belonged to the body; not only was it possible to suture them in place but the ears, one attached to the body and one to the separated fragment, matched perfectly. Having shown conclusively that the separated portion belonged to the particular body it was possible to make a dental identification of that body.

### Wall Charts

I have found a wall chart as advocated by Brown, Delaney, and Robinson (1952) a most useful means of monitoring the progress of the task of identification. A main chart is prepared with a list of the crew and passengers known to be on board down the left-hand side; the adult males are listed first in alphabetical order, then the adult females; male and female children are then grouped either alphabetically or according to age as seems best in view of their numbers and age distribution. It is helpful to annotate each name with the person's age as soon as this is known. The numbers to be accorded to the bodies are written across the top of the chart and an open crossword puzzle is thus available.

As identifications are accepted the appropriate square relating identified body to passenger is filled in; on the extreme right of the chart a brief note can be made of the means by which each identification was made. As the puzzle is gradually completed fewer bodies remain to be identified in each group; it can be seen at a glance, for example, which passenger an unidentified female body could belong to. As the field for consideration is narrowed, attention is often directed quickly to a particular feature that, if followed up, may lead to a quick identification. To take but one simple example, if the bodies of 8 female passengers have not been found and 7 of them were under 30 years of age and one 65 years of age, then a female body found to have greying hair would probably be that of the elderly female. It might be possible to follow-up this clue by seeking information quickly from a relative as to whether the 65-year-old had had three laparotomies ('three children born by operation', perhaps) to match the surgical scars found on the abdomen of the grey haired body.

### Comparison of the Recorded Data about the Cadavers with the Information supplied about the Crew and Passengers

If one has adequate clerical assistance, a clerk can be given the task of comparing the recorded data on cadavers with the information about the known persons. In the early stages this is quite simply done, especially with the record sheets readily visible through transparent file covers. The prepared documents of tentative matches can be put to one side by the clerk for later careful assessment by the police and pathologists to determine whether the evidence is sufficiently strong for an identification to be accepted. In practice I have found that there is rarely sufficient clerical assistance for this to be done during the main part of a working day. All the clerical assistance available is used in recording the findings in the cadavers as dictated by the pathologists, the details of clothing and personal property as discovered by the police and in dealing with the constant stream of information about the passengers and crew that is received.

After some eight to ten hours of work in the autopsy room it is usually essential to pause. Ancillary staff such as post-mortem room attendants, embalmers, and photographers do not always have reliefs available and it is rarely practicable to continue the examinations of bodies day and night. It is possible after a short rest, for a pathologist and clerical assistant to continue with the work of comparing records. Whenever I have investigated a large accident I have found it necessary to work from sixteen to eighteen hours each day, much of this time being in the autopsy room, the remainder either in continuing the paper work part of identifying the bodies or in consultation with the British accredited representative and the other investigators over matters pertaining to the accident investigation itself. Possibly the hours it is necessary to work on these occasions are excessive but, as already explained, there are pressures from many quarters for the completion as quickly as possible of the pathological part of the investigation. The only way in which long hours of work could be avoided would be the provision of several teams of police, pathologists, and dentists; but this would only be of value when the mortuary and autopsy room facilities available would permit more than one team to work at a time—and I find this is rarely so.

## *Chapter 24*

# CERTIFICATION OF DEATH AND THE DISPOSAL OF THE DECEASED

THESE are matters which are not normally of concern to the pathologist but they may involve him in certain circumstances when he is investigating an aircraft accident abroad; he should have a knowledge therefore, of the relevant regulations.

In the United Kingdom a Coroner or a Procurator-fiscal issues disposal orders and death certificates when satisfied as to the identities and causes of death of the accident victims; the deaths are registered by the registrar of the subdistrict in which the accident has occurred. Abroad, the local legal authorities issue death certificates upon being satisfied about the identifications and causes of death.

Following an aircraft accident the deaths are not registered by the local British consul as normally are deaths of British subjects abroad. The Civil Aviation Act, 1949, required that a return be sent to the Minister of Civil Aviation (now the President of the Board of Trade) of deaths of all travellers killed in an accident to a British registered aircraft outside the United Kingdom (Polson, Brittain, and Marshall, 1962). The informant is usually an official of the airline concerned, and a copy of his return is sent to the Registrar-General who enters the deaths in 'the air register books of deaths'; if the deceased person at the time of death usually resided in Scotland a copy is sent to the Registrar-General for Scotland.

The Registrar-General then issues death certificates and it is these certificates which are required by the relatives for the settlement of the deceased's affairs. It should be noted that issue of these death certificates is not dependent upon the recovery and individual identification of the bodies of the persons concerned and thus they effectively provide declarations of presumption of death where, on the basis of the evidence of the informant, there is good reason to believe that certain persons have died in an accident. These certificates are effective immediately upon issue; there is no statutory delay before presumption of death becomes effective such as occurs in certain other countries when an individual body is not recovered and identified (Chapter 20).

If relatives desire local disposal abroad, then the appropriate order is obtained locally and there is no problem. If the relatives wish a body to be repatriated for disposal in Britain, its import into Britain is straightforward on the basis of the foreign death certificate. If it is to be buried, it is only necessary for the relatives to have the foreign death certificate and a certificate of 'non-liability to register' from the registrar of the district in which burial is to take place.

If, however, relatives desire cremation it will usually be difficult or impossible for them to obtain the usual certificates to satisfy the medical referee. The Cremation Regulations, 1930, provide that the Secretary of State, 'if satisfied that the case is one in which cremation may properly take place, may by order under his hand authorize the medical referee to allow cremation'. The provision by a British pathologist of a certificate to the effect that he has satisfied himself as to the identity of a body and the cause of death has been of considerable help in recent years as a document to support the foreign death certificate and satisfy the Secretary of State that the case was one in which he might reasonably authorize cremation.

*Chapter 25*

# FINAL CONCLUSIONS

FROM this study of 74 fatal civil aircraft accidents, almost all of which were investigated by pathologists with special interest in the work, a number of conclusions are drawn:—

1. A comprehensive pathological investigation may reveal a probable medical cause of an aircraft accident when that cause would otherwise be unsuspected or have, at best, insubstantial evidence to point to it. Accident number 261 (Chapter 4), where there was intoxication of the crew of an airliner by carbon monoxide, accident number 243 (Chapter 11) where there was intoxication of the pilot of a light aircraft by alcohol and accident number 119 (Chapter 15) where there was incapacitation of the pilot of a glider from epilepsy are examples.

2. A full pathological investigation may exclude, or at least provide strong evidence against a possible cause of an accident. In accident numbers 151 and 241 (Chapter 5) there were strong suspicions of sabotage; the pathologists' evidence helped to exclude this in both cases.

3. A pathological investigation of a fatal aircraft accident cannot be considered adequate unless full autopsies on the bodies of the crew are supplemented by histological examination of the major organs, in particular the brain (accident number 225—Chapter 10) the heart (accident numbers 152, 219, and 260—Chapters 3 and 15) and lungs (accident numbers 152 and 244—Chapters 7 and 10). Pathological changes in these organs may be incidental (accident number 219—Chapter 3) or their association with the cause of the accident may be equivocal (accident number 225—Chapter 10); at least having found the changes, it is possible to give them due consideration and significance in the final analysis.

4. Because a medical cause may not be suspected immediately after an accident has occurred, it is essential that the medical and pathological investigation of aircraft accidents should be on a routine basis. Full autopsies should be followed by routine histological and toxicological examinations in the laboratory and a routine investigation into a pilot's medical history. The detailed and comprehensive nature of this medical and pathological investigation must be matched by the caution with which the findings, both positive and negative, are interpreted; accident numbers 152 and 219 (Chapter 3) illustrate this with particular force.

5. The need for routine medical participation in fatal accident investigation is emphasized in particular by those cases in which the pathological evidence has had a bearing upon a non-medical cause of an accident and has helped to reconstruct events in flight prior to the accident (accident number 187—Chapter 6 and Mason's case quoted in Chapter 5). The occasions on which this will prove possible cannot be predicted.

6. It may be held that aviation is not inherently dangerous. Although this may be true, the air, even to a greater extent than the sea, is very unforgiving of human deficiency. A high standard of medical fitness is required of pilots of powered aircraft; a similar

but perhaps slightly lower standard is necessary for glider pilots. A detailed pathological study of those pilots killed in aircraft accidents is not the only, nor indeed the prime means by which medical selection and surveillance of pilots can be judged—records of invaliding or retirement on medical grounds provide most evidence on the subject. Autopsies, nevertheless, provide an important source of information and no opportunity to tap it should be missed.

The number of accidents investigated by the Department that have involved pilots of powered aircraft is insufficient for anything other than tentative conclusions but there is no indication that the medical selection and control either of professional or private pilots is deficient.

On the other hand the study of over half of the relatively few fatal gliding accidents that have occurred in recent years, positively supports the contention that the medical standards now imposed by the British Gliding Association are satisfactory; that the introduction of a government sponsored medical certification system would be unlikely materially to affect the safety record of this form of aviation. But the trends in fatal accident rates for gliding show that there must be no relaxation by the B.G.A. of its medical standards or other safety measures.

7. Since aircraft accidents will not be completely preventable in the foreseeable future, it is important that no reasonable means of improving the chance of a passenger's survival in an accident should be overlooked. Only from a routine study of fatalities can patterns of injury and their causes be discovered and preventive measures taken. The circumstances of two accidents are never quite the same; a measure which might be life-saving in one instance might be potentially lethal in another. Only by the assessment of safety and survival aspects of every accident can sufficient evidence be collected to justify specific safety measures.

Furthermore, it may be that repetitive presentation of evidence on a given subject is required before executive action will be taken. An example is the continuing failure of the controlling authorities to make regulations requiring manufacturers to provide full harnesses for all occupants of light aircraft.

8. The medical and pathological investigation of a fatal aircraft accident which proves to have been valueless is a rarity. Even if the importance of the exclusion of hypothetical causes for an accident and the contribution made by the pathologist in the identification of the dead are discounted, it can still be claimed that there were medical and pathological findings of significance in at least 6 of the 18 public transport accidents, in 8 of the 42 light aircraft accidents and 8 of the 14 glider accidents—almost 30% of the total accidents investigated. If the importance of each investigation into a light aircraft accident with regard to the analysis of the relationship between the lack of safety equipment and death in this type of flying is taken into account, then the proportion of accidents in which there was pathological evidence of value is very much higher.

9. A full and comprehensive medical and pathological investigation of a glider accident or a light aircraft accident with but few casualties is not a major task. The investigation of a large airliner disaster, its casualties numbered in tens today and probably in hundreds tomorrow, is, and will continue to be a major undertaking. It can be successfully completed only if there are experienced pathologists organized and

constantly ready to accompany an investigation team to an accident site; if local police and legal authorities are briefed about the importance of a thorough accident investigation and about their roles in ensuring it; if an information service such as that described in Chapter 23 is always available and can be put into operation with the minimum of delay after an accident has occurred.

10. At the present time there are between 20 and 30 fatal flying accidents each year in Britain or involving British registered civil aircraft abroad. A single department such as that at the Royal Air Force Institute of Pathology and Tropical Medicine has shown that it can deal with a work load of this magnitude, and it is logical that a country the size of Britain should have only one such highly specialized unit to deal both with military and civil cases.

If, however, the volume of all types of civil aviation continues to rise without a corresponding improvement in fatal accident rates it may be that the total number of accidents each year will justify the establishment of a civilian section to the department. It may be that in a few years the number of fatal civilian accidents will so outnumber the military ones that the department will become a civilian unit with a responsibility for military accident investigation—the reverse of the present situation. It would, in my opinion, be a retrograde step for a separate civilian unit to be established; much of the value of the single specialized unit such as at present exists at Halton lies in the fact that many accidents are investigated by relatively few, highly motivated, and experienced personnel.

The time for re-organization, however, has not yet come—perhaps it never will. It is to be hoped that the combined efforts of all whose common cause is the promotion of safety in aviation will belie the pessimistic forecasts that have been made of the number of accidents and deaths to be expected in the future.

# *APPENDIX*

## GLIDING: DETAILED STATISTICS 1950–68

THERE are no official statistics concerning the volume of gliding in Britain. Wills (1966) published figures from the British Gliding Association's records which showed that the total number of accidents per annum increased much more slowly during the period 1959–68 than did the volume of gliding activity. In that decade only 938 accidents occurred, only 180 of these were sufficiently serious to be legally reportable, but a total of over 1·6 million flights were made. These figures would suggest that gliding is a safe sport and has been getting slowly safer during recent years.

So far as can be ascertained no previous attempts have been made to collect figures with a view to calculating a fatal accident rate for gliding which could provide a further guide to trends in safety in this sport. Two fatal accident rates have been calculated from the figures presented in *Table XIII*; a comment about the sources of these figures is necessary.

There are, in general, three groups of people who engage in gliding in Britain; they are the private civilian clubs, the Armed Services' clubs, and the Air Cadets. Most of the civilian clubs are members of the British Gliding Association (B.G.A.) and most complete for the B.G.A. an annual return of activities in terms of launches made and hours flown. These figures are published in the B.G.A.'s magazine *Sailplane and Gliding*. Since gliding is a sport, club officials are leisure-time enthusiasts and the returns are not compulsory, it is not surprising that the returns are occasionally not made or, more frequently, are made late; thus the figures that appeared in *Sailplane and Gliding* in the April issue of any year, and related to the previous year, have frequently been incomplete. However, in the April issues of the magazine in subsequent years, when gliding activites over a period have been reviewed, corrected totals have been published. Hence the figures recorded in *Table XIII* are those which, from a study of all the reports in *Sailplane and Gliding*, appear to be the most accurate.

The Services' Gliding Associations are affiliated to the B.G.A.; the individual clubs in these associations make 'official' returns of their gliding activities to their parent associations and 'unofficial' returns to the B.G.A. The B.G.A. has published the operational statistics of the Royal Air Force Gliding Associations separately from those of the civilian clubs in most of their annual reports; until recent years most of the Army's gliding was done at Lasham and its operations were included with those of the civilian clubs at Lasham. In 1968 the Army Gliding Association's figures for 1967 were published in the total attributed to 'combined Services'; in 1969 the figures for 1968 were given in detail. For simplicity the Army figures for 1967 and 1968 were included with the relevant civilian figures in the second column of *Table XIII* to preserve the pattern of the figures given for previous years.

The secretaries of the Royal Air Force and Naval Gliding Associations were able to supply accurate figures of the operations of their clubs in recent years; they differ

## *Table XIII.*—Gliding Operations in Britain and Fatal Accident Rates for Gliders: 1950–68

| | Hours Flown | | | | | Launches Made | | | | | Total | Fatal Accident | |
|---|---|---|---|---|---|---|---|---|---|---|---|---|---|
| *Year* | *Civilian*[1] | *R.N.G.S.A.* | *R.A.F.G.S.A.* | *Air Cadets* | *Total* | *Civilian*[1] | *R.N.G.S.A.* | *R.A.F.G.S.A.* | *Air Cadets* | *Total* | *Fatal Accidents* | *per 10,000 hrs* | *Rates per 100,000 launches* |
| 1950 | 7560 | 300[2] | 150[3] | 8800[4] | 16,810 | 42,518 | 3450 | 2500[3] | 105,614 | 154,082 | 3 | 1·79 | 1·95 |
| 1951 | 7834 | 100[3] | 250[3] | 5500 | 13,684 | 42,613 | 1000[3] | 4000[3] | 88,498 | 136,111 | 1 | 0·73 | 0·74 |
| 1952 | 8223 | 100[3] | 354 | 5203 | 13,880 | 49,836 | 1000[3] | 5097 | 92,692 | 148,625 | 2 | 1·44 | 1·35 |
| 1953 | 9967 | 100[3] | 619 | 7346 | 18,032 | 53,692 | 1000[3] | 7594 | 96,649 | 158,935 | 1 | 0·55 | 0·63 |
| 1954 | 10,586 | 106 | 759 | 7497 | 18,948 | 59,249 | 1234 | 9493 | 99,575 | 169,551 | 0 | 0·00 | 0·00 |
| 1955 | 13,381 | 515 | 1389 | 7194 | 22,479 | 77,719 | 6823 | 15,082 | 95,476 | 195,100 | 1 | 0·44 | 0·51 |
| 1956 | 13,596 | 125 | 1815 | 5186 | 20,722 | 75,594 | 1500 | 19,465 | 65,200 | 161,759 | 1 | 0·48 | 0·62 |
| 1957 | 17,996 | 125 | 2365 | 4538 | 25,024 | 96,139 | 1300 | 22,585 | 64,659 | 184,683 | 0 | 0·00 | 0·00 |
| 1958 | 17,798 | 64 | 3664 | 4586 | 26,112 | 99,448 | 907 | 34,719 | 71,713 | 206,787 | 2 | 0·78 | 0·97 |
| 1959 | 22,937 | 250[3] | 5332[5] | 8536[4] | 37,005 | 121,196 | 3000[3] | 39,911[5] | 102,434 | 266,541 | 1 | 0·27 | 0·38 |
| 1960 | 19,136 | 448[6] | 6732[5] | 9600[4] | 35,916 | 122,013 | 3965[6] | 48,111[5] | 115,203 | 289,292 | 1 | 0·28 | 0·35 |
| 1961 | 24,564 | 521[6] | 7421[5] | 10,695[4] | 43,201 | 139,826 | 6322[6] | 54,094[5] | 128,339[7] | 328,581 | 2 | 0·46 | 0·61 |
| 1962 | 30,546 | 901[6] | 7639[5] | 11,310[4] | 50,396 | 162,998 | 7377[6] | 53,433[4] | 135,725[7] | 359,533 | 2 | 0·40 | 0·56 |
| 1963 | 27,523 | 1264[6] | 6635[5] | 11,362[4] | 46,784 | 152,676 | 7512[6] | 47,469[5] | 136,345[7] | 344,002 | 2 | 0·43 | 0·58 |
| 1964 | 33,225 | 1786[6] | 9339[5] | 15,307[4] | 59,657 | 171,806 | 11,613[6] | 59,217[5] | 183,693[7] | 426,329 | 4 | 0·67 | 0·94 |
| 1965 | 37,617 | 1540[6] | 10,083[5] | 15,167[4] | 64,407 | 183,527 | 13,719[6] | 57,962[5] | 182,001[7] | 437,209 | 4 | 0·62 | 0·91 |
| 1966 | 38,494 | 1881[6] | 9,921[5] | 15,131[4] | 65,427 | 201,881 | 12,787[6] | 59,646[5] | 181,576[7] | 455,890 | 3 | 0·46 | 0·66 |
| 1967[8] | 44,942[9] | 1977 | 13,844[5] | 13,508[4] | 74,271 | 201,684[9] | 15,352 | 71,147[5] | 162,082 | 450,265 | 5 | 0·67 | 1·11 |
| 1968 | 54,733[9] | 1881 | 15,117 | 15,720[4] | 87,451[10] | 223,775[9] | 12,869 | 78,219 | 188,641 | 503,504[10] | 6 | 0·69 | 1·19 |

One fatal accident only occurred in the first six months of 1969.

Except where annotated, figures were published in, or calculated from those published in, *Sailplane and Gliding*.

1. Figures include most but not all Army Gliding Club operations.
2. Estimated on the basis of launches made (*see* column 8); published in *Sailplane and Gliding*.
3. No records traceable: estimated on the basis of annual trends.
4. Air cadet gliding consists mainly of teaching cadets to make a safe launch circuit and landing. Hours flown are estimated from the numbers of launches made, on the basis of an average of 5 minutes per flight.
5. From Secretary, R.A.F.G.S.A.
6. From Secretary, R.N.G.S.A.
7. From Officer Commanding, Air Cadets.
8. Figures for first 9 months only—change in administrative year to October/September.
9. Calculated to include most Army Gliding Club operations; details from Secretary, B.G.A.
10. Gliding activities—especially long-distance flights affecting hours more than launches—were restricted for some months due to an epidemic of foot-and-mouth disease.

but little from those published by the B.G.A. The figures published in *Sailplane and Gliding* were accepted for the earlier years.

*Sailplane and Gliding* also reported in most years the total operations of the Air Cadets (formerly the Air Training Corps) for the previous year; these were the only figures available for the 1950's but the Officer Commanding, Air Cadets, supplied details of the launches made since 1960. For some time the Air Cadets have kept records only of the launches made; the type of gliding activity which they undertake consists essentially of a launch, a circuit, and a landing; the total hours flown can be estimated reasonably on the basis of an average of 5 minutes per flight.

The amount of civilian gliding carried on in Britain by groups who are not members of the B.G.A. is negligible. Any inaccuracies in the figures presented in *Table XIII* arise therefore either because of incomplete returns to the B.G.A. by member clubs or because estimates have been made where figures have not been available; these inaccuracies are almost certainly so small as not to affect the calculated fatal accident rates.

The figures for total fatal glider accidents have been obtained from the annual surveys of aircraft accidents published by the Ministry of Aviation or the Civil Aviation Department of the Board of Trade, from the secretaries of the Services' Gliding Associations, and from the Officer Commanding, Air Cadets. There is every reason to believe that these are completely accurate. The numbers of fatal accidents each year are too small for trends to be assessed on an annual basis; however, the calculation of quinquennial statistics (*Table XI*, Chapter 14) gives some indication of the safety of gliding during the period reviewed.

# REFERENCES


ACOCK, G. Accidents Investigation Branch, Board of Trade (1967), personal communication.

*Aerospace Medicine* (1969), 'Protective Smoke Hoods for Emergency Use by Passengers and Crew Members', **40**, 326.

AIR MINISTRY (1925), 'Report on the Accident to Imperial Airways DH34, G-EBBY, which occurred on 24 December, 1924', Command Paper No. 2351.

AIR REGISTRATION BOARD (1968), 'Maintenance of Cockpit and Cabin Combustion Type Heaters and Associated Exhaust Systems', ARB Notice No. 41. Issue 1. April 16.

AKSNES, E. G. (1954), 'Effect of Small Doses of Alcohol upon Performance in a Link Trainer', *J. Aviat. Med.*, **25**, 680

AMOËDO, O. (1899), 'Identification of Bodies by the Expert Dentist', *Dent. Cosmos*, **41**, 444.

ANDERSON, G. H. (1919), *Medical and Surgical Aspects of Aviation*. London: Hodder & Stoughton.

ANDERSON, I. H. (1968), 'Aeromedical Investigation of Fatal Aircraft Accidents', *Aerospace Med.*, **39**, 617.

ARMSTRONG, J. A., FRYER, D. I., STEWART, W. A., and WHITTINGHAM, H. E. (1955), 'Interpretation of Injuries in the Comet Aircraft Disasters', *Lancet*, **1**, 1135.

ASVALL, J. E. (1961), 'Post-mortem Absorption of Carbon Monoxide in Rats', *Scand. J. clin. Lab. Invest.*, **13**, 32.

*Aviation Week and Space Technology* (1967), 'F.B.I. Probing Blast on American Flight', 20 November, p. 30.

— — — — (1968), '707 Lands Safely after Blast, Fire', 25 November, p. 24.

BAENSCH, W., and FIEDLER, A. (1900), 'Über Acute Interstitielle Myokarditis', *Zentbl. inn. Med.*, **21**, 212.

BAROLDI, G. (1965), 'Acute Coronary Occlusion as a Cause of Myocardial Infarct and Sudden Coronary Heart Death', *Am. J. Cardiol.*, **16**, 859.

— — and MANION, W. C. (1967), 'Microcirculatory Disturbances and Human Myocardial Infarction', *Am. Heart J.*, **74**, 173.

BEARD, R. R., and WERTHEIM, G. A. (1967), 'Behavioural Impairment associated with Small Doses of Carbno Monoxide', *Amer. J. publ. Hlth.*, **57**, 2012

BEDDOE, H. L. (1956), 'Methods of Investigation in the Identification of Human Remains', *J. forens. Sci.*, **1**, 47.

BENNETT, D. R. (1964), 'Epilepsy in Aircrew', *Aerospace Med.*, **35**, 153.

BENSON, A. J. (1965), 'Spatial Disorientation in Flight', in *A Textbook of Aviation Physiology* (ed. GILLIES, J. A.), pp. 1086–1129. London: Pergamon.

BENSON, O. O. (1937), 'Coronary Artery Disease: Report of a Fatal Attack in a Pilot while Flying', *J. Aviat. Med.*, **8**, 81.

BERRY, F. B., and STEMBRIDGE, V. A. (1958), 'The Human Element in Aircraft Accidents', *Ann. Surg.*, **147**, 590.

BEZREH, A. A. (1963), 'Helicopter versus Fixed-wing Crash Injuries', *Aerospace Med.*, **34**, 11.

BIRKE, G., LILJEDAHL, S., and TROELL, L. (1957), 'Studies on Burns', *Acta chir. scand.*, Suppl. 228.

BLACKMORE, D. J. (1967), Unpublished report to the Officer-in-Charge, Department of Aviation Pathology, R.A.F. Institute of Pathology, Halton.

— — (1968), 'The Bacterial Production of Ethyl Alcohol', *J. forens. Sci. Soc.*, **8**, 73.

— — (1969), 'Determination and Interpretation of Carbon Monoxide in Decomposing Blood and Tissue', paper given at the Fifth International Meeting of Forensic Sciences, Toronto, Canada, June.

— — (1970), 'The Determination of Carbon Monoxide in Blood and Tissue', *Analyst*, in press.

BOARD OF TRADE (1966), CAP 265, 'A Survey of the Accidents to Aircraft of the United Kingdom in 1965', London: H.M.S.O.

— — (1967), CAP 290, 'Accidents to Aircraft on the British Register/1966', London: H.M.S.O.

— — (1968a), CAP 307, 'Accidents to Aircraft on the British Register/1967', London: H.M.S.O.

— — (1968b), CAP 305, 'Report on the Accident to Comet Series 4B G-ARCO, 12 October 1967', London: H.M.S.O.

— — (1970), CAP 327, 'Accidents to Aircraft on the British Register/1968', London: H.M.S.O.

BONNICHSEN, R., HALSTRØM, F., MØLLER, K. O., and THEORELL, H. (1953), 'Development of Ethanol in Blood Samples and Human Organs during Forensic Chemical Practice', *Acta pharmac. tox.*, **9**, 352.

BORKENSTEIN, F., CROWTHER, R., SHUMATE, R. P., ZIEL, W. B., and ZYLMAN, R. (1964), 'The Role of the Drinking Driver in Traffic Accidents', Indiana University: Department of Police Administration.

BOWDEN, C. H., and WOODHALL, W. R. (1963), 'The Determination and Significance of Low Blood Carboxyhaemoglobin Levels', *Med. Sci. Law*, **4**, 98.

BOWDEN, K. M., and MCCALLUM, N. E. (1949), 'Alcohol Content: Some Aspects of its Post-mortem Uses', *Med. J. Aust.*, **2**, 76.

BRITANNICA BOOK OF THE YEAR (1963) (ed. ARMITAGE, J.), 'Events of 1962. Disasters', p. 160. London: Encyclopaedia Britannica.

— — — (1964), 'Events of 1963', *Ibid.*, p. 149.

## REFERENCES


BRITANNICA BOOK OF THE YEAR (1965), 'Events of 1964', p. 166. London: Encyclopaedia Britannica.
——— (1966), 'Events of 1965. Disasters', p. 239. (ed. GOETZ, P.) Chicago: William Benton.
——— (1967), 'Events of 1966. Disasters', p. 238. (ed. DELL, W. R.) Chicago: William Benton.
——— (1968), 'Events of 1967', *Ibid.*, p. 286.
——— (1969), 'Events of 1968', *Ibid.*, p. 286.

BRITISH MEDICAL ASSOCIATION (1964), *Accidents in the Home*, London.
——— (1965a), 'Accident Services of Great Britain and Ireland, Second Report of the Review Committee', London.
——— (1965b), 'The Medicolegal Investigation of the Drinking Driver. Report of the Special Committee', London: British Medical Association.

*British Medical Journal* (1966), *News and Notes*, 'Epidemiology', *Br. med. J.*, **1**, 808.
——— (1968), 'Cadaveric Kidneys', *Ibid.*, **1**, 784.

BROOKS, P. W. (1966), 'British Light Aviation', *Jl R. aeronaut. Soc.*, **70**, 270.

BROWN, T. C., DELANEY, R. J., and ROBINSON, W. L. (1952), 'Medical Identification in the "Noronic" Disaster', *J. Am. med. Ass.*, **148**, 621.
—— and LANE, J. C. (1966), 'The Australian Civil Aviation Pathology Programme', Paper read at the International Meeting on Aviation and Space Medicine, Sydney, Australia, December.

BROWN, V. (1966), 'The Story of Air Accident Investigation by a One-time Inspector', *Jl R. aeronaut. Soc.*, **70**, 243.

BRYAN, A. C. (1967), 'Discussion of Canadian Experience in the DC8, Ste. Therese, Quebec', Paper presented at Sixth Scientific Session, *Jt. Comm. Aviat. Path.*, Ottawa, September.

BULEY, L. E. (1967), 'Human Factors in "Jet Upset" ', Paper presented to the 16th International Congress on Aviation and Space Medicine, Lisbon, September.
—— (1969), 'Incidence, Causes, and Results of Airline Pilot Incapacitation while on Duty', *Aerospace Med.*, **40**, 64.

CAMPBELL, H. E. (1960), 'The Case for Rear-facing Seats in Commercial Aircraft', *Clin. Med.*, **7**, 2529.

CAMPS, F. E. (1963), 'Hypoglycaemia in Motor Vehicle Drivers', in *Alcohol and Road Traffic: Proceedings of the Third International Conference* (ed. HAVARD, J. D.), p. 116. London: British Medical Association.

CARROLL, T. B., and GRUBER, F. H. (1968), 'Seat Belt Fractures', *Radiology*, **91**, 517.

CATLETT, G. F., and KIDERA, G. J. (1968), 'Glaucoma in Commercial Pilots', *Aerospace Med.*, **39**, 1329.

CIVIL AERONAUTICS BOARD (1956), 'Accident Investigation Report, File No. 1—0143, United Air Lines, Inc., Douglas DC-6B, N-37559, 1 November, 1955'.
——— (1958), 'Accident Investigation Report, File No. 1—0065, Western Air Lines, Inc., Convair 240-1, N-8406 H, 25 July, 1957'.
——— (1960), 'Aircraft Accident Report, SA.352, File No. 1—0002, National Airlines, Inc., Douglas DC-6B, N-8225H, 6 January, 1960'.
——— (1962), 'Aircraft Accident Report, File No. 1—0003, Continental Air Lines, Inc., Boeing 707-124, N-70775, 22 May, 1962'.
——— (1964), 'Aircraft Accident Report, File No. 1—0007, Pacific Air Lines, Inc., Fairchild F27, N2770R, 7 May, 1964'.
——— (1967), 'Aircraft Accident Report, SA 392, File No. 1—0001, American Flyers Airline Corporation, Lockheed Electra-L188C, N183H, 22 April, 1966'.

CLARK, B., and GRAYBIEL, A. (1956), 'Report No. NM 001 110 100.43, U.S. Naval School of Aviation Medicine: Pensacola'.
—— and NICHOLSON, M. A. (1954), 'Aviator's Vertigo: A Cause of Pilot Error in Naval Aviation Students', *J. Aviat. Med.*, **25**, 171.

CLAWSON, B. J. (1928), 'Myocarditis', *Am. Heart J.*, **4**, 1.

COBURN, R. F., WILLIAMS, W. J., and KAHN, S. B. (1966), 'Endogenous Carbon Monoxide Production in Patients with Haemolytic Anaemia', *J. clin. Invest.*, **45**, 460.

CORBY, C. (1960), 'Isolated Myocarditis as a Cause for Sudden Obscure Death', *Med. Sci. Law*, **1**, 23.

CULBERT, W. L., and LAW, F. M. (1927), 'Identification by Comparison of Roentgenograms', *J. Am. med. Ass.*, **88**, 1634.

CUNHA, C. (1952), 'Identificao des Cadaveres', *Revta méd. Aeronaút.*, **3**, 49.

CURRY, A. S., Home Office Central Research Establishment, Aldermaston (1966), personal communication.

DALITZ, G. D. (1962), 'Age Determination of Adult Human Remains by Teeth Examination', *J. forens. Sci. Soc.*, **3**, 11.

DAVIS, G. L. (1968), 'Alcohol and Military Aviation Fatalities', *Aerospace Med.*, **39**, 869.

DEMY, N. S. (1963), 'Radiologic Identification in Murder, Wilful Injuries and Mass Disaster', Paper presented at Third International Meeting in Forensic Immunology, Medicine, Pathology and Toxicology. Abridged Proceedings, International Congress Series No. 80, p. 82. Amsterdam: Excerpta Medica Foundation.

## REFERENCES


DENISON, D. M., LEDWITH, F., and POULTON, E. C. (1966), 'Complex Reaction Times at Simulated Cabin Altitudes of 5000 ft. and 8000 ft.', *Aerospace Med.*, **37**, 1010.

DEPARTMENT OF CIVIL AVIATION, AUSTRALIA (1958), 'Disorientation in Flight', *Aviation Safety Digest*, No. 16.

— — — — (1962), 'Accident to DC4, Brisbane', *Ibid.*, No. 29.

— — — — (1968), 'Aircraft Accidents and Aviation Safety', *Australia and New Zealand Civil Aviation News Letter*, 1 March, 1968. p. 11.

DEPARTMENT OF TRANSPORT, CANADA (1965), 'Accident Report No. 2628, Canadian Pacific Airlines, Douglas DC-6B, CF-CUQ, 8 July 1965'.

DILLE, I. R., and MOHLER, S. R. (1969), 'Drug and Toxic Hazards in General Aviation', *Aerospace Med.*, **40**, 191.

— — and MORRIS, E. W. (1967), 'Human Factors in General Aviation Accidents', *Ibid.*, **38**, 1063.

— — and PEI, C. T. (1964), 'In-flight Loss of Consciousness', *Ibid.*, **35**, 579.

DODD, B. E., Department of Forensic Medicine, London Hospital Medical School (1966), personal communication.

DOMINGUEZ, A. M. (1962), 'Problems of Carbon Monoxide in Fire', *J. forens. Sci.*, **7**, 379.

— — CHRISTENSEN, H. E., GOLDBAUM, L. R., and STEMBRIDGE, V. A. (1959), 'A Sensitive Procedure for Determining Carbon Monoxide in Blood or Tissue utilizing Gas-solid Chromatography', *Toxic. appl. Pharmac.*, **1**, 135.

— — HALSTEAD, J. R., and DOMANSKI, T. J. (1964), 'The Effect of Post-mortem Changes on Carboxyhaemoglobin Results', *J. forens. Sci.*, **9**, 330.

DOUGHERTY, J. D. (1965), 'Lakefront Airport: an Epidemiological Approach', *Aerospace Med.*, **36**, 558.

— — and HARPER, C. R. (1968), 'Physical Defects of Civilian Pilots related to Aircraft Accidents: a New Look at an Old Problem', *Ibid.*, **39**, 521.

DOYLE, B. C. (1968), 'Aeromedical Investigations of Civil Aircraft Accidents', in *Medical Investigation of Aviation Accidents*, pp. 38–58. Chicago: College of American Pathologists.

DRESSLER, R. F. (1966), 'New Approach to Air Safety Statistics', paper presented at the Flight Safety Foundation's Annual International Air Safety Seminar, Madrid, November.

DREW, G. C., COLQUOUN, W. P., and LONG, H. A. (1958), 'Effect of Small Doses of Alcohol on a Skill resembling Driving', *Br. med. J.*, **2**, 993.

DUBOIS, E. F. (1952), 'Safety-belts are not Dangerous', *Ibid.*, **2**, 685.

DUDGEON, A. C. (1947), 'The Case for the Backward-facing Seat', *Aeroplane*, **72**, 131.

ELLIS, J., Chairman, Safety Panel, British Gliding Association (1969), personal communication.

FEDERATION OF RHODESIA AND NYASALAND (1962), 'Report of the Commission on the Accident Involving Aircraft SE-BDY', C.Fed.202, p. 23'.

FIEDLER, A. (1899), 'Über Acute Interstitielle Myokarditis', paper presented at a meeting to celebrate the 50th anniversary of the Dresden-Freiderichstadt Hospital.

FINCK, P. A. (1966), 'Exposure to Carbon Monoxide: Review of the Literature and 567 Autopsies', *Milit. Med.*, **131**, 1513.

FISH, J., and WRIGHT, R. H. (1965), 'The Seat Belt Syndrome—Does it exist?' *J. Trauma*, **5**, 746.

FISHER, R. S., SPITZ, W. U., BREITENECKER, R., and ADAMS, J. E. (1965), 'Techniques of Identification applied to 81 Extremely Fragmented Aircraft Fatalities', *J. forens. Sci.*, **10**, 121.

FITZGIBBON, G. M. (1967), 'Coronary Heart Disease in Aircrew—a Cardiologist's Impression', paper presented at Sixth Scientific Session, Jt. Comm. Aviat. Path., Ottawa, September.

— — (1969), 'Coronary Angiography Evaluation of Aircrew Problems', *Aerospace Med.*, **40**, 774.

FLAHIFF, T. (1960), 'Flight 108—to Murder', *Reader's Digest*, 76 (pt 6), 39.

FLIGHT SAFETY (1968), Abstracts: *Federal Air Surgeon's Medical Bulletin*, 2 (pt 2), 42.

FLUX, M., and DILLE, J. R. (1969), 'In-flight Spontaneous Pneumothorax: a Case Report', *Aerospace Med.*, **40**, 660.

FORNARI, A. (1955), 'Le Lesione Corporee Risconstrate Sulle Persone a Bordo del Comet Nell'incidente Aereo a sud Dell'isola d'Elba', *Riv. Med. aeronaut. spaz.*, **18**, 250.

FRACHE, G., CARELLA, A., MURINO, P., and FUCCI, P. (1954), 'L'indagine Gruppospecifica nella Ricomposizione delle Vittime di un Disastro Aereo', *Ibid.*, **17**, 163.

FRANKS, W. R. (1959), 'The Summation of some Physiological Factors leading to Incidents in the Air', in *Medical Aspects of Flight Safety*, (ed. EVRARD, E. and colleagues), p. 40. London: Pergamon.

FRYER, D. I. (1958), 'Aircraft Passenger-Seat Design and Crash Survival', Flying Personnel Research Committee Report No. 1055. London: Air Ministry.

— — (1959), 'Passenger Survival in Aircraft Crashes', *Aeronautics*, Lond., 40 (pt 2), 31.

— — (1961), 'Pathological Findings in Fatal Subatmospheric Decompression Sickness', *Med. Sci. Law*, 2, 110.

— — (1965a), 'Accident Statistics', in *A Textbook of Aviation Physiology* (ed. GILLIES, J. A.), p. 1142. London: Pergamon.

FRYER, D. I. (1965b), 'The Results of Accidents', in *A Textbook of Aviation Physiology* (ed. GILLIES, J. A.), p. 1171. London: Pergamon.

—— (1965c), 'The Preventive Medicine of Accidents', *Ibid.*, p. 1207.

FRYKHOLM, K. O. (1956), 'Identification in the "Ormen Friske" Disaster', *Acta odont. scand.*, **14**, 11.

—— and LYSELL, L. (1962), 'Different Systems for the Recording of Teeth and Teeth Surfaces', *Int. dent. J. Lond.*, **12**, 194.

FUCHS, H. S. (1967a), 'Idiopathic Spontaneous Pneumothorax and Flying', *Aerospace Med.*, **38**, 1283.

—— (1967b), 'Spontaneous Pneumothorax in "Healthy" Aircrews', *Ibid.*, **38**, 1286.

—— (1967c), 'Idiopathic Spontaneous Pneumothorax in Apparently Healthy Military Personnel. Review 4–67', Brooks A.F.B. Texas: U.S.A.F. School of Aerospace Medicine.

FULLY, G., COBLENTZ, A., DESSERTINE, A., and DÉROBERT, L. (1965), 'Solution Proposée au Problème de l'Identification des Victimes d'Accident d'Avion (Trafic international)', *Annls Méd. Lég. Crimin. Police scient.*, **45**, 257.

GAVSHON, A. L. (1963), 'The Last Days of Dag Hammarskjöld', p. 239. London: Barrie & Rockliff with Pall Mall Press.

GEDYE, J. L. (1964), 'Transient Changes in the Ability to Reproduce a Sequential Operation Following Rapid Decompression', Report No. 271. London: R.A.F. Institute of Aviation Medicine. Ministry of Defence (Air).

GENSINI, G. G. (1963), 'Coronary Angiography', *Progr. cardiovasc. Dis.*, **6**, 155.

GERRITSEN, R., FROBESE, A. S., and PEZZI, P. J. (1966), 'Unusual Abdominal Injuries due to Seat Belts', *J. A. Einstein med. Cent.*, **14**, 63.

GETTLER, A. O., and FREIMUTH, H. C. (1940), 'The Carbon Monoxide Content of the Blood under Various Conditions', *Am. J. clin. Path.*, **10**, 603.

GIBBONS, H. L., ELLIS, J. W., and PLECHUS, J. L. (1966), 'Medical Factors in 1964/1965 Fatal Aircraft Accidents in the Southwest', *Aerospace Med.*, **37**, 1057.

—— PLECHUS, J. L., CHANDLER, E. H., and ELLIS, J. W. (1966), 'Alcohol-induced Hypoglycaemia as a Factor in Aircraft Accidents', *Ibid.*, **37**, 959.

—— —— and MOHLER, S. R. (1967), 'Investigation of Volitional Acts in Aircraft Accidents', *Ibid.*, **38**, 1057.

GIBBS-SMITH, C. H. (1967), 'A Brief History of Flying', pp. 23–33. London: H.M.S.O.

GIFFORD, H., and TURKEL, H. W. (1956), 'Diffusion of Alcohol through the Stomach Wall after Death', *J. Am. med. Ass.*, **161**, 866.

GILSON, J. C., STEWART, W. K., and PEKAREK, Z. (1943), 'Prevention of Injury in Aircraft Crashes', Flying Personnel Research Committee Report No. 556. London: Air Ministry.

GISSANE, W. (1966), A paper presented at the Office of Health Economics Symposium 'Alive to 45', College of General Practitioners, London, 27 November. Quoted in *Br. med. J.*, **2**, 1449.

GLAISTER, J. (1962), *Medical Jurisprudence and Toxicology*, 11th ed., p. 21. Edinburgh: Livingstone.

GORDON, I. (1967), 'The Mechanism of Death', *J. forens. Med.*, **14**, 125.

—— (1968), 'The Biological Definition of Death', *Ibid.*, **15**, 5.

GORDON-BURGE, H., Accidents Investigation Branch, Ministry of Aviation (1960), personal communication.

GORE, I., and SAPHIR, O. (1947), 'Myocarditis: a Classification of 1042 Cases', *Am. Heart J.*, **34**, 827.

GORMSEN, H. (1954a), 'Yeasts and Production of Alcohol Post Mortem', *J. forens. Med.*, **1**, 170.

—— (1954b), 'Alcohol Production in Dead Body—Further Investigations', *Ibid.*, **1**, 314.

—— (1955), 'Sudden Unexplained Death due to Myocarditis', *Acta path. microbiol. scand.*, Suppl., **105**, 30.

GRANT, E. A., PRENDERGAST, W. K., and WHITE, E. A. (1952), 'Dental Identification in the "Noronic" Disaster' *J. Can. dent. Ass.*, **18**, 3.

GRATTAN, E., HOBBS, J. A., and EAST, A. (1967), 'Mechanisms of Injury to Motor Vehicle Occupants; a Preliminary Study', Road Research Laboratory Report LR 109. London: Ministry of Transport.

—— and JEFFCOATE, G. O. (1968), 'Medical Factors and Road Accidents', *Br. med. J.*, **1**, 75.

GREULICH, W. W. (1960), 'Skeletal Features Visible on the Roentgenogram of the Hand and Wrist which can be used for Establishing Individual Identification', *Am. J. Roent.*, **83**, 756.

GULLBRING, B., and STRÖM, G. (1956), 'Changes in Oxygen-carrying Function of Human Haemoglobin during Storage in Cold Acid-citrate-dextrose Solution', *Acta med. scand.*, **155**, 413.

GUSTAFSON, G. (1947), 'Microscopic Examination of Teeth as a Means of Identification in Forensic Medicine' *J. Am. dent. Ass.*, **35**, 720.

—— (1950), 'Age Determinations on Teeth', *Ibid.*, **41**, 45.

—— (1966a), *Forensic Odontology*. London: Staples Press.

—— (1966b), *Ibid.*, pp. 21, 31.

—— (1966c), *Ibid.*, pp. 27–28.

—— (1966d), *Ibid.*, p. 105.

—— (1966e), *Ibid.*, pp. 118–39.

HADDAWAY, G. E. (1963), 'Why Pilots Fail', *Flight Mag.*, **52** (pt 5), 13.

HALEY, J. L., TURNBOW, J. W., MACRI, S., and WALHOUT, G. S. (1966), 'Helmet Design Criteria for Improved Crash Survival, U.S.A.A.V.LABS. Technical Report No. 65–44. Fort Eustis, Virginia: U.S. Army Aviation Material Laboratories.

HALLBERG, L. (1955), 'Blood Volume, Haemolysis and Regeneration of Blood in Pernicious Anaemia: Studies based on the Endogenous Formation of Carbon Monoxide and Determination of the Total Amount of Haemoglobin', *Scand. J. clin. Lab. Invest.*, **7**, Suppl., 16.

HALPIN, E. H. (1969), 'Vital Statistics', in *Britannica Book of the Year—Events of* 1968 (ed. DELL, W. R.), p. 797, Chicago: William Benton.

HAMILTON, J. A. (1967a), *British Railways Accidents of the Twentieth Century*, p. 40. London: Allen & Unwin.

— — (1967b), *Ibid.*, p. 62.

HARPER, C. R. (1964), 'Physical Defects in Civilian Pilots related to Aircraft Accidents', *Aerospace Med.*, **35**, 851.

— — and ALBERS, W. R. (1964), 'Alcohol and General Aviation Accidents', *Ibid.*, **35**, 462.

HARVEY, W. (1966), 'Identity by Teeth and the Marking of Dentures', *Br. dent. J.*, **121**, 334.

HASBROOK, A. H., and DILLE, J. R. (1964), 'Structural and Medical Analysis of a Civil Aircraft Accident', *Aerospace Med.*, **35**, 958.

HAVARD, J. D. (1960), *The Detection of Secret Homicide*, p. 146. London: Macmillan.

DE HAVEN, H., and HASBROOK, A. H. (1952), 'Shoulder Harness: Its Use and Effectiveness. Crash Injury Research Report', New York: Cornell University Medical College.

— — TOURIN, B., and MACRI, S. (1953), 'Aircraft Safety Belts: Their Injury Effect on the Human Body. Crash Injury Research Report', New York: Cornell University Medical College.

HAWKES, R. (1956), 'Air Crash Death or Injury may be prevented by Sound Detail Design', *Aviat. Week*, **65**, (pt 19), 61.

HEGGIE, R. M., Cunard Line Limited, Southampton; formerly of Northampton General Hospital (1968), personal communication.

HELPERN, M. (1957), 'Identification of Incinerated Human Remains', paper presented at the International Meeting in Forensic Pathology, Brussels. July.

H.M. CHIEF INSPECTOR OF FACTORIES (1966), 'Report for 1965', London: H.M.S.O.

— — — — — (1967), 'Report for 1966', London: H.M.S.O.

HERNER, B., SMEDBY, B., and YSANDER, L. (1966), 'Sudden Illness as a Cause of Motor-vehicle Accidents', *Br. J. ind. Med.*, **23**, 37.

HILL, R. (1933), 'Oxygen Affinity of Muscle Haemoglobin', *Nature, Lond.*, **132**, 897.

HOBBS, S. A. (1967), 'The Work of the Road Accident Injury Group', Road Research Laboratory Report LR 108. London: Ministry of Transport.

HOWARD, P. (1965), 'The Physiology of Negative Acceleration', in *A Textbook of Aviation Physiology* (ed. GILLIES, J. A.), pp. 692, 693. London: Pergamon.

HUMBLE, B. H. (1933), 'Identification by Means of Teeth', *Br. dent. J.*, **54**, 528.

INTERNATIONAL CIVIL AVIATION ORGANIZATION (1957), Accident No. 20. Aircraft Accident Digest No. 7. I.C.A.O. Circular 50-AN/45, p. 108. Moutreal

— — — — (1962), Personnel Licensing. Annex 1 to the Convention of International Civil Aviation, pp. 12 and 32. Montreal.

— — — — (1963), Accident No. 32. Aircraft Accident Digest No. 12. I.C.A.O. Circular 64-AN/58, p. 162.

— — — — (1969), Annual Report of the Council to the Assembly.

JACKSON, J. R. (1962a), 'Potentially Disabling Lesions in Aircrew: Findings in a Series of Fatal Aircraft Accidents', *Med. Servs J. Can.*, **18**, 165.

— — (1962b), 'The Relation of Cardiovascular Disease and Disorder to Aircraft Accidents', paper presented at the Third International Conference of Aviation Cardiology. National Defence Medical Center, Ottowa. June.

JAKOBSEN, J. (1967), 'Physiological Melanin Pigmentation in the Oral Mucosa', paper presented at the Third Meeting of the Scandinavian Society of Forensic Medicine. Ahrus, Denmark, June.

JERMAN, A. C., and MILLER, C. D. (1968), 'Denture Identification', Review 6–68. U.S.A.F. School of Aerospace Medicine: Brooks A.F.B. Texas.

JONES, F. H. (1962), 'Accident to BEA Comet G-ARJM at Ankara, Turkey 21 Dec. 1961: Examination of Director Horizons from Pilots' Instrument Panels', unpublished report, Structures A4/11246/14/FHJ, Royal Aircraft Establishment, Farnborough, Ministry of Aviation. April 1962. London: H.M.S.O.

JONES, G. M. (1957), 'A Study of Current Problems associated with Disorientation in Man-controlled Flight' Flying Personnel Research Committee Report No. 1021. London: Air Ministry.

JONSSON, E., and SUNDGREN, N. (1969), 'Essential Hypertension in Airline Pilots', *Aerospace Med.*, **40**, 70.

*Journal of the American Medical Association* (1954), 'Postmortem Blood Alcohol Determinations', **155**, 803.

KALANT, H. (1968), 'Interpretation of Post-mortem Ethanol Concentrations', *Aerospace Med.*, **39**, 633.

KEIL, F. W., and BLUMBERG, J. M. (1963), 'Survey of Rotary Wing Accidents', *Aerospace Med.*, **34**, 42.
KEISER-NIELSEN, S. (1963), 'Dental Investigation in Mass Disasters', *J. dent. Res.*, **42**, 303.
—— (1967), Scand. Soc. forens. Odont. Newsletter No. 5, p. 3.
—— FRYKHOLM, K. O., and STRØM, F. (1964), 'Identification of Unknown Bodies', *Int. dent. J.*, **14**, 317.
KELMAN, G. R., CROW, T. J., and BURSILL, A. E. (1969), 'Effect of Mild Hypoxia on Mental Performance assessed by a Test of Selective Attention,' *Aerospace Med.*, **40**, 301.
KILLICK, E. M. (1940), 'Carbon Monoxide Anoxaemia', *Physiol. Rev.*, **20**, 313.
KLEMIN, A., SAYRE, D. C., and RASPET, A. W. (1963), 'Gliding', in *Encyclopaedia Britannica* (ed. ASHMORE, A. S.), Vol. 10, p. 428. Chicago: William Benton.
KNIGHT, B. (1965), 'The Post-mortem Demonstration of Early Myocardial Infarction', *Med. Sci. Law*, **5**, 31.
—— (1967), 'Early Myocardial Infarction', *J. forens. Med.*, **14**, 101.
KNOTT, N. J. (1967), 'Identification by the Teeth of Casualties in the Aberfan Disaster', *Br. dent. J.*, **122**, 144.
KREFFT, S., Flugmedizinischen Institute der Luftwaffe, Fürstenfeldbruck (1967), personal communication.
*Lancet* (1957), 'Cars and Drivers', **2**, 627.
LEEPER, C. K. (1968), 'The Development of Aviation Pathology and the Joint Committee on Aviation Pathology', in *Medical Investigation of Aviation Accidents* (ed. REALS, W. J.), p. 71. Chicago: College of American Pathologists.
LILIENTHAL, J. L., and FUGITT, C. H. (1946), 'The Effect of Low Concentrations of Carboxyhaemoglobin on the "Altitude Tolerance" of Man', *Am. J. Physiol.*, **145**, 359.
*Lloyd's List and Shipping Gazette* (1948), 'Aviation Casualties', 19 July, p. 9, and 20 July, p. 9.
———— (1949a), 'Aviation Casualties, P1-C-98', 10 May, p. 9, and 17 June, p. 11.
———— (1949b), 'Aviation Casualties, CF-CUA', 12 September, p. 11.
———— (1952), 'Aviation Casualties, XA-GUJ', 27 September, p. 7.
———— (1953), 'Aviation Casualties, PI-C-38', 7 February, p. 9.
———— (1957), 'Aviation Casualties, F-BAVH', 21 December, p. 9.
———— (1959), 'Aviation Casualties, XA-', 10 September, p. 12.
———— (1964), 'Aviation Casualties, CP-639', 10 December, p. 13 and 18 December, p. 13.
———— (1965), 'Aviation Casualties, CP-639', 1 January, p. 13.
———— (1966), 'Aviation Casualties, CU-', 30 March, p. 7.
———— (1967), 'Aviation Casualties, Bogota May 30', 1 June, p. 13.
— *Weekly Casualty Reports* (1966), 'Aden Airways, Douglas DC3, VR-AAN', 29 November, p. 378.
LOWE, R. B., and BROUGHTON, A., R.A.F. Institute of Pathology and Tropical Medicine, Halton (1965), Case A130/65, personal communication.
MCCANN, J. P., and SCHULZE, V. E. (1963), 'In-flight Pilot Incapacitation', *J. Am. med. Ass.*, **183**, 1088.
MCDOWELL, F. H. (1959), 'Spontaneous Subarachnoid Haemorrhage', in *Cecil-Loeb Textbook of Medicine* (ed. BEESON, P. B., and MCDERMOTT, W.) p. 1622. Philadelphia: Saunders.
MCFADDEN, E. B., REYNOLDS, H. I., and FUNKHOUSER, G. E. (1968), 'Protective Passenger Smoke Hood' *Aerospace Med.*, **39**, 177.
MCFARLAND, R. A. (1953), *Human Factors in Air Transportation*, p. 190. New York: McGraw-Hill.
—— ROUGHTON, F. J., HALPERIN, M. H., and NIVEN, J. I. (1944), 'The Effects of Carbon Monoxide and Altitude on Visual Thresholds', *J. Aviat. Med.*, **15**, 381.
MANGOS, J. F. (1941), 'The Healing of Extraction Wounds', *N.Z. dent. J.*, **37**, 4.
MANION, W. C. (1966), 'Myocarditis: A Review of the Development of the Concept', *Med. Ann. Distr. Columbia*, **35**, 405.
MANT, A. K., Department of Forensic Medicine, Guy's Hospital Medical School (1966), personal communication.
MARSHALL, O. R. (1963), 'Theobald on Wills', pp. 688–90. London: Stevens.
MARSHALL, T. K. (1968), 'Changes after Death', in *Gradwohl's Legal Medicine*, 2nd ed. (ed. CAMPS, F. E.), p. 93. Bristol: Wright.
MARTIN, E., Civil Aviation Department, Board of Trade (1967), personal communication.
MARTIN, J. F., and JONES, G. M. (1965), 'Theoretical Man-machine Interaction which might lead to Loss of Aircraft Control', paper presented at 36th Annual Scientific Meeting, Aerospace Medical Association, New York, April.
MARTIN, P., and MASON, J. K. (1969), 'Commorientes: Some Legal and Medical Observations', *New Law J.*, **119**, 325.
MASON, J. K. (1962a), *Aviation Accident Pathology*. London: Butterworths.
—— (1962b), *Ibid.*, p. 206.
—— (1962c), *Ibid.*, p. 192.
—— (1962d), *Ibid.*, p. 148.
—— (1962e), *Ibid.*, p. 178.

REFERENCES


Mason, J. K., (1962f), *Aviation Accident Pathology*. p. 288. London: Butterworths.

— — (1962g), *Ibid.*, p. 46.

— — (1963a), 'Acute Coronary Insufficiency while at the Controls of an Aircraft: a Report of Two Cases', *Med. Sci. Law*, **3**, 194.

— — (1963b), 'Asymptomatic Disease of Coronary Arteries in Young Men', *Br. med. J.*, **2**, 1234.

— — (1967), personal communication.

— — (1968a), 'Pulmonary Fat and Bone-marrow Embolism as an Indication of Ante-mortem Violence', *Med. Sci. Law*, **8**, 200.

— — (1968b), 'Transportation Accidents', in *Gradwohl's Legal Medicine*, 2nd ed. (ed. Camps, F. E.), p. 395. Bristol: Wright.

— — (1969), personal communication.

— — and Tarlton, S. W. (1965), 'Multiple Disinterments in Equatorial Africa', *Aerospace Med.*, **36**, 636.

— — — — (1969), 'Medical Investigation of the Loss of the Comet 4B Aircraft, 1967', *Lancet*, **1**, 431.

— — Townsend, F. M., and Jackson, J. R. (1963), 'Death from Coronary Disease while at the Controls of an Aircraft', *Aerospace Med.*, **34**, 858.

Mercer, J. O., Reid, J. D., and Uttley, K. F. (1954), 'The Identification of Exhumed Bodies: A Brief Report of the Unidentified Dead after the Tangewai Railway Accident', *N.Z. med. J.*, **53**, 329.

Midda, M. (1969), 'A Disclosing Solution for Synthetic Fillings', *Br. dent. J.*, **127**, 519.

Milčinski, J. (1965), 'Einige Erfahrungen aus der Technik und Taktik der Identifizierung bei Katastrophen', in Proceedings of a Symposium, Aktuelle Fragen der gerichtlichen Medizin, Halle, Germany, October 1964, (ed. Mäde, A.) p. 108. Halle Wittenburg: Martin-Luther-University.

Miles, A. E. (1963), 'The Estimation of Age from the Dentition', Third International Meeting in Forensic Immunology, Medicine, Pathology, and Toxicology. Abridged proceedings. International Congress Series, No. 80. p. 35. Amsterdam: Excerpta Medica Foundation.

Millikan, G. A. (1936), 'The Kinetics of Muscle Haemoglobin', *Proc. R. Soc. B.*, **120**, 366.

— — (1939), 'Muscle Haemoglobin', *Physiol. Rev.*, 19, 503.

Ministry of Aviation (1961), CAP 169, 'Report of the Committee on Civil Aircraft Accident Investigation and Licence Control', p. 28. London: H.M.S.O.

— — (1962), CAP 181, 'A Survey of the Accidents to Aircraft of the United Kingdom in 1961', London: H.M.S.O.

— — (1963), CAP 193, 'A Survey of the Accidents to Aircraft of the United Kingdom in 1962', London: H.M.S.O.

— — (1964), CAP 211, 'A Survey of the Accidents to Aircraft of the United Kingdom in 1963', London: H.M.S.O.

— — (1965), CAP 240, 'A Survey of the Accidents to Aircraft of the United Kingdom in 1964', London: H.M.S.O.

— Civil Aviation (1950a), 'Report on the Accident to Tudor V, G-AKBY, which occurred on 12 March, 1950 at Sigginstone, Glamorganshire', M.C.A.P. 88. London: H.M.S.O.

— — — (1950b), 'Report on the Accident to Viking IB G-AIVL which occurred on 13 April, 1950 in Flight about 30 miles South-east of Hastings', M.C.A.P. 86. London: H.M.S.O.

— — — (1953), 'Report on the Accident to Auster V, G-ALBW which occurred on 24 July, 1952 at Booker Airfield, Bucks', M.C.A.P. 108. London: H.M.S.O.

— Transport (1965), 'Railway Accidents', London: H.M.S.O.

— — (1967), 'Railway Accidents', London: H.M.S.O.

Mohler, S. R., Bedell, R. H., Ross, A., and Veregge, E. J. (1969), 'Aircraft Accidents by Older Persons', *Aerospace Med.*, **40**, 554.

— — Berner, W. H., and Goldbaum, L. R. (1968), 'Alcohol Question in Aircraft Accident Investigation', *Ibid.*, **39**, 1228.

Moore, R. L. (1962), 'How Crash Helmets save Life', *New Scient.*, **16**, 288.

Morland, N. (1950), *An Outline of Scientific Criminology*, p. 287. London: Cassell.

Moseley, H. G. (1955), 'Injuries incurred in Aircraft Accidents', *Milit. Med.*, **116**, 440.

— — Townsend, F. M., and Stembridge, V. A. (1958), 'Prevention of Injury and Death in Aircraft Accidents', *Archs ind. Hlth*, **17**, 111.

— — Zeller, A. F. (1958), 'Relation of Injury to Forces and Direction of Deceleration in Aircraft Accidents', *J. Aviat. Med.*, **29**, 739.

Moser, R. (1969), 'Spatial Disorientation as a Factor in Accidents in an Operational Command', *Aerospace Med.*, **40**, 174.

Muehlberger, D. W. (1954), 'Medicolegal Aspects of Alcohol Intoxication', in *Legal Medicine* (ed. Gradwohl, R. B.), p. 794. St. Louis: Mosby.

## REFERENCES


NATIONAL TRANSPORTATION SAFETY BOARD, U.S.A. (1969a), 'A Preliminary Analysis of Aircraft Accident Data, U.S. Civil Aviation, 1968', Washington: N.T.S.B.

— — — — — (1969b), 'Safety Information Release SB 69–38'. (202) 382–7273.

NEAVES, R. A. (1968), Safety Panel Report, *Sailpl. Gliding*, **19**, 147.

NEILSON, D. B. (1958), 'Sudden Death due to Fulminating Influenza', *Br. med. J.*, **1**, 420.

NELSON, E., and HAYMAKER, W. (1957), 'Colloid Cyst of the Third Ventricle in Flyers', *J. Aviat. Med.*, **28**, 356.

NEWMAN, H. W. (1947), 'Variability in Tolerance to Depressive Drugs', *Stanford med. Bull.*, **5**, 12.

NEWTON, J. A. (1951), 'The Human Factor in Aircraft Accidents', *Jl R. aeronaut. Soc.*, **55**, 110.

NICHOLLS, L. C. (1960), 'A Modified Cavett Method for the Determination of Alcohol in Body Fluids', *Analyst*, **85**, 840.

NUTTALL, J. B., and SANFORD, W. G. (1959), 'Spatial Disorientation in Operational Flight', in *Medical Aspects of Flight Safety* (ed. EVRARD, E., and colleagues), p. 73. London: Pergamon.

OGDEN, F. W., JONES, Q. W., and CHAPPELL, H. R. (1966), 'Disorientation Experiences of Army Helicopter Pilots', *Aerospace Med.*, **37**, 140.

OSMOND-CLARKE, H. (1967), Proceedings of the B.M.A. Annual Scientific Meeting. Quoted *Br. med. J.*, **3**, 230.

PAUL, G. C. (1959), 'Accident Analysis for 1958', *Sailpl. Gliding*, **10**, 75.

— — (1960), 'Accident Analysis for 1959', *Ibid.*, **11**, 83.

PAYNE, B. F. (1962), 'Glaucoma as an Aviation Hazard', *Aerospace Med.*, **33**, 1328.

PEARSON, R. G. (1961), 'Impact-injury Relationships in Lightplane Accidents 1942–1952', *Archs envir. Hlth*, **3**, 514.

— — (1962a), 'Relationship between Tie-down Effectiveness and Injuries sustained in Lightplane Accidents 1942–52', *Aerospace Med.*, **33**, 50.

— — (1962b), 'Determinants of Injury Severity in Lightplane Crashes', *Ibid.*, **33**, 1407.

— — (1963), 'Human Factor Aspects of Lightplane Safety', Civil Aeronautical Research Institute Report No. 63–35.

PEATFIELD, R. (1966), 'Safety-belts', *Br. med. J.*, **2**, 305.

PEDERSEN, P. O., and KEISER-NIELSEN, S. (1961), 'Retsodontologi', *Tandlaegebladet*, **65**, 585.

PEFFERS, A. S., Air Corporations Joint Medical Service, London Airport (1961), personal communication.

— — (1964), personal communication.

PLUECKHAHN, V. D. (1967), 'The Significance of Blood Alcohol Levels at Autopsy', *Med. J. Aust.*, **2**, 118.

— — (1968), 'Alcohol Levels in Autopsy Heart Blood', *J. forens. Med.*, **15**, 12.

POLSON, C. J., BRITTAIN, R. P., and MARSHALL, T. K. (1962), *The Disposal of the Dead*, 2nd ed., p. 90. London: English Universities Press.

PORTER, S. D., and GREEN, E. W. (1968), 'Seat Belt Injuries', *Archs Surg., Chicago*, **96**, 242.

VON POST-LINGEN, M. L. (1964), 'The Significance of Exposure to Small Concentrations of Carbon Monoxide', *Proc. R. Soc. Med.*, **57**, 1021.

PRESTON, F. S. (1968a), 'Twelve Year Survey of Airline Pilots', *Aerospace Med.*, **39**, 312.

— — (1968b), 'An Outbreak of Gastro-enteritis in Aircrew', *Ibid.*, **39**, 519.

PURCHASE, W. B., and WOLLASTON, H. W. (1957a), 'Jervis on Coroners', 9th ed., p. 131. London: Sweet & Maxwell.

— — — — (1957b), *Ibid.*, p. 158.

— — — — (1957c), *Ibid.*, p. 103.

— — — — (1957d), *Ibid.*, p. 18.

'R. B.' (1954), 'On going Forwards Backwards', *Flight*, **66**, 91.

REALS, W. J., DAVIDSON, W. H., and KARNITSCHNIG, H. H. (1964), 'Pathology of Light Aircraft Accidents', *Aerospace Med.*, **35**, 133.

— — MOHLER, S. R., DOYLE, B. C., and GIBBONS, H. (1968), 'Aeromedical Investigation of Civil Aircraft Accidents', *Ibid.*, **39**, 82.

REGISTRAR-GENERAL (1965), 'Statistical Review of England and Wales for the Year 1964', London: H.M.S.O.

— (1966), 'Statistical Review of England and Wales for the Year 1965', London: H.M.S.O.

REID, R. (1884), 'On the Application of Dental Science to the Detection of Crime', *J. Br. dent. Ass.*, **5**, 556.

REIGHARD, H. L., and MOHLER, S. R. (1968), 'Sudden Cardiovascular Incapacitation in Airmen', *Aerospace Med.*, **38**, 1273.

ROAD RESEARCH LABORATORY (1963), 'Research on Road Safety'. London: H.M.S.O.

— — — (1965), 'Annual Report: 1964', p. 85. London: H.M.S.O.

ROBERTS, G. B. (1957), 'Fulminating Influenza', *Lancet*, **2**, 944.

ROBIE, R. R., LOVELL, F. W., and STEMBRIDGE, V. A. (1959), 'Pre-existing Disease in Aircraft Accident Fatalities', paper presented at 30th Annual Meeting, Aeromedical Association, Los Angeles, April.

ROBINSON, A. E., Department of Forensic Medicine, London Hospital Medical School (1965), personal communication.

## REFERENCES


Roche, J. (1933), 'Recherches sur les Globins: Sur le Rôle des Hématine et des Globins dans la Spécificité des Pigments Hématiniques', *Bull. Soc. Chim. biol.*, **15**, 110.

Rook, A. F. (1947), 'Fainting and Flying: An Analysis of Five Hundred Cases of Impairment of Consciousness in Pilots and Aircrew', *Jl. Med.*, **16**, 181.

Roughton, F. J., and Root, W. S. (1945), 'The Fate of CO in the Body during Recovery from Mild Carbon Monoxide Poisoning in Man', *Am. J. Physiol.*, **145**, 239.

Ruff, S. (1950a), 'Brief Acceleration: Less than One Second', in *German Aviation Medicine—World War II*, vol. 1, p. 589. Washington: U.S. Air Force.

— — (1950b), *Ibid.*, p. 588.

Saphir, O. (1942), 'Myocarditis: General Review with Analysis of 240 Cases', *Archs Path.*, **33**, 88.

Scheinman, H. Z. (1968), 'Coronary Atherosclerosis in Military Pilots: I, Relationship to Flying and Aviation Accidents', *Aerospace Med.*, **39**, 1348.

Schirnding, H. (1934), 'The Teeth and their Significance in Forensic Medicine, with Special Regard to the Identification of Corpses', *Dent. Cosmos*, **76**, 853.

Scholander, P. F., and Roughton, F. J. (1943), 'Microgasometric Estimation of Blood Gases: Carbon Monoxide', *J. biol. Chem.*, **148**, 551.

Schuller, A. (1943), 'A Note on the Identification of Skulls by X-ray Pictures of the Frontal Sinuses', *Med. J. Aust.*, **1**, 554.

Schulte, J. H. (1963), 'The Effects of Mild Carbon Monoxide Intoxication', *Archs envir. Hlth*, **7**, 524.

Schwartz, C. J., and Mitchell, J. R. (1962), 'The Relation between Myocardial Lesions and Coronary Disease 1. An Unselected Necropsy Study', *Br. Heart J.*, **24**, 761.

Scott, R. W., and Saphir, O. (1929), 'Acute Isolated Myocarditis', *Am. Heart J.*, **5**, 129.

Seipel, J. H., and Wentz, A. E. (1963), 'Unsuspected Neurologic Disease in Aviation Personnel: Survival following Seizures in Flight', *Aerospace Med.*, **34**, 552 and 758.

Sellentin, L. (1904), 'Acute Isolierte Interstitielle Myokarditis', *Z. klin. Med.*, **54**, 298.

Shapiro, H. A. (1967), 'Organ Grafting in Man', *J. forens. Med.*, **14**, 41.

— — (1968), 'Heart Grafting in Man', *Ibid.*, **15**, 1.

Shaw, R. R. (1956), 'Relative Comfort in Forward and Backward-facing Seats', Aeronautical Engineering Report SM18, Issue 2. Civil Aviation Department, Australia.

Siegel, P. E., and Mohler, S. R. (1969), 'Medical Factors in U.S. General Aviation Accidents' *Aerospace Med.*, **40**, 180.

Simpson, C. K. (1939), 'Coronary Thrombosis', *Lancet*, **1**, 635.

— — (1947), 'Pathology of Sudden Death', *Ibid.*, **2**, 745.

— — (1951), 'Dental Evidence in the Reconstruction of Crime', *Br. dent. J.*, **91**, 229.

— — (1953), *Modern Trends in Forensic Medicine*, p. 53. London: Butterworths.

— — (1965), *Taylor's Principles and Practice of Medical Jurisprudence*, 12th ed., Vol. 1, p. 114. London: Churchill.

— — (1967), 'Moment of Death. Abbottempo, Book 3', p. 22. Amsterdam: Abbot Universal.

Sims, B. G. (1968a), 'Identification by the Teeth and Jaws and other Aspects of Forensic Odontology', in *Gradwohl's Legal Medicine*, 2nd ed. (ed. Camps, F. E.), p. 155. Bristol: Wright.

— — (1968b), *Ibid.*, p. 161.

Singleton, A. C. (1951), 'The Roentgenological Identification of the Victims of the "Noronic" Disaster', *Am. J. Roentgenol.*, **66**, 375.

Sjöstrand, T. (1951), 'Endogenous Formation of Carbon Monoxide', *Acta physiol. scand.*, **22**, 137.

— — (1952), 'The in-vitro Formation of Carbon Monoxide in Blood', *Ibid.*, **24**, 314.

Sobernheim, J. F. (1837), *Praktische Diagnostik der inneren Krankheiten mit vorzuglischer Rucksicht auf Pathologische Anatomie*, p. 117. Berlin: Hirschwald.

Stamm, W. P. (1968), 'Aviation Pathology', *Proc. R. Soc. Med.*, **61**, 1075.

Stanojlovic, B. R. (1967), 'Air Safety', in *Britannica Book of the Year: Events of* 1966 (ed. Dell, W. R.), p. 751. Chicago: William Benton.

Stapp, J. P. (1953), 'Crash Protection in Air Transports', *Aeronaut. Engng Rev.*, **12** (pt 4), 71.

— — (1966), Contribution to a Conference on Trauma, NIH Bethesda, Maryland, February. Quoted in *J. Trauma*, 1968, **8**, 115.

Stevens, P. J. (1963), 'Fatal Aircraft Accidents and Disease of Aircrew', *Aerospace Med.*, **34**, 450.

— — (1965a), 'Practical Problems arising in the Investigation of Airline Disasters Abroad', *Ibid.*, **35**, 641.

— — (1965b), 'Identification in Aviation Pathology', *Milit. Med.*, **130**, 653.

— — (1966a), 'The Role of the Air Force Pathologist in Accident Investigation', *Zentbl. Verk.-Med.*, **12**, 28.

— — (1966b), 'Identification of a Body by Unusual Means', *Med. Sci. Law*, **6**, 160.

— — (1968a), 'The Pathology of Fatal Public Transport Accidents', *Ibid.*, **8**, 41.

STEVENS, P. J. (1968b), 'Fatal Accidents involving Light Aircraft: A Review of U.K. Experience 1956–1966', *Aerospace Med.*, **39**, 622.

— — and TARLTON, S. W. (1963), 'Identification of Mass Casualties: Experience in 4 Civil Air Disasters', *Med. Sci. Law.*, **3**, 154.

— — — — (1966), 'Medical Investigation in Fatal Aircraft Accidents: the Role of Dental Evidence', *Br. dent. J.*, **120**, 263.

STEWART, W. K., SPELLS, K. E., and ARMSTRONG, J. A. (1955), 'Lung Injury by Impact with a Water Surface', *Nature, Lond.*, **175**, 504.

STRØM, F. (1935), 'Tannlaegevidenskapeni Rettsmedisinens og Politiets Tjeneste', *Norske Tandlaegeforen. Tid.*, **45**, 394.

— — (1954), 'Dental Aspects of Forensic Medicine', *Int. dent. J.*, **4**, 527.

— — and TOVERUD, G. (1940), 'Die Brandkatastrophe in Oslo 1938 und die Ergebnisse der zahnartzlichen Mitarbeit bei der Identifizierung der Verungluckten', *Dt. Zahn-Mund- u. Kieferheilk.*, **7**, 720.

TANNENBAUM, C. S. (1958), 'The Relationship of Concomitant Disease to the Occurrence and Management of Trauma', *Am. J. Surg.*, **95**, 897.

TEARE, D. (1951), 'Post-mortem Examinations on Aircraft Victims', *Br. med. J.*, **2**, 707.

THEORELL, A. H. (1934), 'Kristalinisches Myoglobin. IV. Mitteilung. Myoglobin im Gleichgewicht mit Sauerstoff und Kohlenoxyd', *Biochem. Z.*, **268**, 64.

THOMPSON, A. H. (1897), 'Identification by Means of Teeth', *Dent. Cosmos*, **39**, 227.

TONGE, J. I., Department of Health, Brisbane, Australia (1968), personal communication.

TOWNSEND, F. M., and STEMBRIDGE, V. A. (1958), 'Modern Concepts in the Investigation of Aircraft Fatalities', *J. forens. Sci.*, **3**, 381.

TURKEL, H. W., and GIFFORD, H. (1957), 'Erroneous Blood Alcohol Findings at Autopsy: Avoidance by Proper Sampling Technique', *J. Am. med. Ass.*, **164**, 1077.

TWEEDIE, P. G. (1963), 'Investigating Air Accidents', *New Scient.*, **17**, 83.

UNITED NATIONS ORGANIZATION (1962a), Report of the Commission of Investigation into the Conditions and Circumstances Resulting in the Tragic Death of Mr. Dag Hammarskjöld and of Members of the Party accompanying him. Document A/5069, issued 24 April, 1962. pp. 65, 66.

— — — (1962b), *Ibid.*, Add. 1, Annex vii, p. 6.

U.S. PUBLIC HEALTH SERVICE (1966), Report: Conference on Trauma. Publication No. 1565. Quoted in *J. Trauma*, 1968, **8**, 113.

URSCHEL, D. L. (1963), 'Medical Factors in Non-fatal Aircraft Accidents', *Aerospace Med.*, **34**, 547.

VAN LEEUWEN, M. (1948), 'Post-mortem Examination of Teeth and Supporting Structures to aid in Personal Identification', *Archs Path.*, **46**, 119.

VINACKE, W. E. (1947), 'Illusions experienced by Aircraft Pilots while Flying', *J. Aviat. Med.*, **18**, 308.

— — (1948), 'Aviator's Vertigo', *Ibid.*, **19**, 158.

VIVIAN, M. H. (1967), 'Setting the Scene', *Flight Safety Bull.* (Gen. Aviat. Safety Comm. U.K.), **1**, 4.

WARREN, R. C., Accidents Investigation Branch, Board of Trade (1967), personal communication.

WHITE, M. S. (1940), 'Coronary Thrombosis occurring in a Pilot while in Flight in a Single Seat Aircraft', *J. Am. med. Ass.*, **115**, 447.

WHITEHEAD, R. (1965), 'Isolated Myocarditis', *Br. Heart J.*, **27**, 220.

WHITEHEAD, T. P., and WORTHINGTON, S. (1961), 'The Determination of Carboxyhaemoglobin', *Clin. chim. Acta*, **6**, 356.

WICK, R. L. (1965), 'A Five Year History of Sailplane Accidents', *Aerospace Med.*, **36**, 269.

WILLIAMS, J. S., LIES, B. A., and HALE, H. W. (1966), 'The Automotive Safety Belt: In Saving a Life may Produce Intra-abdominal Injuries', *J. Trauma*, **6**, 303.

WILLS, P. A. (1966), 'Gliding', *Jl R. aeronaut. Soc.*, **70**, 273.

WOLTHERS, H. (1958), 'Undersøgelser over postmortel Alkoholdannelse', Academic Dissertation. Copenhagen: Christtreus Bogtrykkeri.

WYCKOFF, R. D. (1957), 'Personal Identification by Means of the Teeth', *U.S. arm. Forces med. J.*, **8**, 500.

YOUNG, J. W. (1966), 'Recommendations for Restraint Installation in General Aviation Aircraft', Report AM 66–33, Federal Aviation Agency: Oklahoma City, Oklahoma.

# INDEX


ACCIDENT(S), epidemiological aspects, 1
— Investigation Branch (A.I.B.), 2
— — — aero-medical specialists of, 6
— rates, fatal, for gliders, 99, 189
— — — light aircraft, 62
— — — public transport aircraft, 7
— research into, 2
— trends, glider, 98
— — in light aircraft flights, 62
— — public transport flights (*Figs.* 1, 2), 7
Acrylic crowns, identification of (*Figs.* 89–91), 167
Aero-medical specialists, 6
Aerospace Pathology, Department of, U.S., 6
Age, assessment of (*Fig.* 98) 170, 174
A.I.B. (*see* Accidents Investigation Branch)
Air Cadets, gliding by, 189, 191
Aircraft accident(s) inquiries, international, Standards and recommended practices for, 123
— — major, in perspective, 121
— — — organization of investigation into, 122
— — mortality, 1
— breaking up in air, evidence from remains (*Fig.* 19), 46
— crew, shooting of, 42
— metal, fused pieces of (*Fig.* 18), 45
— seats, increasing strength of, 58
Airline, interest of, in cause of accident, 132
Airliner accident as example of mass disaster, medico-legal aspects (*Figs.* 60–102), 121–188
— — major, illustrative case histories (*Figs.* 60–64), 133
Air Navigation Act, 1920, 2
— — (Investigation of Accidents) Regulations, 1922, 2
— register books of deaths, 184
— transportation standards and recommended practices adopted by I.C.A.O., 123
Alcohol, consumption as cause of accident, incidence, 81
— as contributory factor in accident, 4
— impaired efficiency of pilot due to 29, 79, 85
— level in blood affecting flying skill, 80
Altitude, effects of, in conjunction with carbon monoxide contamination (*Figs.* 11, 12), 37, 38
Amphetamine taken before flight, 76
Amplivox/Stadium universal-fitting protective helmet (*Fig.* 42), 93
Aneurysm, cerebellar, in pilot, (*Fig.* 27), 70
Angina pectoris in pilot, possible effect on angle of flight, 21
Annex 13 of Chicago Convention, 123
Appendicitis, acute suppurative, causing sudden incapacitation, 25
Ardmore, Oklahoma, accident through illness at, 13, 14
Army Gliding Association, 189
Asphyxiation due to post-crash fire (*Figs.* 25, 26), 55, 56
Assumed death, verdict of, 130
Australia, aviation pathology service in, 6
— safety harness required in light aircraft in, 95
Autopsy on bodies of all killed, as basis of medical investigation, 11
— pilot, early case of, 3
— room, need for adequately equipped, 129
Aviation fuel, post-mortem changes in skin soaked in (*Fig.* 19), 47
— pathology, aims, 11, 63
— — in other countries, 6
— — Joint Committee on, 6
— — Royal Air Force Department of, 5
— safety statistics (*Fig.* 1), 7, 62
'Aviator's vertigo', 50

BACTERIAL production of ethyl alcohol, research into, 30
Blood grouping as aid to identification, 151
Bodies, on-site examination, 129, 135, 136
— removal from scene of accident, 129 (*Fig.* 61), 134, 137
— — precipitous, from scene of accident, 128, 133
Bomb in luggage, sabotage through, 42, 43
Bone-marrow emboli, as evidence of antemortem injury, 20, 49, 56
Boom microphone, 93
Breathing apparatus for cabin crew, 55
Britain, history of civil aircraft accident investigation in, 2
— National Commission of Inquiry in, 125
British Gliding Association (B.G.A.), 97, 189
— — — declaration of physical fitness required by (*Fig.* 59), 117
Bronchopneumonia and pneumonitis in pilot (*Fig.* 33), 74
Brown, Air Commodore Sir Vernon, 3
Bullets found in incinerated bodies (*Figs.* 15–18), 44

CANADA, aviation pathology in, 6
Carbon monoxide as cause of impaired efficiency of pilot (*Figs.* 10–14), 31–41
— — contamination of cockpit, 4, 186
— — effects on higher cerebral function, 35
— — intoxication in pilot of light aircraft, 82
— — production, post-mortem, 32
— in trachea as evidence of death from asphyxiation from fire (*Fig.* 7), 20
Cerebellar aneurysm in pilot (*Fig.* 27), 70
Certification of death and disposal of deceased, 184
Check-list for collection of information about those believed killed (*Fig.* 99), 177
Chief Inspector of Accidents, 3, 125
Circumstantial clues to identity, 141, 144
Civil aircraft accident(s) due to disease in crew (*Figs.* 3–9), 12–28, 65–78, 100–110
— — — investigation, history, 2
— Aviation (Investigation of Accidents) Regulations, 1951 and 1969, 3, 125
Clothing as aid to identification (*Figs.* 65–67, 70), 143, 144
Cockpit(s) heater, defective, causing carbon monoxide poisoning 34 (*Figs.* 13, 14), 39

Cockpit(s) of light aircraft, carbon monoxide contamination of, 82
— open, value of safety belts in aircraft with, 87
Comet I aircraft disasters, 1954, 5
'Commorientes, Rule of', 131
Concussion, safety helmets and, 87
Consciousness, sudden loss of, in flight, possible causes, 25
Convair 580, accident to, at O'Hare International Airport, crash survival study, 58
Co-pilot, case of focal myocarditis in (*Fig.* 3), 18
Coronary artery disease, difficulties of detection of presence of, 28
— — — in glider pilot(s) (*Figs.* 43, 46), 100, 101, 102, 103, 105
— — — pilot(s), 5, 13, 27
— — — — of light aircraft, 65, 67
Coroner's function in fatal accident investigation, 125
Count of bodies recovered, 175
Cremation of victim of air disaster, authority for, 184
Crew seats, evidence from, in stalled aircraft (*Fig.* 24), 54, 55
Cumulo-nimbus cloud, delay in opening parachute in, 113

DARK adaptation, failure of, as cause of accident, 4
'Dark night take-off phenomenon', 50
Data about bodies, recording of (*Figs.* 100–102), 179
Death certificate, identification of body and, 130
— certification of, and disposal of deceased, 184
— relative timing of, possible importance of, 130
Deceleration, vertical and forward, in aircraft stalled on take-off, 55, 57
Deduction, validity of identification by (*Figs.* 97, 98) 173
Dental evidence of age, 170
— — as aid to identification (*Figs.* 65–67), 141, 142, (*Figs.* 73–96), 152–172
— nomenclature, 153
— prostheses and restorations, distinctive (*Figs.* 84–88), 163
— racial characteristics, 158
— radiographs (*Figs.* 89–95), 167
— records and radiographs, collection of, 177
— — comparison with dental evidence in bodies (*Figs.* 73, 95), 154
— — inconsistencies in (*Figs.* 76–82), 157
Dentist, value of, in pathological team, 152, 172
Dentures, complete, difficulty in identification, 164
Descent due to loss of control, evidence relating to, 49
Director horizon, faulty, as likely cause of accident (*Figs.* 8, 9), 23, 24
Disclosing solution for revealing dental restorations, 167
Disease, natural, as contributory cause of accident, 26
— — in glider pilot(s) (*Figs.* 43–51), 100
— — incidence in airline pilots, 27
— — — of accidents to light aircraft caused by, 77
— — main cause of accident (*Figs.* 3–9), 12
— — in operating crew (*Figs.* 3–9), 12–28
— — pilots of light aircraft (*Figs.* 27–33), 65–78
— — private pilots, incidence of, 77
Disorientation of pilot as cause of accident (*Fig.* 20), 49, 75
Documents as aid to identification (*Figs.* 65–67), 146
Drugs as possible cause of impaired efficiency, 31, 74, 76, 81

EMBOLI, fat, as evidence of antemortem injury, 20, 49, 56
— bone-marrow as evidence of antemortem injury, 20, 49, 56
— as clue to epilepsy in glider pilot, 109
Emergency exits, position of, in relation to escape (*Fig.* 23), 54
Encephalitis, in pilot of light helicopter, 72
England and Wales, local legal authority's investigation in, 126
Epilepsy as cause of sudden incapacitation, 25
— in glider pilot (*Fig.* 51), 109
Escape from aircraft after accident, 52
— — glider in flight, failed attempt (*Figs.* 53–58), 112
Ethyl alcohol, post-mortem production of, 29,79
Evidence, problems of preservation of, 110, 128, 133
— relative value of types of, in identification of bodies (*Figs.* 65–67), 141
Exclusion, process of identification by (*Figs.* 97, 98), 173

FAT emboli, as evidence of antemortem injury, 20, 49, 56
Fatty liver in glider pilot, 102
Finger-prints as aid to identification, 150
Flight path reconstruction, in case of carbon monoxide intoxication of crew (*Fig.* 10), 35
— recorder, evidence from, 49
Flying Tiger Airlines Constellation, disappearance of, over Pacific, 42
Foreign death certificate, 184
Forensic odontology, 152, 166
Funeral Director's information service (*Fig.* 99), 176, 177

GAS chromatographic technique to estimate alcohol in tissues, 29, 30
— — — — carbon monoxide in tissues, 31, 32
Germany, aviation pathology in, 6
Glaucoma, acute, as cause of sudden incapacitation, 25
Glider accident(s) (*Figs.* 43–58), 97–120, 189
— — rates, fatal, 189
— — reconstruction of events during (*Figs.* 52–58), 111
— — trends, 98, 189
— pilots, medical standards for 162 (*Fig.* 59), 117
— — natural disease in (*Figs.* 43–51), 100
— survival and safety equipment of, 116
Gliding, detailed statistics (1950–68), 189
— history of sport, 97
Gravity vector, apparent, identified with real (*Fig.* 20), 50
Ground impact, evidence that death followed (*Fig.* 7), 20, 24

HADERUP system of dental nomenclature, 154
Hammarskjöld, Dag, accident causing death of 6, (*Figs.* 15–18) 44
Head injuries sustained with lap belt restraint, 58
Heart attack suffered by pilot in flight, 13, 66
Heater, cockpit, faulty, as cause of accident, 39–41
Helicopter accident 63, (*Figs.* 28–32), 74
Helmet, protective, availability of (*Fig.* 42), 93
— — effectiveness of (*Figs.* 39–41), 90, 91, 96

Helmet, protective, for glider flying, 116
Humerus, assessment of age by examination of (*Fig.* 98), 174
Hypoglycaemia as cause for loss of consciousness in flight, 25
Hypoxia as cause of accident, 4
— due to carbon monoxide and altitude (*Figs.* 11, 12), 37, 38

IDENTIFICATION of bodies (*Figs.* 65–102), 140–183
— — legal importance of, 130
— — by local legal authority, 126, 127
— — — pathologist, 128, 138
— — difficulties in way of, 133, 134, 136
— by exclusion, process of (*Figs.* 97, 98), 173
— organization of information service to assist in (*Fig.* 99), 176
— protocol (*Figs.* 100, 101), 179
— relative value of means of (*Figs.* 65–67), 140
Impact, events at, and immediately after accident (*Figs.* 21–26), 52
— in light aircraft accident, reconstruction of events at (*Figs.* 34–42), 84–95.
Imperial Airways DH34, 3
Incinerated bodies, evidence from bullets found in (*Figs.* 15–18), 44
Incompetence of pilot as cause of accident, 68, 74
Infection, acute, causing sudden incapacitation, 24
Information service, organization (*Fig.* 99), 176
Inspector of Accidents, 3, 125
Insurance fraud through aircraft sabotage, 42
International Civil Aviation Organization (I.C.A.O.), 123
'Intestacy, Rule of', 131
Intoxication, impaired efficiency of pilot due to (*Figs.* 10–14), 29–41, 79
Intra-abdominal injuries caused by use of lap belt (*Figs.* 37, 38), 87, 88
Investigating Officer, 3, 125
Investigation into major aircraft disaster, organization of, 122, 139
— — — — — various authorities, etc., concerned in, 122, 123–139
Irresponsibility as cause of accident, 4

JET transport aircraft, disorientation of pilot of, 50
Jewellery as aid to identification (*Figs.* 65–67) 142, 147

LAP belt(s), 58
— — injury potential of, in light aircraft (*Figs.* 37, 38), 85, 87
— — relative inefficiency of, 90, 92
— — ruptured aortae due to flexion over, 5
Law of Property Act, 1925, 130
Light aircraft accidents (*Figs.* 27–42), 62–96
— — — association between lack of safety equipment and death in, 90
— — — injury from use of lap belts in, 59
— — — reconstruction of events at impact (*Figs.* 34–42), 84–95
— — impaired efficiency of pilot of, due to intoxication, 79
— — need for fitted safety harness in, 95
Lightning, glider struck by, 112
Local legal authority's inquiry into fatal accident, 125
— — authorities, issue of death certificates by, 184

MANUAL of Aircraft Accident Investigation, 124, 129
Mass disaster, major aircraft accident as, 121
Medical evidence of identity (*Fig.* 72), 148
— fitness, public transport pilot's and co-pilot's certificate of, 12, 28
— — glider pilots, 117
— — private pilots, 65
— investigation of transportation accidents 3, 124, 186
— standards for airline pilots, 28
— — glider pilots, 102, (*Fig.* 59), 117, 187
Medicolegal aspects of fatal airliner accidents (*Figs.* 60–102), 121–188
Meteorological conditions causing accident, 48
Migraine in pilot, 71
Molars, difficulties encountered with (*Fig.* 82), 161
Mortuaries, buildings available for, 129
Myocardial fibrosis in pilot (*Fig.* 28), 72
— infarct in pilot, as cause of accident, 14
Myocarditis in airline pilots, 27
— focal, in glider pilot (*Fig.* 45), 102
— — in public transport co-pilot, 18
— — — — pilot, as possible cause of accident, (*Figs.* 3–7), 19
— — pilot of light helicopter (*Figs.* 29, 30), 72
— isolated focal, as cause of accident (*Figs.* 3–7), 15
— — — as an incidental finding, 17, 18

OBESITY in glider pilot, 102
Occupant restraint system, failures of, in relation to survival and injury, 58
Odontology, forensic, 152, 166
Operating crew, natural disease in (*Figs.* 3–9), 12–28
Organization, pre-planned, of investigation into airliner disaster, 124, 139

PARACHUTE, glider pilot's failure to use (*Figs.* 53–58), 112
— harness box, injury to thigh from (*Figs.* 57, 58), 115
Passengers' lap belts, limited efficacy of, 58
Passport photograph as help to identification, 143
Pathological evidence of events prior to accident (*Fig.* 20), 49, 107
Pathologist's investigation, aims, 11, 63
— local, and their facilities, 129
— report on relative timing of death, wording, 132
Personal property, identification by (*Figs.* 70, 71), 141, 144, 147
Physical fitness, declaration of, by glider pilots (*Fig.* 59), 117
Pilot(s), airline, incidence of natural disease in, 27
— and crew, autopsy on, after accident, 3, 186
— case of focal myocarditis in (*Figs.* 4–6), 19
— disorientation of, as cause of accident (*Fig.* 20), 49
— fatigue as cause of accident, 4
— illness of, as cause of accident, 3, 5, 12, 186
— impaired efficiency of, due to intoxication (*Figs.* 10–14), 29–41, 79
— of light aircraft, natural disease in (*Figs.* 27–33), 65–78
— public transport aircraft, natural disease in (*Figs.* 3–9), 12–28
— reduced efficiency of, through disease, contributing to cause of accident, 26
Pneumothorax, spontaneous, causing sudden incapacitation, 25
— — history of, in gliding pupil, 108
Police and initial rescue operation, 128
— pre-planning and equipment required for dealing with mass disaster, 139

Post-crash fire causing deaths of survivors from asphyxiation, 55
Post-mortem examination(s) after accident, 3, 11
— — ordered by Coroner, 126
Post-mortem production of carbon monoxide, 32
— — ethyl alcohol, 29
— skin desquamation ('skin slip') (*Fig*. 19), 47
Procurator-fiscal, function of, in fatal accident investigation, 127
Public transport aviation accident(s) (*Figs*. 1–26), 7–61
— — — — association of 'pilot error' and, 26
— — — — disease in operating crew (*Figs*. 3–9), 12–28
— — — — impaired efficiency of pilot due to intoxication (*Figs*. 10–14), 29–41
— — — — non-medical cause for (*Figs*. 15–19), 42
— — aviation, improving safety in, 9
— — — increased volume accompanied by increased fatalities (*Fig*. 2), 10
Pulmonary oedema as evidence of death from asphyxiation (*Fig*. 7), 20

Radiography as aid to identification (*Fig*. 71), 148
— dental (*Figs*. 89–95), 167, 170
Rearward-facing seats, arguments against, 59
— — in relation to survival, 57, 58, 59
— — recommendations for, 5, 59
Recorded data, comparison with information supplied, 182
Recording of data about bodies (*Figs*. 100–102), 179
Recovery of bodies, counting after, 175
Refrigeration facilities, 130
Registrar-General, return of deaths from air accidents abroad sent to, 184
Relatives of deceased, 130
Repatriation of body to Britain, 184
Rescue operation, initial, police and, 128
Respiratory allergy in airline pilots, 27
Road accidents, injuries due to seat belts in, 88
Road traffic accidents, 1, 2, 12, 28
Royal Air Force Department of Aviation Pathology, 5
— — — Gliding Association, 189
— — — Institute of Pathology and Tropical Medicine, 5, 188
— — — transport aircraft, rearward-facing seats of, 59

Sabotage, 42, 76
— accidents requiring consideration of (*Figs*. 15–19), 44
Safety equipment, 58
— — of glider, 116
— — question of adequacy of, in light aircraft, 89, 90, 187
— — and belts, failure to fasten, 55, 57
— and survival in light aircraft accident (*Figs*. 34–38), 84
*Sailplane and Gliding*, 189, 190
Salicylates in urine, testing for, 31
Scandinavia, forensic odontology in, 152
Scotland, local legal authority's investigation in, 127
Seat(s) attachments, failure of, in light aircraft (*Fig*. 36), 85
— orientation of, in relation to survival, 59
Seating positions in relation to survival and escape (*Fig*. 23), 52
Serology as aid to identification, 151
Services' Gliding Associations, 189
Shoulder harness, availability of, 94
— — effectiveness of (*Fig*. 39), 88, 90, 96
— — failure to fasten, 55
Skin desquamation, post-mortem, following soaking with aviation fuel (*Fig*. 19), 47
'Skin slip', 47
Smoke hood for use in emergency, 55
Sodium amytal, prescribed for pilot, 71
Spatial disorientation of pilot as cause of accident (*Fig*. 20), 49, 75
Spinal fracture sustained with lap belt restraint, 59
Stage-flight, fatal accident rate per, 8
Stall and recovery demonstration in glider, crash during (*Figs*. 47–51), 107
Stalling on take-off, accident due to (*Figs*. 4–7), 19, (*Figs*. 21–26), 52
Structural failure of glider, cause (*Fig*. 52), 111
Subconjunctival haemorrhages in crashed glider pilot (*Fig*. 52), 111
Suicide motive for light aircraft crash, 76
Survival aspects of light aircraft accidents, analysis of, 89
— and escape (*Figs*. 21–26), 52
— fastening of safety harness in relation to, 55, 57
— safety equipment of glider, 116
Survivorship, question of, 130

Time-bomb in causation of accident, 42, 43, 48
Tooth (teeth), anatomical abnormalities of (*Fig*. 83), 162
— extraction, recent, evidence from, 162
Toxicological screening, routine, value of, 31, 81
Toxicology research unit, Home Office/R.A.F., 30
Train accidents, 1, 121
Transportation accidents, 1
— — medical investigation, 3
Transvestism complicating identification of body (*Fig*.72), 149
Triominic tablets taken before flight, 74, 75
Tudor 5 aircraft disaster, 1950, 5
Turbulence, use of lap belts in, 58

Undertaker's information service (*Fig*. 99), 176, 177
United States, aviation pathology in, 6
— — citizens, identification by finger-prints, 150
— — dentistry and British (*Fig*. 88), 166
— — glider accidents in, 120
— — incidence of light aircraft accidents due to alcohol, 81
— — suppliers of light aircraft, and shoulder harness provision, 94
Urine, alcohol in, 30

Vertigo in pilot, 71
Visual identification (*Figs*. 68, 69), 142
— —relative value of (*Figs*. 65–67), 141

Wall charts, 182

Zsigmondy's system of dental nomenclature, 153